Digital Humour in the Covid-19 Pandemic

"Cast in the mould of the Shakespearean fool, *Digital Humour in the Covid-19 Pandemic* is a compendium deserving our critical and entertaining attention. From the clown who exhibits a rustic and uneducated disposition thereby provoking laughter with his/her ignorance, to the courtly fool or jester in whom wit and pointed satire reposes, the volume demonstrates the numerous ways the global pandemic has elicited humorous responses from the Global South. From WhatsApp memes and Hashtags to subaltern humoring of political elites, the volume underscores the power of laughter as a music of the soul and a much-needed balm in the age of digital social media."

—Prof Olufemi Abodunrin, *University of Limpopo*

"'Even the scary moment of Covid-19 pandemic which has caused panic across the world could not inhibit the humorous trait and indeed laughter of coping mechanisms, with disasters. This message is delivered meticulously by this groundbreaking volume which takes the subjects of humour and laughter to higher level of scholarship, drawing from the rich social media archive.'"

—Sabelo J. Ndlovu-Gatsheni, Professor and Chair of Epistemologies of the Global South and member of the Africa Multiple Cluster of Excellence, *University of Bayreuth, Germany*

"This is an impressive and timely collection. Like the coronavirus, the contributors argue, jokes and memes related to the epidemic have infected our minds and travelled between regions, creating a greater awareness of our globally connected identities. Unique for its ambitiously broad geographical coverage, the collection includes case studies from across the global South: including on India, Zimbabwe, Brazil, Nigeria, Kenya and South Africa.

The authors draw on the protocols of a wide range of disciplines and approaches. Some of these are familiar to humour discussions such as discourse analysis, but there is a wealth of new interventions here too, including engaging with Bollywood, the creeping virus-like infection of political misrule, dark humour as quotidian coping mechanism, on COVID-19 and its similarity to Big Brother Naija, silly citizenship that made everyone with a mobile phone a potential journalist, the challenges and affordances of doing digital ethnography during lockdown, and feminist stand-up comics' responses to the pandemic.

The scholarship contained in this collection will have a reach beyond this current contagion, as the chapters bring fresh insights and new questions to the scholarship on humour and social media."

—Carli Coetzee Editor, *Journal of African Cultural Studies*

Shepherd Mpofu
Editor

Digital Humour in the Covid-19 Pandemic

Perspectives from the Global South

palgrave
macmillan

Editor
Shepherd Mpofu
University of Limpopo
Polokwane, South Africa

ISBN 978-3-030-79278-7 ISBN 978-3-030-79279-4 (eBook)
https://doi.org/10.1007/978-3-030-79279-4

This Palgrave Macmillan imprint is published by the registered company Springer Nature Switzerland AG.
The registered company address is: Gewerbestrasse 11, 6330 Cham, Switzerland

About the Book

This book project is a culmination of shared talks and dreams with some academic colleagues from different parts of the world. I remain thankful for their encouragement and seeing a possibly scholarly contribution in this endeavour. This book project would not have been successful had it not been for various contributors whose chapters make up this work. They worked through tough times under restrictive circumstances as different governments and institutions tried to contain and arrest the spread of the COVID-19. Some authors were directly affected, as they suffered from the virus or lost loved ones. Our sympathies go to them and, in the same vein, would like to dedicate this work to all those who succumbed, survived and were in the frontline against the virus. I extend my gratitude to the staff at Palgrave Macmillan, especially Mala Sanghera-Warren, Emily Wood and Md Saif for working with me till the end of the project. Mala was the first person I contacted with the proposal and has been enormously supportive and helpful since then until the competition of the project. Thad Metz has been a generous mentor and adviser, and for that, I remain thankful. I also thank Prof Olufemi Abodunrin, from whose interactions some of my ideas were sharpened. Drs Tawanda Nyawasha, Trust Matsilele and Metji Makgoba, and Profs Martin Ndlela and Sabelo Ndlovu-Gatsheni have challenged me and pushed me to do better. Our families as editor and contributors to this volume deserve some special mention. I thank my wife Vera and our children Maka and Lelo for their support and encouragement. Last but not least I thank the South African National Research Foundation, University of Limpopo Research Director and Vice Chancellor for research, my departmental colleagues and Ms. Semang Mathobela for their assistance and support in this and other projects.

Contents

Notes on Contributors

Nassir Mohammed Abba-Aji is a senior lecturer and the incumbent Head of Department at the Department of Mass Communication, University of Maiduguri, Nigeria. He has a PhD in Mass Communication. He has also published quite a number of articles in reputable journals and books.

Aje-Ori Agbese is an associate professor at the University of Texas Rio Grande Valley's Department of Communication. Her research focuses on Nigerian media, media history, journalism and communication.

Edeanya Agbese has a Master's in Public Health and is a research project manager in the Department of Public Health Sciences at the Penn State College of Medicine. Her research interests include access to care, the effects of healthcare financing on service use for families of children with autism, mental health research and treatment patterns for substance use disorders.

Gloria Chimeziem Ernest-Samuel is a senior lecturer in the Department of Theatre Arts, IMO State University, Owerri. She holds a PhD in Media Studies from the University of the Witwatersrand, Johannesburg, South Africa. She has published widely in many peer-reviewed journals and books. Her most recent essay appeared in *The Literature and the Arts of Niger Delta* (2021), edited by Tanure Ojaide and Enajite.

Keziah Wangui Githinji is a PhD scholar in Film Studies and a film/ communication trainer. Keziah is the Executive Director of Gwira Communications. She is an accomplished filmmaker and a mentor with

Yanibes Mentorship Program in Stockholm, Sweden. She has spoken in various forums such as African Women in Media Conference (AWiM-19) and African Studies Association of Africa (ASAA) 2019. She is a member of the Association of Media Women in Kenya (AMWIK), Kenya Scriptwriters Guild, in which she is the Secretary, and the Kenya Film and Television Professionals Association. She is a TED talk presenter on the Art of Story Telling (2020).

Adamkolo Mohammed Ibrahim is pursuing a PhD in a Mass Communication programme at Bayero University, Kano, Nigeria. He received his master's degree in Development Communication from Universiti Putra Malaysia (UPM) in 2017. In 2007, he received his first degree (BA Mass Communication) from the Department of Mass Communication, University of Maiduguri, Nigeria.

Adelina Mbinjama is a lecturer in the Department of Media Studies at the Cape Peninsula University of Technology in Cape Town, South Africa. Her teaching and research interests are in social media communications, cyber-ethics, black feminism and representation of women in the media. She holds a doctoral degree in Media Studies from the Nelson Mandela University.

Shepherd Mpofu is Associate Professor in Media and Communications at the University of Limpopo. He holds a PhD in Media Studies from the University of the Witwatersrand. He is also an African Humanities Programme fellow. His research interests include digital media; media, elections, protests and democracy; new media, diaspora, race and identity; media, violence and genocide. In 2020 he co-edited his latest book *Mediating Xenophobia in Africa* (with Dumisani Moyo). He has published several book chapters and journal articles in reputable local and international publications on the above-mentioned areas. He has also offered media commentary to local and international media around issues that fall within his expertise.

Mbongeni Jonny Msimanga is a PhD candidate in the Department of Communication at the University of Johannesburg. His research interests are in digital cultures, satire, identity constructions and political communication.

Mphathisi Ndlovu is a research fellow in the Journalism department at Stellenbosch University. He holds a PhD in Journalism from the same university. He is concurrently a lecturer in the Department of Journalism and Media Studies at the National University of Science and Technology (Zimbabwe). His research interests include cultural studies, digital cultures, collective memory, identity politics and critical discourse analysis. He has published in peer-reviewed journals such as *African Journalism Studies*, *Nations and Nationalism*, *Critical Arts*, *Communicatio* and the *Journal of African Cultural Studies*.

Nonhlanhla Ndlovu is a postdoctoral research fellow in Journalism and Media Studies at Rhodes University. She has researched in the areas of gender and the media, reception analysis and tabloidisation. Her research interests are in critical textual analysis and issues of identity and social belonging as related to online media.

Joyce Omwoha is a lecturer in the Department of Journalism and Media Studies at the Technical University of Kenya. Through her research interests, Joyce has won international grants and fellowships which have enabled her to carry out research on: media, citizenship and identity, media and peacebuilding, gender studies, development communication (health and advocacy) and the analysis of the social media culture in Kenya and beyond. Joyce holds a fellowship by the Global Minds Fund at Ghent University, working on a project titled "The Intricacy of Adolescent Contraception Policy as Depicted and Portrayed in the Kenyan Media". She is also exploring digital citizenship and how using social media and technology can promote peace and sustainable development.

Imran Parray is an assistant professor at the Department of Communication and Journalism, Institute of Home Economics, University of Delhi, India. He was the Indian Council of Social Science Research (ICSSR) doctoral candidate at the Centre for Culture, Media and Governance, Jamia Millia Islamia, New Delhi, India. A recipient of the International Committee of the Red Cross–Press Institute of India Award (2013) for covering under-reported issues, he has been a journalist in Kashmir. His research interests include media history, media anthropology, postcolonial media theory and new media.

Millie Phiri is a University of Johannesburg postdoctoral fellow. Her specialisation is in social media, digital technologies, media, journalism, freedom of expression, gender-based violence and health information focusing on infodemics. She is also a Zimbabwean award-winning journalist who has worked extensively in various media organisations in Southern Africa. She also spearheaded the setting up of the Pan African Network of Women

Journalists under the auspices of the Graca Machel Trust and setting up its publishing platform Swenga.org.

Mvuzo Ponono is a Xhosa man from the Eastern Cape. He is based at the University of the Free State, where he is a lecturer in Communication Science. His research interests include audience and postcolonial studies. His MA examined the influence of a township family context on the interpretation of a health education television programme. His recently completed PhD research is an ethnographic study of the interpretation of mainstream news by township youth. He will continue conducting research focused on townships until practical application of theory benefits the lives of those involved, or he will die trying.

Lungile Augustine Tshuma is a PhD candidate in the Department of Journalism, Film and Television at the University of Johannesburg. His research interests are in political communication, visual culture and collective memory.

Phuong Thi Vi holds a master's degree in Media Journalism from the famous Vietnamese media training institute, the Institute of Journalism and Communication, National University of Vietnam. She is Lecturer of Journalism and Media Studies at the Thai Nguyen University of Science, Vietnam. Her research interests include media culture, journalism history, public press/media, online multimedia, electronic newspaper journalism, public opinion, as well as journalism, media and public relations.

Alexandre Werneck is a professor at the Department of Sociology and the Graduate Program in Sociology and Anthropology (PPGSA), both at the Federal University of Rio de Janeiro (UFRJ). He is also a research coordinator at the Centre for Studies on Citizenship, Conflict, and Urban Violence (Necvu). He was a postdoctoral fellow at UFRJ. He has a PhD (2009) in Sociology from PPGSA/UFRJ (with stage doctoral at the École des Hautes Études en Sciences Sociales, EHESS, Paris, France), producing a work that deserved an Honourable Mention in the 2010 Capes National PhD Work Award and which resulted in the book *The Excuse: Circumstances and Morals of Social Relations* (2012).

List of Figures

CHAPTER 1

Social Media and COVID-19: Taking Humour During Pandemics Seriously

Shepherd Mpofu

Introduction

At the end of 2019, the world was engulfed by the coronavirus disease (COVID-19) that interrupted life as we had known it. The virus was believed to have originated from a Chinese district of Wuhan in the Hubei province. As the pandemic swept across the globe, people made different readings of its spread, effects and control. An *infodemic* ensued whereby some people discussed its cause, treatment and impact by sharing news, disseminating fake news, conspiracy theories and humorous memes. Most citizens in the Global South have experienced different kinds of crises such as leadership, environmental issues due to climate change, electoral violence, economic crises and corruption, among others. To negotiate some of these challenges gossip, fake news, conspiracy theories, ridicule and humour in the form of jokes and satire have been critical. This humour could be spread through cartoons in mainstream media or through alternative social media platforms (wo)maned by citizens now empowered to

S. Mpofu (✉)
University of Limpopo, Polokwane, South Africa
e-mail: shepherd.mpofu@ul.ac.za

S. Mpofu (ed.), *Digital Humour in the Covid-19 Pandemic*,
https://doi.org/10.1007/978-3-030-79279-4_1

create, package and distribute content without the intervention of trained media professionals but with the risk of political leaders pouncing on deviants even in these clandestine public spheres.

'Coronavirus ain't no joke' warned the Daily Show host, Trevor Noah, a South African comedian based in the United States of America, reprimanding young people whose images were shown on social media at some American beaches as the numbers of infections rose in America and globally. But this statement by Noah was helping cast light on the gravity of the pandemic across the globe, and not necessarily that people should not make jokes about the pandemic. Besides, we should take humour seriously as it is part of human communication and adaptation to our environment (Palmer, 1994). Noah used his show to lampoon society's behaviour and attitudes towards the virus, critique governments and politicians' management of the pandemic.

Dark humour, jokes and laughter on and about illnesses and pandemics are treated as grave, tasteless, offensive and therefore no laughing matter. Dark humour and laughing during pandemics and making fun of those who are affected, killed or deformed invites psychic censorship and is treated as taboo in many societies that find the reality of facing one's death or deformation unfathomable. Dark humour or morbid humour is that type of comedy that makes light of events that are otherwise traumatic, serious and painful to face and discuss. There have been jokes around traumatic and deadly events and pandemics. Dundes (1989) has done some work on humour around the HIV/AIDS pandemic. Smyth (1986) has also discussed how people made jokes out of the Space Shuttle disaster of 1986 where seven Americans died on a trip to space. Some scholars have also looked at the humour surrounding terrorism and the French (Nice) terrorist attacks (Dynel & Poppi, 2018; Kuipers, 2005). The Cholera pandemic of 1831–1832 (Park & Park, 2010), the Spanish Influenza of 1918 and the Swine Flu scare of 2009–2010 (Rosa, 2012) are among pandemics which, despite frowns from some quarters in society, have elicited humour in the way they were represented and engaged with by the media and everyday people. This humour served different purposes. Not all dark humour should be seen in the negative as this type of humour makes fun of a tragic situation 'even if it is inspired by them and relevant to them' (Dynel & Poppi, 2018, 384). Dark humour during pandemics, illnesses and death has been essential in relieving tension and pain. Dark humour, for Dundes (1989, 73), helps as a mental hygiene defence mechanism 'that allows people to cope with the most dire of disasters'.

Humour can alleviate poor health as some writers like Robert Frost, Lord Byron, Charles Dickens and researchers such as Dillon and Totten (1989), Carroll and Schmidt (1992), Abel (2002), Kuiper and Martin (1993), among others, have argued. However, some scholars argue that having a good sense of humour does not translate into being a healthy person (Kuiper et al., 2004; McClelland & Cheriff, 1997; Martin & Dobbin, 1988). They suggest it is one of the cheapest medicines in times of illness. Added to that, humour 'produces a spiritual equipoise' critical in the 'management of psychological and instinctual forces that threaten equilibrium…a form of ethological integration [that] aids social bonding' (Palmer, 1994, 58). Humour also has an extended function of group identity preservation as joking 'is a rule-bound activity, it has the characteristics of ritual, the common acceptance of which is a means of forming group identity' (Palmer, 1994, 58). The coronavirus pandemic, in a way, created a global group identity as it was a definer of human relations and experiences as a shared common denominator.

Ridicule and humour, while helping reduce anxiety, making people laugh and make sense of their circumstances and at times appreciating their conditions of existence or even pushing them to make alterations—as a capacitor for change—has been one of the accessible ways for coping or bringing about change or understanding our predicaments in society. At the same time, humour has proven to be a sophisticated avenue into accessing people's thoughts about crises or pandemics, interpretation of the same and views on society in general. Social media has created alternative avenues where ordinary citizens, unbounded by time and geographic boundaries, interact among themselves and the political elite where power is differently negotiated, operationalized and imagined.

Social Media, Community and Humour

That humour should be taken seriously cannot be overstated. The use of social media to generate humorous reflections on the COVID-19 pandemic should not be read as idleness or silly playfulness, but this has to be seen as speaking to the current socio-political and economic factors and fears. Chiodo et al. advised us to 'Use technology to spread smiles' (2020, 164) during the pandemic. Of course, with the world on lockdown and social distancing a new normal for demonstrating a duty of care, social media platforms such as Facebook, Twitter, Weibo (Chinese version of Twitter that is highly censored by the state), YouTube, Instagram,

MySpace, Telegraph, TikTok to mention the most common, 'have replaced witty dad jokes' (Chiodo, 2020, 264) and been used to share humour and laughter during the pandemic.

But what are social media? Social media cannot be well understood outside the terms Web 2.0 and User Generated Content (UGC). Web 2.0 is a term first introduced by Tim O'Reilly in 2005 to describe the novel way in which software developer in the World Wide Web and internet users used platforms in a communal and co-creative collaborative manner. The term User Generated Content was propounded in 2005 and, as Kaplan and Haenlein say, 'can be seen as the sum of all ways in which people make use of social media...describe(s) the various forms of media content that are publicly available and created by end users'. UGC has to fulfil the following criteria to be referred to as such: 'first it needs to be published either on a publicly accessible website or on a social networking site accessible to a selected group of people; second, it needs to show a certain amount of creative effort; and finally, it needs to have been created outside of professional routines and practices' (2010, 61). Web 2.0, according to Kaplan and Haenlein, 'represents that ideological and technological foundation', while UGC 'can be seen as the sum of all ways in which people make use of Social Media' (2010, 61). Therefore, social media could be defined as 'a group of internet-based applications that build on the ideological and technological foundations of Web 2.0, and that allow the creation and exchange of User Generated Content' (Kaplan & Haenlein, 2010, 61). Mpofu magnifies this thus:

> Social media are characterised by their broad reach, flexibility in terms of access, composition, editing, uploading and consumption of content, easy accessibility where there is readily available internet, speedy communications and allowing many people to interact at the same time especially on public-facing platforms such as Facebook, blogs, listservs, WhatsApp, Twitter, Instagram and the like. (2019, 110)

These social media platforms are a critical cog in the information ecosystem. These could be added to extend the definition of what is labelled as pavement radio or *radio trottoir* by Stephen Ellis (1989). For Ellis pavement radio was almost like the bush telegraph, even though he went on to say about it: 'this is unsatisfactory in that is an old-fashioned metaphor: the telegraph superseded decades ago, whereas the radio has for some 30 years been Africa's favorite news medium' (1989, 321). Of course, the radio remains predominant in Africa, especially in rural settings where the penetration of the internet, mobile cellular phone connectivity, satellite television, electrification, literacy and accessibility of other news media such as newspapers remain low compared to urban areas. Social media, as news gathering, editing, sharing and consumption sites, are riddled with distrust because of ethical problems associated with the whole sociology of news production and dissemination within these platforms. But this is not enough to dismiss them easily as they are laden with socio-political and economic meanings in the life of any society. Besides, as Ellis suggests, the bush which was a platform for bush telegraph no longer exists and has been replaced by the 'urban pavement, bar, markets, living room or taxi-park' (1989, 321). New media technologies have added and altered, rather than replaced these as sites of news and gossip sharing making them an all-important aspect in the societal communicative regime. What is crucial with pavement radio especially in the Global South, largely, is that it is trusted and exists not because they are vaults of truths and verified information but because:

> Its subject matter are issues of public interest about which there has not been an official announcement, or where official information cannot be trusted. Widespread corruption in post-apartheid South Africa has not done much to improve citizens' respect for official narratives. They know what it feels like to be lied to (Wasserman, 2020)

Besides, social media platforms, just like tabloid newspapers whose consumption is communal, help build sharing communities since communication and information sharing rituals happen within a context of community and communalism in sharing and interpretation (Wasserman, 2020).

The digital media platforms have become spaces where people adopt different persona, share information and co-exist as members of an imagined community with humour as of the unifying rituals. Humour helps unify people so they do not feel 'isolated in a lonely time' (Chiodo et al., 2020, 164). In that existence, the sharing 'practices illustrate how the conviviality of ... societies also influence their media use. Similarly, joking about the coronavirus may be a way for people to say "it is all very absurd, but we're in this together"' (Wasserman, 2020).

Indeed, the COVID-19 pandemic brought people together through driving them apart, social distancing. Thus, while social distancing became the norm, humans shared fear, empathy, hope, hopelessness and aspirations for a better future when the virus would be eradicated, with good health and economies. Fundraising campaigns were done where people donated money and food to fellow citizens some of whom they did not know. That people saw humorous side of things during this period is instructive and worthy of intellectual interrogation. Humour serves various socio-eco-political and pyscho-social purposes. The coverage of the pandemic showed lack of leadership in some contexts, magnified the dangers of the pandemic, instilled panic and fear in the hearts and minds of citizens and laughter and humour to navigate life. Humour was variously used to critique society, calm fear, spread fake news and perform invincibility. In a context where most people do not trust authority, especially politicians, pharmaceutical and technology companies, some people found it helpful to share and trust social media posts, fake and authentic, than mainstream media or officialdom. As Wasserman expounds, 'political disillusionment with the current government(s) and feelings of frustration have also proven to be fertile ground for rumours and conspiracy theories that provide more plausible explanations of people's current circumstances than political, economic or scientific authorities' (2020). The *colonization* of the Global South by new technologies has caused some tensions: political, cultural, economic and social. For instance, when one looks at the resistance towards the e-hailing transport services such as Taxify and Uber by traditional transport operators and subsequent deadly fights between the two generations of transport operators, one gets a sense of what technology has done in terms of disrupting traditions. Politically, citizens can ridicule, engage and insult their leaders, a transposition of how power and big mannism have been understood in political spheres in some Global South contexts where citizens respect, fear and do not challenge big men in authority. Also, digital media, while making leaders accessible, have also empowered them to share humour with their constituencies. In essence, the ethics of communication that guide traditional media and even cultural ways of communication between the ruled and the rulers or elders and youngsters are disrupted and left to renegotiation.

Social media have been, before the COVID-19, central in human communication. The dawn of the pandemic created a situation whereby people relied more on digital connectivity for various socialization and working appointments. In the process, to keep sane, social media were used to share jokes. There has been a growing body of research on humour in social media (Dynel & Poppi, 2020; Davis et al., 2018; Demjén, 2016, Duerringer, 2016). *Digital Humour in the Covid-19 Pandemic: Perspectives from the Global South*, as already intimated, makes that important and unique intervention in that it deals with a novel issue—the world in lockdown due to a pandemic, something a larger percentage of the citizens in the globe are experiencing for the first time—and breaks new ground in researching an area and phenomenon that is relatively new: world of COVID-19 pandemic and social media humour. The book project looks at this pandemic through the lens of social media humour and in so doing adds new dimensions in the discussion of humour and pandemics. These include COVID-19 humour and pandemics; comparative analyses between countries such as Ghana, Senegal, Pakistan and Ethiopia; gender, identity humour and the pandemic humour; fear and loathing during the pandemic; humour, curfews and politics, among others. Online humour and associated participatory rituals are 'indicative of the *polyvocality of participatory culture* which is the hallmark of social media' (Dynel & Poppi, 2020, 3).

COVID-19, Mediatization and Datafication of Society

COVID-19 did not only become a health crisis, but also a political, social and economic one of big proportions. The media were central in magnifying the ramifications of the pandemic. It is through the media that society looks at itself. The media 'serve for observing and influencing developments and events from different viewpoints' (Nguyen, 2020, 1). One implication of the COVID-19 pandemic was that of mediatization and datafication. When the world health experts were asked to come up with possible solutions to the pandemic, lockdowns were suggested and implemented across the globe. The media played an important role in informing and convincing the public to follow regulations so that the pandemic could be contained. This had implications on how people performed work (Microsoft Teams), dating and other social and family relations (Facebook, Zoom, WhatsApp), schooling (Google Meet, Black Board Collaborate and Skype) and other service provisions. The digital economy and technology companies' dominance and centrality in these contexts were magnified (Nguyen, 2020).

Digitization and mediatization accelerated datafication of society leading to, among other things, the spread of fake news, conspiracy theories around human data corporate and government control. Governments in countries such as the Austria, Australia, Belgium, Brazil, Brunei, Canada, South African, Singapore, South Korea, Germany, Dutch, Ecuador, Britain, China and others made use of corona-apps which guided their control of the spread of the virus. There were also fears that using technology in the combating of the virus meant people had to give away their data and bio-information to tech-companies, government and other systems, and this led to questions of 'privacy, data surveillance, data ownership, which can influence citizens' willingness to use them' (Nguyen, 2020, 2). Not that citizens were not creating too much data and giving them to corporates and the government already through using apps, walking in the city streets with CCTV surveillance and volunteering information to supermarkets and via shopping apps and medical information to the doctors before, but there seems to be dangers associated with a situation where data is ***demanded*** by the political elite for governance purposes because *we are under attack*. This has given to fear which has led to a phenomenon of data vigilantism whereby citizens collectively take offence, outrage and take it upon themselves to photograph and distribute images of fellow citizens who infringe on lockdown or any other rules, making them subject to possible harm, public scorn, ridicule and shame.

Digital or data vigilantism, according to Trottier 'is a process where citizens are collectively offended by other citizen activity, and coordinate retaliation on mobile devices and social platforms. The offending acts range from mild breaches of social protocol to terrorist acts and participation in riots' (2017, 55). Data vigilantism is justified by those who participate in it by arguing that they are trying to protect the legally constituted order 'so the appearance and diffusion of vigilantism in the Coronavirus emergency seems inevitable'(Milan & Di Salvo, 2020). The net effect of this self-righteous behaviour is that 'a lasting and invasive impact on the privacy of the accused, as well as inciting aggression and a desire for revenge' (Milan & Di Salvo, 2020). The breaking of coronavirus lockdown rules was more observable than proven. In some instances, *law breakers* are seen, and there is no proof they are breaking lockdown laws as some might be going to hospital, or work in critical services or going to get supplies from the shops. In some cases, digital vigilantism has potential to demarcate society between the bad and good guys with devastating consequences for social cohesion. Related to this is the idea of privacy and normalization of surveillance.

That COVID-19 pandemic accelerated datafication, justified and normalized citizen surveillance cannot be understated. A critical question to be asked is: What role does privacy have in a pandemic and what's more, a datafied setting? In an attempt to curb the spread of the virus, dictatorial countries such as South Korea, China and Singapore made advances towards surveillance and digitally monitoring citizens. In South Africa, for example, a visit to a restaurant, supermarket, bar, university or hotel meant that you had to leave your details on some registration form or app, and in most cases, there was no disclaimer or statement on how the information could be used in future. Will the technologies of surveillance and accompanying infrastructure be creatively used and adapted to the post-COVID-19 world needs, or will they be destroyed? For Yuval Noah Harari (2020), writing in the *The New York Times*, it is difficult to imagine the latter as 'short-term emergency measures will become a fixture of life'. For instance, Israel Security Agency was authorized to 'deploy surveillance technology normally reserved for battling terrorists to track coronavirus patients' (Harari, 2020) by Benjami Netanyahu, the Prime Minister who forcibly gave orders after a parliamentary sub-committee shot down the idea. In some countries there has been a rise in the use contact tracing apps, and again, these lead us into question: What are the rights of the citizens in such a context? Usually the debate leads to what Milan and Di Salvo (2020) call a 'false dichotomy between privacy and the defense of public health, as if the former is an insurmountable challenge to the latter'.

Why the Global South?

What is the Global South and why does it matter? I seek to address this question in this short section. According to Nour Dados and Raewyn Connell, the term Global South functions as more than a metaphor for underdevelopment. The term is used to reference 'an entire history of colonialism, neo-imperialism, and differential economic and social change through which large inequalities in living standard, life expectancy, and access to resources are maintained' (2012, 130). The Global South is both a political and geographic location, a collection of countries formerly known as the Third World. In academic circles, the Global South has not been looked at with the same lens as the West, the Global North: it has been exoticized and has been part of the world where Euro-Americans or Westerners 'projected most forcefully and fancifully their own pride and prejudice' (Chabal, 2009, 20). This geographic and political location has been in the Western gaze for a long time and comprises of countries and continents once colonized by the West, in some cases, currently having a colonial hangover and yearning for decolonial exorcism (Ndlovu-Gatsheni, 2013; Quijano, 2000a, 2000b; Robins, 2013, Mbembe, 2017; Maldonado-Torres, 2007).

It is no secret that in the Global North technology has been appropriated to an extent that it is used in spaces that the Global South only currently dreams of. For example, electronic voting or vote counting is used in a handful of Global South countries compared to the Global North. In addition, the current Fourth Industrial Revolution seems more advanced in the West than in the Global South where, in some cases, resistance to these technologies have led to citizen-citizen violence and even violations of human rights of citizens by the state still stuck in old technologies. Resistance is partly informed by the fear that the benefits of technology will be accessed by a few members of the society, while more will be made poorer and excluded (Juma, 2016). The Global South is not a homogeneous geographic, ideological, commercial or social space. There are hierarchies even within this space where, for instance, the Chinese and Indians are seen as 'racist' towards other members of this geographic region such as Africans.

The focus on Global South does not mean that there are no shared experiences with the West. They could well be, but this sub-region has not been treated as a site of intellectual production (Hegel, 1956) and therefore we have to make deliberate efforts to do empirical studies and present knowledge from the sub-region. In many instances, the region and its peoples have been used as sites of data production and collection by Western scholars and then the analyses are done in Western universities and research centres. Katie Bryant helps us see the bigger picture here when she says:

> that editors and reviewers of international journals demand that findings from studies situated in the Global South and being done by Southern researchers must have greater global generalizability than findings coming from studies situated in the Global North; and… that Southern researchers doing research in particular geographic locations in the Global South struggle more than their Northern counterparts to have their research questions and findings deemed important enough to contribute to the conversations taking place in their international research communities. (2014, 230)

A journal article about Trump's administration is accepted as global enough in some global journals, while a similar one on Ian Khama is rejected for lacking that global appeal, flair and contribution to important conversations. It is therefore important to write from experience and context where there is no imagined superior other. The superior other is that context whereby every form of knowledge production, theory and analysis has to draw from, follow a certain template and suit the requirements set therein. Not that we are arguing for sloppy scholarship. No! The argument here is that the Global South can have and has data, scholarship and intellectual traditions and lenses, theories, methodologies, scholars and analysts who can analyse and produce academic works without the need of using Western theories, methods and so on as a final and ultimate arbiter of and for that particular scholarship for it to be acceptable as rigorous intellectual work. The intellectual strength and contribution of this volume lies in that.

The Global South political space is admittedly one of worry and challenges. The aftermath of the pandemic and datafication of society cannot make one hopeful of the future. This is so because in some contexts, the pandemic found already fragile nation-states, economies characterized by disease, violence, conflict, maladministration, poverty and poor political leadership in general. In most cases, during lockdown in the Global South, especially in Africa, many cases were reported where governments used the lockdown and weaponized COVID-19 as an excuse to curtail their citizens' rights. In others, security forces killed citizens for breaking COVID-19 laws. Some of these countries switch off the internet during protests and there will be nothing stopping them for using the biometric surveillance systems beyond the COVID-19 pandemic. Given a choice between privacy and health, ordinary people are likely going to choose health, because, even though they can share jokes about death and pandemics on social media, health remains everyone's ideal. After all data influences how 'societies make sense of, try to overcome and behave in crisis' (Nguyen, 2020, 4). But in a context where data illiteracy levels are high, especially in the Global South, abuse of bio-data by corporates and governments remains higher and much more worrisome. But people laugh and laughed while the pandemic lasted.

Humour and Pandemics

There has been a considerable body of academic work done globally in the area of humour in health communication (Wooten, 1993; Wanzer et al., 2005; Hendriks & Janssen, 2018) and most of this has been academic journals. Interestingly, the COVID-19 pandemic is the first of such a pandemic in the last 100 years and has rightfully elicited a lot of interrogation from academics focusing on varied aspects such as Black Twitter: coping with the pandemic while black in America (Outley et al., 2020), coping with stress (Savitsky et al. 2020), health and conspiracy theories (Ahmed, 2020). Few articles have focused on humour during the pandemic (Amici, 2020; Chiodo et al., 2020; Thelwall & Thelwall, 2020). Most of these studies emanate from the Global North. Amici's study found that humour was used to spread positivity while distancing oneself from negativity. In some instances, humour was used to enhance social cohesion. Chiodo et al's intervention advocates the use of gallows humour that 'includes jokes, irony and humorous remarks about frightening topics such as combat or death' because the COVID-19 pandemic 'presents ample opportunity for the use of this form of humour [as it could help others as a] coping mechanism that may also boost camaraderie and morale' (2020, 763–764). Of course, they offer this advice with caution for joking responsibly as 'Corona virus ain't a joke' ☺. Elsewhere, Thelwall and Thelwall observed that humour was used to 'emphasize the threat or seriousness of the pandemic', to express 'fear' and share 'social distancing advice … in the form of comic video messages' (2020).

There is, however, a need to make sense of the pandemic as understood by ordinary people and as engaged with and expressed, from below, using various social media platforms. Besides Slavoj Žižek's book *Pandemic!* (2020), emerging research on the COVID-19 pandemic is in the form of journal articles addressing economic, socio-political, health issues associated with the pandemic, religion and concerns around fake news and moral panics in specific locales.

This volume therefore occupies a different and yet important space, making a worthwhile intervention by exploring the negotiations of the pandemic in the Global South through the use of humour and ridicule on social media from various angles. There are different ways of engaging with strife, stress and health scares in different contexts of the globe. Diseases are not easily spoken about especially when they affect closer relatives. In Africa, the HIV/AIDS pandemic is one such that has been given nicknames in order to easily talk about. In some instances, a person with HIV is said to have been 'beaten by soldiers' or to be suffering from the 'disease of these days'. Disclosing one's status takes courage and is usually accompanied by exclusion and stereotyping. The meanings drawn from making a mockery and finding humour in social media in connection with COVID-19 raise culturally pertinent ethical questions.

The book project currently comprises 15 chapters addressing how humour was used on social media to negotiate the COVID-19 pandemic in the Global South. Citizens and politicians made various interventions in this regard, among others, critiquing governments in how they handled the matter, showing governmentality, attempting to desensitize and downplay the effects and dangers of the pandemic and as therapy to manage through the pandemic. These chapters are grouped into three sections.

The first section focuses on meme-making practices and making sense of the pandemic. Chapters in the section explore how memes were used as socio-political commentary during health disasters and also as a form of health communication (Mpofu and Werneck). Besides, other themes explored are how memes were used for the purposes of stress relief as they were shared for laughter and light-hearted therapeutic moments. In this playfulness, Msimanga et al. suggest, was imbedded some forms of subversion of science as conspiracy theories abound.

The second section largely focuses on gender, race and familial identities. Here feminist humour interrogated. Phiri specifically demonstrates how women owned their narrative and framed these within the broader societal context. Ndlovu looks at how sharing of jokes and laughter brought South Africans together as a nation. Ponono uses decolonial love as lenses to highlight contradictory emotions of laughter and anger as emblematic of structural issues in South Africa.

The third and final s n ectioof the book focuses on humour as weapons of the weak used to undermine political authority. Through a Foucauldian discourses analysis, Mbinjama-Gamatham's chapter casts light on how people made sense of ANC's corruption. Ndlovu, in the next chapter, argues that WhatsApp memes were used as counter-public spheres largely for subversive purposes by the disenfranchised members of society. In a related chapter, Parray studies the use of humour during the pandemic in India. Parray observes that the Janata Curfew memes circulated in India and beyond were largely targeted at the Prime Minister, Modi, after he urged countrymen and women to clap hands and bang plates in honour of frontline workers. The humour that followed blurred the lines of humour, ridicule, comedy, trolling, threats and violence in India's emergent cultures. Wangui and Omwoha's chapter shines a spotlight on how Kenyans used humour was used for communicative, entertainment and political commentary. Mpofu concludes the section and volume with a critical engagement of dark humour as used by politicians and citizens in South Africa and Zimbabwe.

References

Abel, M. (2002). Humor, stress, and coping strategies. *Humor: International Journal of Humor Research, 15(4)*, 365–381.

Ahmed, W. (2020). COVID-19 and the 5G conspiracy theory: Social network analysis of twitter data. *Journal of Medical Internet Research, 24*(5), 1–9.

Amici, P. (2020). Humour in the age of COVID-19 lockdown: An explorative qualitative study. *Psychiatria Danubina, 32(1)*, 15–20.

Bryant, K. (2014). Research from the Global South: The important role of context in international research activities. *McGill Journal of Education, 49(1)*, 227–235.

Carroll, J., & Schmidt, J. (1992). Correlation between humorous coping style and health. *Psychological Reports, 70(2)*, 402.

Chabal, P. (2009). *Africa: The politics of smiling and suffering*. University of KwaZulu Natal Press.

Chiodo, C. P., Broughton, K. K., & Milchalski, M. P. (2020). Caution: Wit and humour during the COVID-19 pandemic. *Foot and Ankle International, 41(6)*, 763–764.

Dados, N., & Connell, R. (2012). The global south. *Context, 11(1)*, 12–13.

Davis, J. L., Love, T. P., & Killen, G. (2018). Seriously funny: The political work of humor on social media. *New Media & Society, 20*(10), 3898–3916.

Demjén, Z. (2016). Laughing at cancer: Humour, empowerment, solidarity and coping online. *Journal of Pragmatics, 101*, 18–30.

Dillon, K., & Totten, M. (1989). Psychological factors, immunocompetence, and health of breast-feeding mothers and their infants. *Journal of Genetic Psychology, 150(2)*, 155–162.

Duerringer, C. M. (2016). Who would Jesus bomb? The republican Jesus meme and the fracturing of ideology. *Social Media + Society, 2*(1), 1–12.

Dundes, A. (1989). At ease, disease: Aids jokes as sick humor. *American Behavioral Scientist, 30(3)*, 72–81.

Dynel, M., & Poppi, F. I. M. (2018). In tragoedia risus: Analysis of dark humour in post-terrorist attack discourse. *Discourse & Communication, 12(4)*, 382–400.

Dynel, M., & Poppi, F. I. M. (2020). Caveat emptor: Boycott through digital humour on the wave of the 2019 Hong Kong protests. *Information, Communication & Society*. https://doi.org/10.1080/1369118X.2020.1757134

Ellis, S. (1989). Tuning in to pavement radio. *African Affairs, 88(352)*, 321–330.

Harari, Y. N. (2020). *Yuval Noah Harari: The world after coronavirus*. https://wwwft.com/content/19d90308-6858-11ea-a3c9-1fe6fedcca75

Hegel, G. W. F. (1956). *The philosophy of history* (J. Sibree, Trans.). Dover.

Hendriks, H., & Janssen, L. (2018). Frightfully funny: Combining threat and humour in health messages for men and women. *Psychology & Health, 33(5)*, 594–613.

Juma, C. (2016). *Innovation and its enemies: Why people resist new technologies.* Oxford University Press.

Kaplan, A. M., & Haenlein, M. (2010). Users of the world, unite! The challenges and opportunities of Social Media. *Business Horizons, 53*(*1*), 59–68.

Kuiper, N. A., Grimshaw, M., Leite, C., & Kirsh, G. (2004). Humor is not always the best medicine: Specific components of sense of humor and psychological well-being. *Humor – International Journal of Humor Research, 17*(*1–2*), 135–168.

Kuiper, N. A., & Martin, R. A. (1993). Humor and self-concept. *Humor: International Journal of Humor Research, 6*(*3*), 251–270.

Kuipers, G. (2005). "Where Was King Kong When We Needed Him?" Public discourse, digital disaster jokes, and the functions of laughter after 9/11. *The Journal of American Culture, 28*(*1*), 70–84.

Maldonado-Torres, N. (2007). On coloniality of being: Contributions to the development of a concept. *Cultural Studies, 21*(*2–3*), 240–270.

Martin, R. A., & Dobbin, J. P. (1988). Sense of humor, hassles, and immunoglobin A: Evidence for a stress moderating effect of humor. *International Journal of Psychiatry in Medicine, 18*(*2*), 93–105.

Mbembe, A. 2017. *Critique of black reason* (L. Dubois, Trans.). WITS University Press.

McClelland, D., & Cheriff, A. (1997). The immunoenhancing effects of humor on secretory IgA and resistance to respiratory infections. *Psychology and Health, 12*(*3*), 329–344.

Milan, S., & Di Salvo, P. (2020). Can Europe make it?: Four invisible enemies in the first pandemic of a "datafied society". https://www.opendemocracy.net/en/can-europe-make-it/four-invisible-enemies-in-the-first-pandemic-of-a-datafied-society/

Mpofu, S. (2019). For a nation to progress victims must 'move on': A case of Zimbabwe's social media discourses of Gukurahundi genocide silencing and resistance. *African Identities, 17*(*2*), 108–129.

Ndlovu-Gatsheni, S. J. (2013). *Empire, global coloniality and African subjectivity.* Berghahn Books.

Nguyen, D. (2020). Mediatisation and datafication in the global COVID-19 pandemic: On the urgency of data literacy. *Extraordinary Issue: Coronavirus, Crisis and Communication, Media International Australia.* https://doi.org/10.1177/1329878X20947563

Outley, C., Shamaya, B., & Harrison, P. (2020). Laughing while black: Resistance, coping and the use of humor as a pandemic pastime among blacks. *Leisure Sciences.* https://doi.org/10.1080/01490400.2020.1774449

Palmer, J. (1994). *Taking humour seriously.* Routledge.

Park, M. P., & Park, R. H. R. (2010). Fear and humour in the art of cholera. *Journal of the Royal Society of Medicine, 103*, 481–483.

Quijano, A. (2000a). Coloniality of power, eurocentrism and Latin America. *Nepantla: Views from the South, 1(3)*, 533–579.
Quijano, A. (2000b). Coloniality of power and social classification. *Journal of World Systems, 6(2)*, 342–386.
Robins, S. (2013). The (third) world is a Ghetto'?: Looking for a third space between 'Postmodern' cosmopolitanism and cultural nationalism. *CODESRIA Bulletin, 2&3*, 18–26.
Rosa, G. P. (2012). The Swine Flu pandemics in Portugal through newspaper humour. *Journalism and Mass Communication, 2(7)*, 735–747.
Savitsky, B., Findling, Y., Ereli, A., & Hendel, T. (2020). Anxiety and coping strategies among nursing students during the COVID-19 pandemic. *Nurse Education in Practice*. https://doi.org/10.1016/j.nepr.2020.102809
Smyth, W. (1986). Journalism and mass communication. *Western Folkore, 45(4)*, 243–260.
Thelwall, M., & Thelwall, S. A. (2020). A thematic analysis of highly retweeted early COVID-19 tweets: Consensus, information, dissent and lockdown life. *Aslib Journal of Information Management*. https://doi.org/10.1108/AJIM-05-2020-0134
Trottier, D. (2017). Digital vigilantism as weaponisation of visibility. *Philosophy & Technology 30*(1), 55–72.
Wanzer, M., Booth-Butterfield, M. & Booth-Butterfield, S. (2005). If we didn't use humor, we'd cry: Humorous coping communication in health care settings. *Journal of Health Communication, 10*(2): 105–25.
Wasserman, Herman. (2020). Laughter in the time of a pandemic: Why South Africans are joking about coronavirus. The Conversation. 15 March 2020. https://theconversation.com/laughter-in-the-time-of-a-pandemic-why-south-africans-are-joking-about-coronavirus-133528
Wooten, P. (1993). Making humor work. *Journal of Nursing Jocularity, 3*(4): 46–47.

PART I

Meme-making Practices and Making Sense of the Pandemic

CHAPTER 2

Social Media Memes as Commentary in Health Disasters in South Africa and Zimbabwe

Shepherd Mpofu

Introduction

Is it okay to meme and laugh during the pandemic? What does laughter mean amidst a crisis? This research attempts to answer these questions by exploring humor during health disasters and pandemics. New media is increasingly shaping the communicative spheres in South African and Zimbabwean communities further influencing socio-political and economic debates especially from below. This study is a comparative case study of how South Africans and Zimbabweans humorously dealt with the COVID-19 pandemic by engaging in meme composing, spreading and consumption. The choice of Zimbabwe and South Africa is informed by that the countries are neighbors and their economies are shared and in some cases the pandemic was transferred across borders leading to a need for cooperatively dealing with the pandemic. In addition, there are a lot of

S. Mpofu (✉)
University of Limpopo, Polokwane, South Africa
e-mail: shepherd.mpofu@ul.ac.za

S. Mpofu (ed.), *Digital Humour in the Covid-19 Pandemic*,
https://doi.org/10.1007/978-3-030-79279-4_2

Zimbabweans based in South Africa leading to citizens sharing information, fears and aspirations across the borders. Moreover, whenever announcements like lockdown regulations were made by South African authorities, these influenced Zimbabwe vice versa. On the analysis of humor and health crises in South Africa, I specifically chose to use the listeriosis case, a foodborne disease which started in late 2017 and was contained around and declared over in September 2018, and COVID-19 pandemic.

Listeriosis caused some health scares, killed 218 people, with 1065 cases confirmed and left some with life-long medical conditions (Whitworth, 2020). It started at a ready-to-eat processed polony meat factory in one of South Africa's provinces, Polokwane. The World Health Organization declared the outbreak 'the largest recorded globally to date' (Grobler, 2020). Listeriosis was not declared a pandemic. At the beginning of March in 2018, South Africa's Minister of Health Aaron Motsoaledi released what became breaking news that day: the finding by scientists that two particular companies were responsible for releasing into the market food that caused listeriosis leading to the death of 180 people and, later, birth of disabled children. While this alarmed and scared a lot of people when they realized that the processed foods they had hitherto been consuming were responsible for the outbreak, some people took to social media to express their views about the health threat. Similarly, when the COVID-19 started spreading across the globe, there were few cases in South Africa and memes raptured the digital sphere where ordinary people expressed their views, some of which were couched on invincibility born out of the fact that they survived Listeriosis. Listeriosis did not affect Zimbabwe, but COVID-19 affected both countries. At the time of writing this chapter, a Google search for 'COVID-19 memes' returned 1,780,000,000 hits in 0.59 seconds.

The novel coronavirus of 2019, which became known as COVID-19, is a respiratory disease caused by the coronavirus, transmitted via droplets that are produced when infected people sneeze, cough or exhale. The subsequent droplets, too heavy to remain floating in the air, land on surfaces and floors, and the virus survives for a considerable amount of time. As of September 30, 2020, the COVID-19 pandemic had infected 34.1 million people with 23.7 million recoveries and 1.02 million fatalities globally. These numbers rose to 107 million infected, 60 million recovered and around three million deaths. A number of scientists are not agreeing on the origin of the virus. Some claim the virus originated in bats and later spread to pangolins and humans. The first person to catch the virus possibly from a pangolin was a 'someone in the now world-famous Huanan seafood market in Wuhan' (Readfearn, 2020). Others argued that 'samples from a Wuhan food market initially suspected as a path for the virus's spread to humans, failed to show links between animals being sold there and the pathogen' with one scientist declaring that 'it now turns out that the market was one of the victims' (Areddy, 2020).

However, evidence suggests that Chinese authorities covered up the outbreak, to an extent of silencing Li Wenliang, a medical doctor who first raised alarm about the virus in December 2019. He died of the virus in February 2020. Prior, police targeted him, leading to his arrest for 'disturbing social order' and 'spreading rumors ...after he posted a warning on social media about a cluster of cases of flu-like disease that had been treated at his hospital [with] symptoms that reminded him of SARS' (Severe Acute Respiratory Syndrome). He was released after signing a statement where he agreed 'not to discuss his concerns in public again' (Graham-Harrison et al., 2020). Li later broke that oath at his hospital bed and said 'If the officials had disclosed information about the epidemic earlier... I think it would have been a lot better. There should be more openness and transparency' (Buckley & Lee Myers, 2020). This cast into the spotlight the Chinese authoritarian regime's control and suppression of freedoms of expression and limited democratic rights extended to citizens. This, later, caused a diplomatic spat between the USA and China, with America's then president Donald Trump threatening to punish China for spreading what he called the 'China virus' to the rest of the world. On the other hand, a Chinese official tweeted that the virus was from America. The pandemic did not only end with diplomatic spats as according to the United Nations Secretary General, 'the pandemic continues to unleash a tsunami of hate and xenophobia, scapegoating and scare-mongering' against Chinese, Asians and people of Asian extract (Human Rights Watch, 2020).

In this chapter I pay focus on health communication via Internet memes by examining the extent to which a national tragedy and an international pandemic were turned mediated through jokes for different purposes. Data for this study were gathered from three social media platforms: WhatsApp, Twitter and Facebook. Data were gathered though digital ethnography whereby the author monitored and collected memes relating to the two diseases and analyzed them using narrative analysis.

Social media platforms are communicative spaces where ordinary people interact without any inhibitions or editorializing as is the case with mainstream media, enhancing freedoms of expression in the process. These platforms become alternative sites of unbounded communication. Central to participation in these platforms is access to the technological hardware and software. Data made available by *Statista* suggests that of South Africa's 59 million people, 36.54 million are Internet users. Of these, 34.93 million use the Internet on mobile devices (2020). Of these 22 million have access and use various social media platforms with 21.56 million said to be actively using social media. Of Zimbabwe's 14.9 million citizens, 8.4 million have access to the Internet (Internet World Stats, 2020). There were 4.8 million Internet users as of January 2020 in Zimbabwe, an increase of 413,000 from the previous year. Around 980,000 used social media, a 6.6% social media penetration rate. According to the official statistics from the Posts and Telecommunications Regulatory Authority of Zimbabwe (Potraz) in 2018, WhatsApp and Facebook are said 'to account for about 35% of internet usage in Zimbabwe ... Mobile telephony companies have intensified bundle offerings and promotions for social media platforms in a bid to secure additional revenue' (Karombo, 2018). A total of 92% of the people who accessed Facebook did so via their mobile phones (72.2%), or both mobile and computers (18.9%) or only via a computer (8.4%). A total of 41.2% of those on Facebook are females; 168,500 are on Twitter and 78% of these are reportedly male (Datareportal, 2020).

Memes Culture as Participatory Culture

Memes are artifacts of participatory communications and cultures that are 'rapidly spread by members of participatory digital culture for the purpose of continuing a conversation' (Wiggins & Bowers, 2015, 1886). Memes in the current communicative ecology play a critical role as versatile multi-contextualizable visual short-hand tools in communication. Sometimes they function alone or, as in other cases, have to be accompanied by written text. Memes are central to communication in the digital world because they are relatable, people easily get attracted to images, they add a funny flavor to communication, they are dynamic and therefore attention grabbing, they can easily be adapted to different contexts without losing meaning and as popular cultural fades, most people are familiar with them. They are a universal language.

The concept of the meme was propounded by evolutionary biologist Richard Dawkins (1976) in his seminal book *The selfish gene*. In this book Dawkins defined a meme as similar to a gene in the biosphere, that is, 'a molecular unit of people's bodies, a biological code holding important information for building and maintaining cells and passing the invaluable hereditary data to offspring. Memes are similar to the genes in that they pass cultural information and ideas between individuals and generations' (Donisova, 2019, 6) in the ideosphere. The word meme came up as a result of Dawkins's adulteration of the Greek word 'mīmēma' because he wanted 'a monosyllable that sounds a bit like "gene"' (Dawkins 1986, 192). For Dawkins memes are:

> tunes, ideas, catch-phrases, clothes fashions, ways of making pots or building arches. Just as genes propagate themselves in the gene pool by leaping from body to body via sperms or eggs, so memes propagate themselves in the meme pool by leaping from brain to brain via a process which, in the broad sense, can be called imitation. If a scientist hears, or reads about, a good idea, he passes in on his colleagues and students. He mentions it in his articles or lectures. If the idea catches on, it can be said to propagate itself, spreading from brain to brain.... (1989, 1920)

In essence memes have a life of their own as they move from brain to brain just like parasites of viruses which, when they get into host bodies replicate and propagate. Imitation, for Dawkins, is the way memes replicate, but, just like genes, some memes may be more successful than others. This is because Dawkins viewed memes as selfish and virulent as they 'sought replication for the purpose of its own survival...competing to infect individual minds and use those minds for replication...' (Wiggins & Bowers, 2015, 1889). There are many ways to measure the popularity and success of the replication of memes. For instance, when it comes to music, the popularity will depend on how many people are heard and even seen singing and dancing to a particular tune. For instance, in 2020, a South African artist, Master KG, became a global sensation with his song *Jerusalema*, which led to people watching and even doing the dance moves copied from the song and posting these online. So popular was the song that the South African president, Cyril Ramaphosa, encouraged South Africans to do the dance challenge and post videos online as a way of celebrating cultural day. This, partly, was a meant as a coping mechanism during the COVID-19 pandemic. A few years back, South Korean singer,

PSY, released a song, Gangnam Style, that became a sensation too, becoming the first clip to surpass 'the one billion-view mark' (Shifman, 2014, 1).

In the media spaces, Hofstadter is probably one of the few scholars who took memes literally and even suggested that they will compete for space in traditional media such as 'radio and television time, billboard space, newspaper and magazine column inches and library shelf-space' (Hofstadter, 1983, 18). Further, Hofstadter, to emphasize the variations and somewhat malleability of memes, adds that 'some memes will tend to discredit others, and some groups of memes will tend to internally self-reinforcing' (1983, 18). Later, he claimed that by 1995 the meme had become real and not metaphorical (Burman, 2012). In the academic circles, the term meme was rejected and dismissed but, as Shifman (2014, 1) observes, it has come back through the Windows (and other operating systems of course) and there is a respectable amount of scholarship around memes to accentuate this fact (Brideau & Charles, 2014, Shifman, 2013, Shifman & Thelwall, 2009, Denisova 2019, Blackmore, 2010).

Dawkins's concept of memes was criticized for various reasons. First, memes are much more complex than being 'direct counterparts in preserving and distributing culture…They are not reliable in delivering accurate information yet are beneficial for the development of ideas: people can fill them with additional details and foster new meaning and style of expression' (Donisova, 2019, 7). Another criticism that has been leveled is that there was no need to come up with a new word, meme, when you have the word 'idea' already (Brown, 2014). Dawkins, according to Disonova (2019, 7), revisited the definitional issues of the meme and suggested that 'users create memes to deliberately hijack the original cultural text; thus, the choice and decisions of people drive memes forward' (see also Dawkins & Marshmallow, 2013). Definitionally, the word meme remains unclear and 'pinning down precise criteria for something counting as a meme is close to impossible' (Knobel & Lankshear, 2007, 205). This includes the setting of boundaries or pinpointing what a meme is. Is the whole video clip or song a meme or only the chorus is? First stanza or any other part? Is the picture including the tag line or caption a complete meme or only the picture alone or tag alone a meme? Memes are different from 'iconic images and viral texts that do not experience much alteration. They are never fixed symbols, stories or icons, but interactive aesthetic artefacts that provide a snapshot of the immediate tendencies of culture and public discourses' which alter in appearance, size and modification (Donisova, 2019, 8).

Some scholars have come to the rescue, suggesting that we need to look at memes as a building blocks, units of cultural production and also 'broader modes of human knowledge and comprise names, relationship patterns, principles of society, choices at a traffic light, information about other planets and solar systems' (Donisova, 2019, 7–8). Netizens have made memes ubiquitous, and academics in media, communication and sociology especially have paid attention to these leading to a growth of scholarship in this regard. These scholars, especially digital media scholars, use the concept of the meme as a metaphor (Shifman & Thelwall, 2009; Shifman, 2013, 2014; Vickery, 2015; Milner, 2016; Wiggins, 2019). It is believed that the first Internet memes were emoticons created by a combination of different characters using a keyboard of a computer or mobile phone [e.g. 😀, 😀]. Internet memes are polysemic and multi-owned as they are communally created and their ownership is not settled to any particular province. As Denisova (2019, 3) expounds, memes are 'empty conduits or layouts that anyone can fill with meaning or commentary. This means that neither elites nor opposition own memes; the autonomous and non-aligned character of memes make them especially worth studying in political research. Memes can change sides and connotation through their journey in the digital space'.

Internet memes are artifacts that anchor participatory digital cultures. Human agency is central to virality of memes through 'distribution, replication and propagation' (Wiggins & Bowers 2015, 1890). As Jenkins suggests, participatory cultures are easily accessible to ordinary people as they have relatively low barriers 'to artistic expression and civic engagement, strong support for creating and sharing one's creations and some type of informal mentorship whereby what is known by the most experiences is passed along to novices' (2009, 3). Vickery is worried about the legal and academic and cultural issues surrounding memes as 'intellectual property and copyright' (2015, 1450). She argues that this needs to be addressed because 'memes are challenging current debates about copyright, sharing, authorship/anonymity, and fair use' (Wiggins & Bowers, 2015, 1451). To this end, Denisova's observation that 'A meme does not belong to any author...[it] belongs to the collective creativity, to the decisions and benevolence of the Internet crowds. Like it or not, this is the memetic logic of our days' (2019, 30). Of critical concern is the skill-sets one has to have in order to engage with the memes and be part of the popular culture at production, circulation and consumption levels. As shown above, technological knowhow, access to enabling technologies and associated sundries are critical in the participation in this digital culture. These form the basis of a creation of an environment of participatory communication since memes, 'as genre are akin to continued conversation between and among members of participatory digital culture' (Wiggins & Bowers, 2015, 1894).

Methodology

The colonization of people's communicative, romantic, working, family and other functions by the digital technologies has opened up new avenues for data gathering. In this research I used digital ethnography to gather data. Ethnography, as a research methodology, 'is about telling social stories' (Murthy, 2008, 838). Ethnography is a research method that is qualitative in nature and involves the researcher immersing herself/himself in a community of interest that s/he may be interested in investigating. This immersion allows for a first-hand experience, observation and interaction with the community's cultures, relations and in-group dynamics, leading to the production of a report thereafter. This report is known as the ethnography. This commitment to understanding and documenting people's lives comes with ethical challenges.

The author used two different datasets, the listeriosis data and the COVID-19 data. I used mainly images and not videos as the latter cannot be reproduced and shared in academic writing. Listeriosis data were gathered from the three above-mentioned social media platforms during the outbreak. I randomly screen grabbed the memes and filed them. About 70 memes were gathered throughout the duration of the disease. I also did the same for the COVID-19 memes where, by way of sampling, I conveniently chose some memes shared by South Africans relating to the pandemic in South Africa and also those that related to Zimbabwe as circulated by Zimbabweans. About 200 memes were obtained and analyzed. Convenience sampling is a nonrandom technique whereby a researcher, without the constraints of theories or set number of items or participants, 'decides what needs to be known and sets out to find people who can and are willing to provide the information by virtue' of having the characteristics and qualities that the researcher is interested in (Etikan et al., 2015, 2). The memes chosen speak to the humor deployed by South Africans and Zimbabweans in their negotiation of the listeriosis (for South Africans only) and COVID-19 for both countries. Usually there was an upsurge of COVID-19-related memes before, during and after presidential announcements and updates which were given by South Africa's president, Cyril Ramaphosa.

Similarly, in Zimbabwe there was an upsurge after South Africa's announcement as Zimbabwe's economy and livelihoods are dependent on South Africa to an extent that some Zimbabweans joked that Zimbabwe was a province of South Africa. What is more, Zimbabwe's lackluster president, Emmerson Mnangagwa, also issued statements soon after Ramaphosa had done so, giving an impression of weak undecided leadership.

Digital ethnography, unlike offline ethnography, is encumbered by unique ethical concerns that are important to note. While some humorous messages shared on social media cannot lead to damages to reputation or, if used by researchers, could not lead to harm to those who post them, it is important to note that the author is aware of possible damages that could be caused through highlighting offensive posts or those that may, in future, be used to identify and or trace subjects or interlocutors (Ferguson, 2017) by re-using them in an academic article. Some issues that I will mention but not magnify are the fair usage policy that users accent to when using these online platforms. In addition, where user accounts are protected, there could be a suggestion of privacy, and therefore researchers might need to ask for consent. Added to that, there are certain questions that one has to ask before using the data they find on these platforms. For example, what does it mean when someone uploads data and later deletes the same? May a researcher use the data?

Theoretical and Conceptual Framework

In most cases in South Africa one notices that black people are usually the first ones to see the humorous side of anything that happens in society, be it disastrous or beautiful. Thus, most memes are manufactured in the *Black Social Media Factory*. Meme creation is a highly participatory endeavor as in most cases it is difficult to tell who the originator is. In some instances, memes are edited, altered, gain new meanings and regain old meaning depending on context and user identities (see Wiggins & Bowers, 2015). The countries under study are largely dominated by blacks. These blacks are not even homogeneous to an extent that they draw different meanings from similar events, and even jokes. Social media offer citizens participatory platforms. Social media are 'web based or mobile based communication channels such as applications, blogs, wikis, social book-markings, social network sites and online games that afford community based in-put in the form of creating content, distributing and even co-authoring content for different ends' (Mpofu, 2019, 68). The idea of imagined community is here strengthened and brought to life as, in some cases, people interact with people they imagine exist even though they would have not met them physically. Robots complicate this concept, but as it is beyond the ambit of this study, I will not pursue the idea further.

Black Social Media is about black witnessing, black discourses, *black* ways of being and black storytelling as expressed through social media platforms such as Facebook, TikTok, Twitter, WhatsApp, among others. In most cases this is done for identity creation, group identity formation or solidification or the provocation of laughter or protests. Black Social Media has been critical in the understanding of current events in most African countries, especially South Africa where memes make part of the staple news diet in mainstream media sites. I draw the concept of Black Social Media from Black Twitter. The definition of Black Twitter dovetails neatly with that of Black Social Media. According to Williams and Domoszlai (2013), Black Twitter has one of the most formidable and unified identities to emerge on Twitter. Black Twitter, according to Mpofu (2019, 68), 'does not in any way suggest that it is only for blacks, nor is it representative of all blacks…the main hallmark of Black Twitter is its diversity as a community of users discussing issues concerning blacks, sometimes in a coded language to which only they can relate'. This demonstrates 'cultural knowledge and insider access' (Williams & Domoszlai, 2013) by way of signifyin'. Signifyin' according to Florini (2014, 223) is performance of 'racial identity online … which deploys figurative language, indirectness, doubleness, and wordplay as a means of conveying multiple layers of meaning [serving] as a powerful resource for performance of Black cultural identity on Twitter'. Signifyn' is used for 'social critique … often [speaking] to shared experiences of Blacks … [it] can be a response for encoding and expressing experiential knowledge about Black identities' (Florini, 2014, 227). In the South African and Zimbabwean contexts which are part of this study, signifyn' relates, among other things, to the critique of the socio-economic and political environments of the two countries. In South Africa there are huge levels of inequality between poor blacks and wealthy privileged whites. Many on Black Social Media also lament the abuse of power and resources by the ruling elite and connected members. In Zimbabwe, race is not a central definer of social relations as is the case in South Africa, but the governing party has visited so much harm to the country pushing many citizens to the margins, and the experiences they then talk about are of those of tribalism and exclusion, neo-colonialism, subjugation and looting of state resources by the ruling elite. In both South Africa and Zimbabwe, there has been the looting of COVID-19 resources through irregular tendering processes that benefit members of the respective ruling parties (Gagné-Acoulon, 2020; Maseko, 2020; Transparency International, 2020a, 2020b).

Listeriosis, Identity and Desensitization

Rossing argues that humor contributes on how we relate in society as it 'constitutes a public pedagogy that teaches social norms, (re)produces ideology, constructs public memory, manages group affiliations and identity boundaries, and much more' (2015, 629). One thing that continues to color relationships in South is the race issue. Hence during health disasters and other moments of crises, commentaries on race abound. For instance, the tweet in Fig. 2.1 is a commentary on the socio-economic conditions

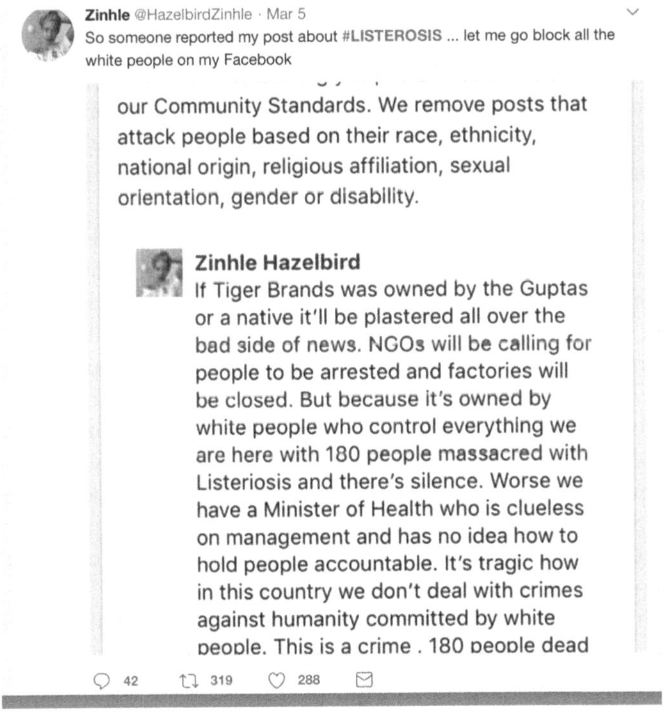

Fig. 2.1 Emancipatory racial humor challenging race relations in South Africa

in South Africa. To be black in South Africa, and indeed in the whole world, is to be a problem and in a state of rage. This rage can only be creatively negotiated through getting by in life via emancipatory humor. The discussant uses emancipatory racial humor as she complains that her post was removed from Facebook. Racial humor can take two directions. It can be retrogressive and advance white superiority and domination (Billig, 2005; Weaver, 2011; Mpofu, 2019). On the other hand, it could be progressive and upset or challenge white domination while advancing the dignity and humanity of the people of color (Walker, 1998).

When one reads the post, one is tickled to laugh, not that it is funny, but at the truthfulness of the country's economic situation and attempts at muzzling commentary that exposes the country and leadership's failures. South Africa has, in recent years, been unwelcoming to immigrants doing business in the townships or menial jobs such as child minding, gardening construction or hailer transport or truck driving. Many have had their small shops vandalized, cars stoned, burnt and looted. The Guptas are Indian brothers who allegedly used their proximity to Jacob Zuma, while he was still president of the country to do business with state departments. They allegedly influenced the president in appointing ministers and strategic personnel in parastatals for business expediency. Emancipatory racial humor 'functions as a vital participant in this struggle over knowledge, identity, power relationships, and agency… [and] proves "emancipatory" because it brings to the forefront perspectives and knowledge that challenge dominant realities, and therefore it bears potential for promoting critical questioning and reflection about racial oppression' (Rossing, 2015, 615). This type of humor fosters a 'critical consciousness about racial identity, racism, and privilege, such humor could help people identify, criticize, and ultimately begin to transform hegemonic racism' (ibid, 2015, 625). The suggestion here is that the case of listeriosis was negligence on the part of Tiger Brands and that, as a white-owned or white-dominated company, they were not punished because whites dominate the South African economy. Thus, there is 'deployment of humor and creation of space where marginalized groups can speak outside of oppressive discourse' (Billingsley, 2013, 20).

The humor departs from the mainstream and official imagining of South Africa in the mainstream public sphere and attempts to offer an alternative and counterhegemonic reading of society. Another meme addressed the issue of class. There was a story in the news that supermarket Woolworths had recalled its rice due to fears that it could have been infected with listeriosis. One meme meant to address this suggested that it was not a big problem if Woolworths's shoppers got the disease as 'all the people who buy food at Woolworths got Medical Aid...So there is nothing to worry about 😂'. Here some blacks use their digital leisure time and spaces to confront systems of power and 'inciting radical thought' (Outley et al., 2020, 3) through the 'strategic use of humour to criticize powerful institutions, to provoke self-reflection and to raise awareness' (Cameron, 2015, 285) about things that should matter in South African society. The humor addresses class and other disparities in South African economy and consumer market. Woolworths is deemed a supermarket where the privileged shop and therefore inaccessible to the poor. The meme suggests also that the poor were at the mercy of the pandemic. While others may argue that joking about poverty is unethical, in this instance, I argue that it is risk worth taking as this helps people find common ground and have public engagements about subjects that matter (Weinberger & Gulas, 1992; Cameron, 2015).

Besides offering incisive commentary on race and class, humor on listeriosis bordered dark humor, that is, on the desensitization of death and suffering. Figure 2.2 is a collection of memes addressing the issues of desensitization to death and health pandemics and also commentary on the citizens' perceptions about the disease and life in general. The humor and laughter prompted by these assists in the release of tension, as argued by Freud who suggested that some humorous moments benefit in the release of energy that is not needed (see Martin, 2007). Death is deprived of its sting and seriousness in the process and acts as a buffer for stress among other health benefits especially for those who are grieving.

The use of a condom as a protective measure employed when eating sausages could be linked to protective measures used in the managing of HIV/AIDS epidemic in South Africa which has killed a lot of black people. Just like the irresistible lure of sex, which is dangerous especially when recklessly practiced, the lure of the sausage seems equally tantalizing such that there is a suggestion to find creative ways of eating it and avoiding contracting the disease. However, not all are agreed that it is ethical to make fun of deathly circumstances as one interlocuter suggests through a meme showing one of South Africa's ministers 'leaving'. The interlocuter decries that despite the death of almost '200 black lives and we have the audacity to find humour in it through nonsensical memes and videos'. But as Kozintsev suggests laughter allows us to engage with certain issues, death included, in a certain way that discounts cultural boundedness and

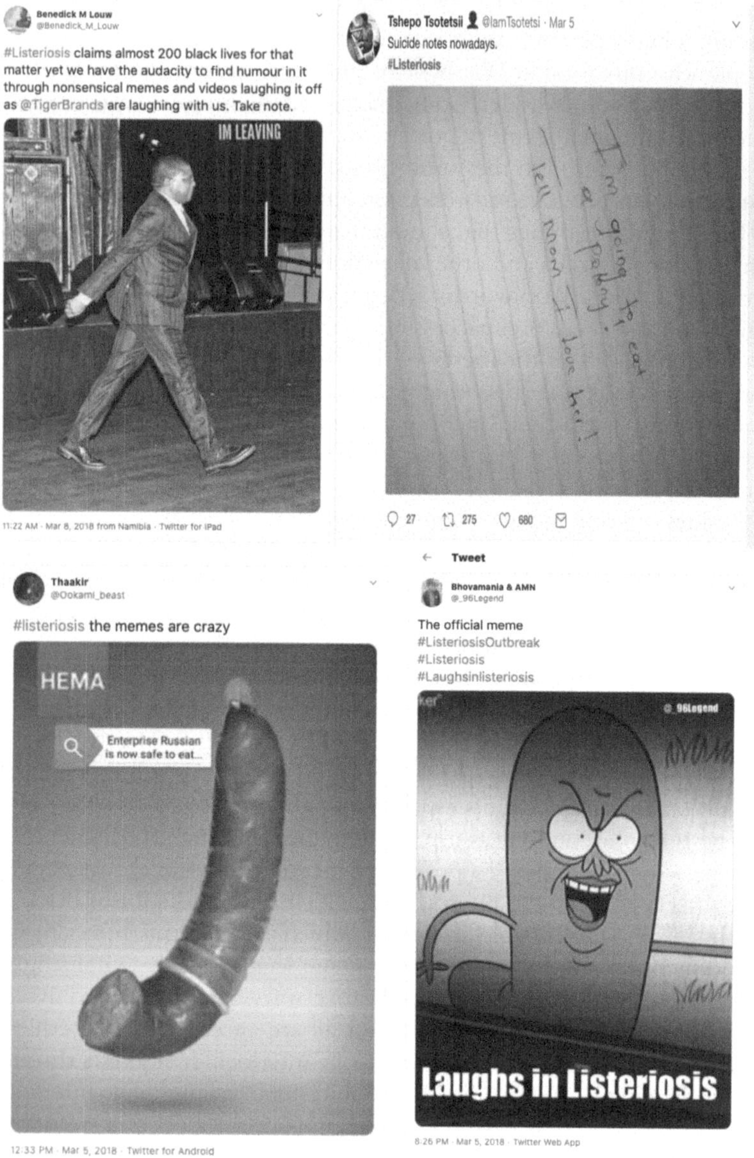

Fig. 2.2 Laughing and contesting laughter in the face of health disasters and death

'liberation from one's own sufferings and the fear of death' (Kozintsev, 2020, 144–145). Whatever the case could be, death, as Freud summarizes human life, 'is the necessary termination of life, that everyone of us owes nature his death and must be prepared to pay his debt, in short, that death was natural, undeniable, and inevitable' (Freud, 1918, 7). Jokes on and about death make death less scary, less powerful and, to a certain extent, less final. The humorous reactions to listeriosis were partly informed by the fact that people have had to contend with HIV/AIDS and have found ways to live with it through medication and using condoms and that emboldened some to believe that listeriosis was also containable. The *management* of these diseases informed attitudes and humorous approaches towards the COVID-19 global pandemic in 2020.

COVID-19 in South Africa

There is no denying that during pandemics and other moments of crisis, humor is critical in the release of humor and stress (Akinola, 2018). Some memes and discussions shared especially on Twitter, while expressing fear that 'this could be virus to eradicate human kind', also suggested the importance of humor as people needed to laugh because 'what else can we do but laugh angusho bathi (translation: *isn't they say*) laughter is the best medicine' (Fig. 2.3).

As Levine (1977) observes, we tend to laugh at our predicament and ourselves in moments of powerlessness and this is indicative of our powerlessness to influence our circumstances for the better. In South Africa humor addressed corruption, signifyin' around presidential announcements and public failures, the excitement of the arrival of the disease in South Africa and various lockdown stages, especially the banning and subsequent permission for the sale of alcohol and cigarettes.

South Africa: Fellow South Africans, Ramabillions, #Coronaviruschallenge

When the first Level 5 total lockdown was announced and national state of disaster declared on March 23, 2020, the president assured the nation that it would last for 21 days. This was in response to the spread of the coronavirus, and the lockdown was 'a decisive measure to save lives of South Africans from infections and to save lives of hundreds of thousands of our people' (Anon, 2020). Lockdown measures were so strict that

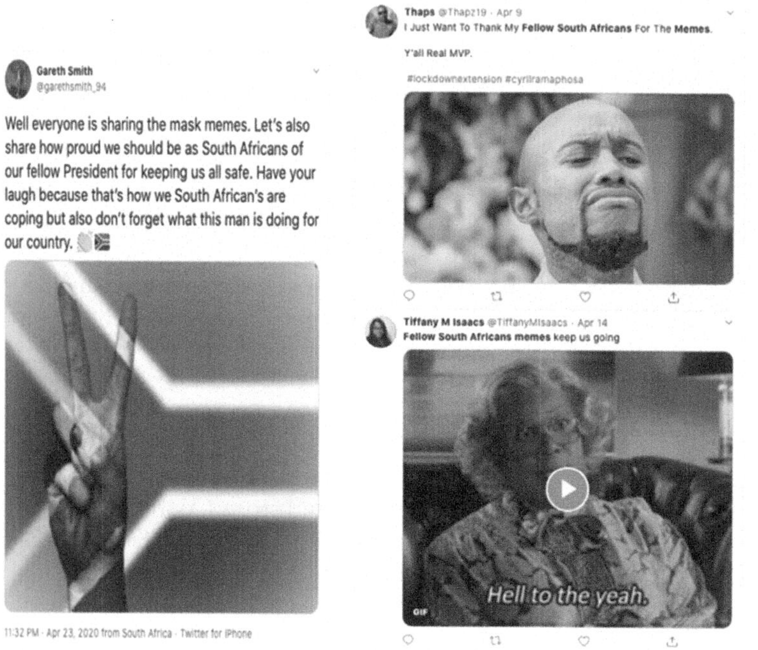
Gareth Smith
@garethsmith_94
Well everyone is sharing the mask memes. Let's also share how proud we should be as South Africans of our fellow President for keeping us all safe. Have your laugh because that's how we South African's are coping but also don't forget what this man is doing for our country.
11:32 PM · Apr 23, 2020 from South Africa · Twitter for iPhone
Thaps @Thapz19 · Apr 9
I Just Want To Thank My Fellow South Africans For The Memes.
Y'all Real MVP.
#lockdownextension #cyrilramaphosa
Tiffany M Isaacs @TiffanyMIsaacs · Apr 14
Fellow South Africans memes keep us going
Hell to the yeah.
GIF

Fig. 2.3 Appreciation of humor a few months after the pandemic came to South Africa and few weeks after the commencement of lockdown at level 5

people had to leave their homes only to seek medical care, buy food, or if they were health care or emergency workers. Soldiers were deployed to reinforce the police in ensuring the public followed the orders. With official unemployment rate at 30%, the president was alive to the fact that the measures announced would have 'a considerable impact on people's livelihoods, on the life of our society and on our economy, the human cost of delaying this action would be far, far greater' (Anon, 2020). The government promised some form of financial cushion to those who lost their livelihoods and the presidency and ministers took salary cuts. Two weeks later, he extended the lockdown and announced that the country had seen an exponential rise of infections from just less than 600 to 340,000 confirmed cases, with, at that time, 1.5 million people confirmed to be COVID-19 positive and 90,000 dead globally. He extended the lockdown by a further two weeks and appealed 'Fellow South Africans. This evening, I stand before you to ask you to endure even longer… I have to ask you to make even greater sacrifices so that our country may survive this crisis and so that tens of thousands of lives may be saved' (Ramaphosa, 2020).

When lockdown started and the wearing of masks enforced, ordinary citizens started a #CoronaVirusChallenge social media hashtag where they 'mocked' the virus by sharing various silly makes of protective masks such as condoms, bras, shoes and so on. Again, we go back to the HIV/AIDS epidemic whereby people thought COVID-19 could be prevented by the same means as HIV. Besides, the suggestion was that listeriosis was conquered, and, since most people live with HIV for long, then COVID-19 was going to be managed. In some instances, referring to it as 'made in China' suggested that, just like cheap Chinese clothes, blankets and electric gadgets that abound in the informal markets and accessed mostly by the poor, the virus was not going to last. One meme that was shared across social media platforms read: 'The Chinese might have the smallest dicks in the world but they managed to f*ck us all Anyway size doesn not matter'. Others had women's pads worn over their nose. These forms of self-deprecating humor not only made fun of the actors but also showed unison in self-mockery. However, these jokes, it would seem, demonstrated the fact that most people had not realized the devastating effects of the COVID-19 pandemic. Of course, some of the bravado was informed by the fact that South Africa managed to eradicate listeriosis and the health sector was 'managing' HIV/AIDS. As time went on, the bravado wore out, and memes became fewer only to reappear around the times of presidential addresses.

During the speeches, South Africans drew some laughter with the President's mode of address such as 'Fellow South Africans' and his demonstration on how to greet using an elbow and his failure to put on a mask on national television. He ended up being referred as *FellowSouthAfricans* and his addresses were code named 'family meetings'. In addition, he promised an economic stimulus of 500 billion Rand, some of which ended up being 'lost' through corruption whose beneficiaries were connected to the ruling ANC. For that he was referred to as *Ramabillion* and this was entertainment-cloaked critique of the possible corruption and mystery surrounding the money as most were sure it was not going to serve its purpose. He was also referred to as *RaMask* and this was a triple-play on his name and parody on his failure to wear a mask and the corruption that involved R500bn. It would seem that Ramaphosa was aware of some of the fun poked at him by the public as he acted on them and started varying, for instance, how he opened his addresses to the nation and calling his national addresses 'family meetings'. He also mentioned some instances where he was made fodder of parody. As Obadare says in disagreeing with

Mbembe's (1992, 2), assertion that humor and ridicule directed towards the *commandment* 'does not do violence to the *commandment* material base' 'it seems plausible that humour actually does perturb the *commandment'* (2009, 248). The memes that were later shared including these formulated and playful names signifyin' many different things showed an understanding of power by ordinary citizens, the subaltern, to caricature the president, 'subvert authority, and in some cases empower themselves' (Obadare, 2009, 245). Thus, ordinary people found creative ways of getting around the curfews and banning of alcohol.

Corruption

As already indicated, citizens did not expect any transparency on the use and allocation of COVID-19 funds, and the labels *Ramabillion* and *RaMask*, among others, were prophetic. And this prophesy was based on how corruption has been banal, institutionalized and normalized (Ashforth & Anand, 2003). When Ramaphosa announced the stimulus packages—the billions—he assured the nation not even a cent will be lost through corruption. By April 2020 there were reports of corruption especially by political leaders involving food parcels for the poor. Not long into the pandemic, the president's spokesperson and her husband were fingered in a R125 million tender fraud for the provision of personal protective equipment (PPE) (Moche, 2020). There were reports of alleged corruption throughout the country, and in most cases some senior ruling party officials were involved. This led to the sharing of memes not only mocking the president for 'pulling a mask over our eyes' as he did on the fateful day when he failed to cover his mouth and nose with a mask and instead got the mask caught over his eyes. People started questioning the sincerity and the trust business, media and ordinary people had shown towards him. This was done in comparison to the former president, Jacob Zuma. One meme read 'South African media is very dangerous, it's a #Propaganda machine on steroids they were very vocal about R250MILLION #Nkandla upgrade now silent when #Ramaphosa blew #R500BILLION while #PravinGordhan's #Eskom blew R4Bln & R149BILLION facilitated by #AndreDeRuyter #JanOberholzer'.

The R250 million the discussant refers to above is the money that was used to upgrade Zuma's rural home, at Inkandla, and this led to him being accused of corruption and he had to pay part of that money to the state. In addition, as one discussant notes, Zuma's alleged handlers, the Guptas, who contributed to what is currently known as State Capture

(Meirotti & Masterson, 2018), #Guptas stole almost R40bn over period of 8 years 😂 #Ramabillions 😂'. This comparison is telling it would seem. The laughing emojis signal the comic nature of politics and laughs at everyone across the board who thought Ramaphosa was a different breed of a leader. Some blamed the president for being slow, hence the snail meme. Previously there has been moments when the president has failed to act on xenophobia, protests, violence and so on timeously despite his campaign themed *Thuma mina* (Send me) (February, 2019). This informed the following meme of him as a snail (Fig. 2.4) and in a way suggested that, even not corrupt himself, he was role modeling corruption by acting slowly (Kelman, 1973; Ashforth & Anand, 2003).

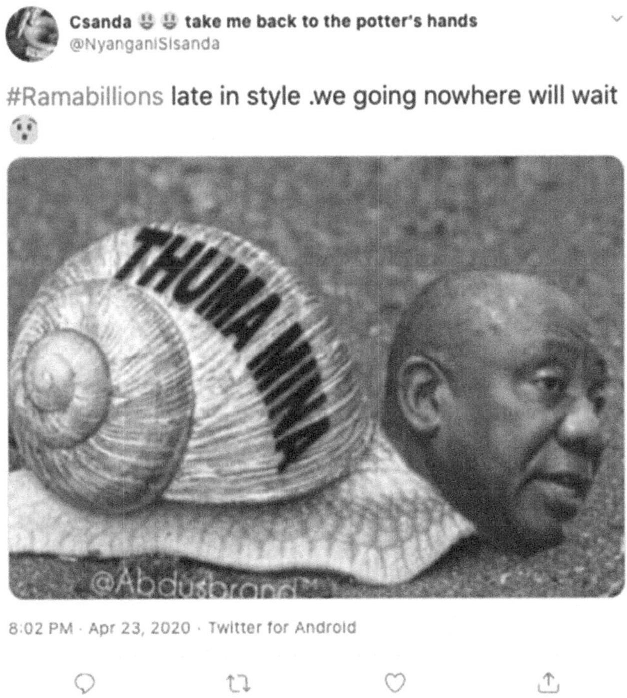

Fig. 2.4 Ramaphosa has been accused of being slightly behind the news and current affairs. Social media commentary suggesting his snail-like pace also alludes to being not pro-active in terms of having plans to curb corruption

Zimbabwe: Humorless State and Protest

When the COVID-19 pandemic started, to spread across the globe and panic abound, Zimbabwe's Defence Minister, among other conspiracy theorists, said the virus was God's punishment of the USA and Europe for imposing sanctions on Zimbabwe. Sanctions were imposed on selected individuals within the ruling Zanu-Pf, and these were as a response by the West to the lack of democracy in Zimbabwe (Ndebele, 2020). However, while some believed COVID-19 would not affect black people in areas where there is hot weather, the coronavirus, it seems, was not limited to race or weather as it affected Zimbabwe and claimed the lives of some political leaders. With the criminalization of fake news around the pandemic, it seems the state would not 'see' humor in citizens' reactions to the pandemic. The reaction to the pandemic, in some cases, especially where lamentations of clueless and uninspiring leadership offered by President Mnangagwa were concerned, bordered on comparing the leadership provided by Ramaphosa to Mnangagwa's. Even though not a meme, but to highlight this point, when Ramaphosa extended lockdown days, one Zimbabwean, Lovemore Zvokusekwa, published a communique to the nation which had the government letterhead and President Mnangagwa's signature purporting to have extended the lockdown by a further 13 days. The police claimed that the 'Accused then disseminated the false press statement on different WhatsApp platforms using his cellphone Huawei 6 Pro serial number 861855030065887 and 861855030082163 with Econet line number 0772103312, yet in actual fact, the President of the Republic of Zimbabwe His Excellency Emmerson Mnangagwa did not make or neither sign that press statement' (Vinga, 2020). Instead of seeing the act as funny and mischievous, Mnangagwa threated: 'That is absolutely nonsense, I have never made such a statement. If we catch this person, it must be exemplary and they must go in for at least at level 14, which is 20 years' imprisonment. That, I think we need to demonstrate that we don't want false news to be circulated' (Aljazeera, 2020).

Zimbabwe's state appears to be humorless and opposed to Thomas Jefferson's advice that a little rebellion by citizens now and then tends to be a good thing. And Zimbabwe's neighbors exercised a healthy dose of this humor. Historically, it seems, poor and repressive states tend to be humorless. Humor is part of freedom of expression and in these states this freedom is curtailed. 'Democracy and humour, as pontificated by Bruner, tend to 'develop when there is persistent and effective balance of powers'

(2005, 151). Conservative states with citizens restricted from humorously engaging with the state that fail to handle ambiguity and dissensus and have monolithic rather than turbulent public spheres are sick and humorless compared to healthy ones where leaders encourage and provide for critical and engaged citizenry (see Bruner, 2005). In oppressive societies like Zimbabwe, history demonstrates that carnivalesque protest can be used to undermine, oppose, challenge, 'or at least temporarily relieve, various forms of oppressive political culture' (Bruner, 2005, 138).

Besides fake news, Zimbabwe had less humorous approach to the pandemic compared to South Africa and reasons could be diverse. Part of the social media memes shared expressed dark humor and violence. The Zimbabwean state is excessively violent as leaders appropriate violence as the only audible language of persuasion and consent. The militarization of the state speaks largely to force rather than other forms of negotiation and coercion. Figure 2.5 shows the reflection of a violent state on society.

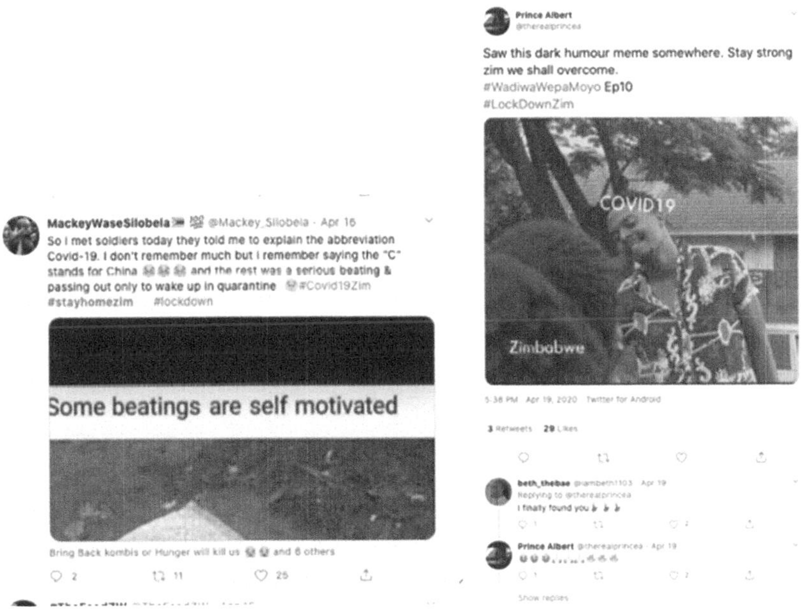

Fig. 2.5 Zimbabwe's dark humor revealed the violent state of affairs during the pandemic

Violence has become so commonplace in the interaction between citizens and the government of the day.

Zimbabweans also critiqued government's lack of preparedness for handling of the pandemic through poor infrastructural development. One meme compared the tents pitched for Zanu-Pf's congress meeting in December to those pitched for the COVID-19 centers. It appears the party's infrastructure was well up to standard compared to the health facilities for the patients suggesting the lack of priorities in the ruling party. In addition, the meme spoke to issues of corruption. Also ridiculed was the health of ministers who were claiming to be COVID-19 negative on social media and some *memeists* composed memes showing the COVID-19 tests and a host of many more ailments for these ministers. For instance, Rey Gwisai Hungwe had his health report composed and shared on Twitter with positive tests on HIV, Syphilis, 'Genital Herps', Gonorrhea, Pubic Lice and others.

Critiques of poor leadership and corruption were also the subject of memes. Interestingly, Mnangagwa seemed to take a cue on addressing the nation from Ramaphosa to an extent that some memes and jokes shared pointed that out and went on to declare Zimbabwe a province of South Africa and Ramaphosa the country's president. President Ramaphosa, even though not a good model of leadership during a crisis compared to others like Germany's Angela Merkel, New Zealand's Jacintha Ardern, Finland's Sana Marin and Taiwan's Tsai Ing-wen, was better than Mnangagwa's clueless, uninspirational, directionless and ineloquent leadership. It could also be true that since Zimbabwe's economy is dependent on South Africa, then citizens were not far off in their commentary and seeing Ramaphosa as their leader. Humor, in this instance, was used to highlight Mnangagwa's shortcomings and drive home a message that Zimbabweans were on their own, leaderless during a crisis. In addition, it also worked as a stress reliever, making people cope with the pandemic and effects of lockdown through laughter.

To highlight corruption at state level, one meme read '3 hours after the World Health Organisation announces that all countries with confirmed cases of COVID-19 will get assistance of 500 million USD from it, Zimbabwe announces its first case of Covid 19 ☺ ☺'. Thereafter there were cases of corruption involving the Minister of Health who was later fired, some businessman and President Mnangagwa's son. The journalists who exposed the corruption were arrested and hunted down by the state security agents. Tawanda Mucheiwa, the nephew of an online newspaper journalist Mduduzi Mathuthu, was abducted and tortured by security agents. The act was caught on camera and no arrests were made by the state despite overwhelming evidence implicate state security agents. Mathuthu went into hiding, while another journalist Hopwell Chino'no was arrested spending a month in maximum prison without trial. This highlights the levels of corruption in a state which has a rapacious appetite for treating the state as a site of eating and self-aggrandizement and use of violence to silence dissenters and those who shine light on the dark corners to expose corruption. In a way, while the memes signaled the coming corruption, when the corruption started it could have been too much to fathom and there were no further memes made and shared laughing at corruption, but protests were organized and quashed by Zimbabwe's military regime.

Conclusion

Internet memes and social media humor are a critical social phenomenon in human conversation about politics, social issues, economy, politics, crises, pandemics and all issues concerning human life. This chapter has touched on the use of humor, as a weapon of the powerless, in South Africa and Zimbabwe during South Africa's listeriosis times and both countries' experiences with the global COVID-19 pandemic. In dealing with both listeriosis and COVID-19, South Africans had to engage with the painful apartheid past and its consequences and corruption from the current ruling elites. Thus, Black Social Media used its digital leisure, spaces and resources to challenge the system, that is, white monopoly capital and industry by critiquing the system under the black government via laughter and uncomfortable memes and commentary (Outley et al., 2020). Besides, ordinary citizens appreciated humor as a way of managing, getting by and enduring their fear of the virus. Both the Zimbabwean and South African citizens dealt with their fears, corruption and challenges of leadership using memes and in some cases this signaled desensitization. Desensitization leads to ordinary people engaging in immoral or violent acts without thinking about their consequences and effects on their subjects and even society. In addition, desensitization numbs moral and humane responses to situations such as sympathy or empathy (Sanchez, 2020). Be that as it may, Internet memes remain a central language in the digitally colonized space of human communication and interaction as it helps society critique, question, desensitize, rebel and correct itself. It also allows power to escape, play along or threaten the subjects and citizens, depending on the depth of a particular citizenship in a given state.

References

Akinola, J. A. (2018). Pragmatics of crisis-motivated humour in computer mediated platforms in Nigeria. *Journal of Language and Education, 4*(3), 6–17.

Aljazeera. (2020). *Zimbabwe president threatens fake news author with 20 years' jail.* https://www.aljazeera.com/economy/2020/4/14/zimbabwe-president-threatens-fake-news-author-with-20-years-jail

Anon. (2020). *South Africans brace for 21-day lockdown as virus cases rise.* aljazeera.com/news/2020/03/24/south-africans-brace-for-21-day-lockdown-as-virus-cases-rise/?gb=true

Areddy, J. T. 2020. *China rules out animal market and lab as coronavirus origin.* https://www.wsj.com/articles/china-rules-out-animal-market-and-lab-as-coronavirus-origin-11590517508

Ashforth, B. E., & Anand, V. (2003). The normalization of corruption in organization. *Research in Organizational Behavior, 25*, 1–52.

Billig, M. (2005). Comic racism and violence. In S. Lockyer & M. Pickering (Eds.), *Beyond a joke: The limits of humour.* Palgrave Macmillan.

Billingsley, A. 2013. *Laughing against patriarchy: Humor, silence, and feminist resistance.* Philosophy Matters Prize Winning Essays, University of Oregon. https://pages.uoregon.edu/uophil/files/Philosophy_Matters_Submission_Marvin_Billingsley.pdf

Blackmore, S. (2010). Dangerous memes: Or, what the Pandorans let loose. In S. Dick & M. Lupisella (Eds.), *Cosmos and culture: Cultural evolution in a cosmic context* (pp. 297–318). NASA.

Brideau, K., & Charles, B. (2014). A brief introduction to impact: 'The Meme Font'. *Journal of Visual Culture, 13*(3), 307–313.

Brown, A. (2014). Serious objections to memes. *The Guardian Religion blog*, 8 July 2009. Available at: www.theguardian.com/commentisfree/andrew-brown/2009/jul/08/religion-atheism

Bruner, M. L. (2005). Carnivalesque protest and the humorless state. *Text and Performance Quarterly, 25*(2), 136–155.

Buckley, C., & Lee Myers, S. (2020). *As new coronavirus spread, China"s old habits delayed fight.* https://www.nytimes.com/2020/02/01/world/asia/china-coronavirus.html

Burman, J. (2012). The misunderstanding of memes: Biography of an unscientific object, 1976–1999. *Perspectives on Science, 20*(1), 75–104.

Cameron, J. D. (2015). Can poverty be funny? The serious use of humour as a strategy of public engagement for global justice. *Third World Quarterly, 36*(2), 274–290.

Datareportal. (2020). *Digital 2020: Zimbabwe.* https://datareportal.com/reports/digital-2020-zimbabwe?rq=zimbabwe

Dawkins, R. (Performer) & Marshmallow, L. (Director). (2013). *Just for hits.* Available at: http://www.youtube.com/watch?v=GFn-ixX9edg

Dawkins, R. (1976/1986). *The selfish gene.* (2nd edn.). Oxford University Press.

Donisova, A. (2019). *Internet memes and society: Social, cultural, and political contexts.* Routledge.

Etikan, I., Musa, S. A., & Alkassim, R. S. (2015). Comparison of convenience sampling and purposive sampling. *American Journal of Theoretical and Applied Statistics, 5*(1), 1–4.

February, J. (2019). *'No Drama' Ramaphosa is missing his opportunities to be presidential.* https://www.dailymaverick.co.za/opinionista/2019-09-24-no-drama-ramaphosa-is-missing-his-opportunities-to-be-presidential/

Ferguson, R. H. (2017). Offline 'stranger' and R online lurker: Methods for an ethnography of illicit transactions on the darknet. *Qualitative Research, 17*(6), 683–698.

Florini, S. (2014). Tweets, Tweeps, and Signifyin': Communication and cultural performance on 'Black Twitter'. *Television and New Media, 15*(3), 223–237.

Freud, S. (1918). *Reflections on war and death.* Moffat, Yard and Company.

Gagné-Acoulon, S. (2020). *Zimbabwe's health minister charged for COVID-19 Corruption.* https://www.occrp.org/en/daily/12594-zimbabwe-s-health-minister-charged-for-COVID-19-corruption

Graham-Harrison, E., Phillips, T., & McCury, J. (2020). *Doctor who blew the whistle over coronavirus has died, hospital says.* https://www.theguardian.com/world/2020/feb/06/whistleblower-chinese-doctor-dies-from-coronavirus

Grobler, R. (2020). *Listeriosis outbreak: How it started, how it was traced, and how it was finally stopped.* https://www.news24.com/news24/southafrica/news/listeriosis-outbreak-how-it-started-how-it-was-traced-and-how-it-was-finally-stopped-20180903

Hofstadter, D. (1983). Metamagical themas: Virus-like sentences and self-replicating structures. *Scientific American, 248*, 14–22.

Human Rights Watch. (2020). *COVID-19 fueling anti-Asian racism and xenophobia worldwide.* https://www.hrw.org/news/2020/05/12/COVID-19-fueling-anti-asian-racism-and-xenophobia-worldwide#

Internet World Stats. (2020). *Africa.* https://www.internetworldstats.com/africa.htm#zw

Jenkins, H. (2009). *Confronting the challenges of participatory culture: Media education for the 21st century.* The MIT Press.

Karombo, T. (2018). *More Zimbabweans engage social networks as OTT dominates.* https://itweb.africa/content/LPwQ5Ml6lWDvNgkj

Kelman, H. C. (1973). Violence without moral restraint: Reflections on the dehumanization of victims and victimizers. *Journal of Social Issues, 29*(4), 25–61.

Knobel, M., & Lankshear, C. (2007). Online memes, affinities and cultural production. In M. Knobel & C. Lankshear (Eds.), *A new literacies sampler* (pp. 199–227). Peter Lang.

Kozintsev, A. (2020). *Mirror of laughter*. Transaction Publishers.
Levine, L. W. (1977). *Black culture and black consciousness: Afro-American folk thought from slavery to freedom*. Oxford University Press.
Martin, R. A. (2007). *The psychology of humor: An integrative approach*. Elsevier.
Maseko, N. (2020). *Coronavirus in South Africa: Misuse of COVID-19 funds 'frightening'*. https://www.bbc.com/news/world-africa-54000930
Mbembe, A. (1992). The banality of power and the aesthetics of vulgarity in the postcolony. *Public Culture, 4*(2), 1–30.
Meirotti, M., & Masterson, G. (Eds.). (2018). *State capture in Africa: Old threats, new packaging*. EISA.
Milner, R. M. (2016). *The world made meme: Public conversations and participatory media*. MIT Press.
Moche, T. (2020). TIMELINE: COVID-19 food parcels, PPE corruption timeline. https://www.sabcnews.com/sabcnews/timeline-covid-19-food-parcels-ppecorruption-timeline/
Mpofu, S. (2019). Jesus comes to South Africa: Black twitter as citizen journalism in South African Politics. *African Journalism Studies, 40*(1), 67–90.
Murthy, D. (2008). Digital ethnography: An examination of the use of new technologies for social research. *Sociology, 42*(5), 837–855.
Ndebele, L. (2020). *Zim minister's bizarre coronavirus claim: 'It's to punish the West for sanctions'*. https://www.timeslive.co.za/news/africa/2020-03-16-zim-ministers-bizarre-coronavirus-claim-its-to-punish-the-west-for-sanctions/
Obadare, E. (2009). The uses of ridicule: Humour, 'infrapolitics' and civil society in Nigeria. *African Affairs, 108*(431), 241–261.
Outley, C., Bowen, S., & Pinckney, H. (2020). Laughing while black: Resistance, coping and the use of humor as a pandemic pastime among blacks. *Leisure Sciences*. https://doi.org/10.1080/01490400.2020.1774449
Ramaphosa. M. (2020). *President Cyril Ramaphosa: Extension of coronavirus COVID-19 lockdown to the end of April*. https://www.gov.za/speeches/president-cyril-ramaphosa-extension-coronavirus-COVID-19-lockdown-end-april-9-apr-2020-0000
Readfearn, G. (2020). *How did coronavirus start and where did it come from? Was it really Wuhan's animal market?* https://www.theguardian.com/world/2020/apr/28/how-did-the-coronavirus-start-where-did-it-come-from-how-did-it-spread-humans-was-it-really-bats-pangolins-wuhan-animal-market
Rossing, J. P. (2015). Emancipatory racial humor as critical public pedagogy: Subverting hegemonic racism. *Communication, Culture & Critique, 9*(4), 614–632.
Sanchez, B. C. (2020). Internet memes and desensitization. *Pathways: A Journal of Humanistic and Social Inquiry, 1*(2), 1–11.
Shifman, L. (2013). Memes in a digital world: Reconciling with a conceptual troublemaker. *Journal of Computer-Mediated Communication, 18*(3), 362–377.

Shifman, L. (2014). *Memes in digital culture.* MIT Press.
Shifman, L., & Thelwall, M. (2009). Assessing global diffusion with web memetics: The spread and evolution of a popular joke. *Journal of the American Society for Information Science and Technology, 60*(12), 2567–2576.
Statista. (2020). *Digital population in South Africa as of January 2020.* https://www.statista.com/statistics/685134/south-africa-digital-population/
Transparency International. (2020a). *Zimbabwe's deadly duo: COVID-19 and corruption: Thousands of citizens report corruption since the start of the pandemic* https://www.transparency.org/en/blog/zimbabwes-deadly-duo-COVID-19-and-corruption#
Transparency International. (2020b). *In South Africa, COVID-19 has exposed greed and spurred long-needed action against corruption.* https://www.transparency.org/en/blog/in-south-africa-COVID-19-has-exposed-greed-and-spurred-long-needed-action-against-corruption
Vickery, J. R. (2015). Memes in digital culture. *Information, Communication & Society, 18*(12), 1450–1451.
Vinga, A. (2020). *Man remanded in custody over fake ED COVID-19 statement.* https://www.newzimbabwe.com/man-remanded-in-custody-over-fake-ed-COVID-19-statement/
Walker, N. A. (1998). *What's so funny? Humor in American culture.* Rowman and Littlefield.
Weaver, S. (2011). Jokes, rhetoric and embodied racism: A rhetorical discourse analysis of the logics of racist jokes on the Internet. *Ethnicities, 11*(4), 413–435.
Weinberger, M., & Gulas, C. (1992). The use of humor in advertising: A review. *Journal of Advertising, 21*(4), 35–59.
Whitworth, J. (2020). *'It ruined my life', says woman infected by Listeria in South African outbreak.* https://www.foodsafetynews.com/2020/02/it-ruined-my-life-says-woman-infected-by-listeria-in-south-african-outbreak/
Wiggins, B. E. (2019). *The discursive power of memes in digital culture: Ideology, semiotics, and intertextuality.* Routledge.
Wiggins, B. E., & Bowers, B. G. (2015). Memes as genre: A structurational analysis of the memescape. *New Media & Society, 17*(11), 1886–1906.
Williams, A., & Domoszlai, D. (2013). *#BlackTwitter: A networked cultural identity.* http://harmony-institute.org/latest/2013/08/06/blackTwitter-a-networked-cultural-identity/

CHAPTER 3

Viral Jokes: Humour and Grace as Critical Devices in Memes About the COVID-19 Pandemic in Brazil

Alexandre Werneck

Introduction

Images like the Fig. 3.1 have become a regular part of Brazilian everyday lives since the start of the COVID-19 pandemic, especially for those of us on social media. The meme[1] has become one of the most habitual signs in contemporary communication (Mina, 2019), and its presence during a period like the coronavirus pandemic would be expected. As I have shown in other texts, even at moments of social commotion surrounding tragedies—as in outbreaks of violence (Werneck, 2020b)—when some

This chapter presents results of the project Ostentatious Moralism: A Study of the Role of Accusatory Critics in Public and Private Worlds, financed by the National Council for Scientific and Technological Development (CNPQ), through its research productivity grant, which I thank for the support.

A. Werneck (✉)
Federal University of Rio de Janeiro (UFRJ), Rio de Janeiro, Brazil
e-mail: av.werneck@ifcs.ufrj.br

S. Mpofu (ed.), *Digital Humour in the Covid-19 Pandemic*,
https://doi.org/10.1007/978-3-030-79279-4_3

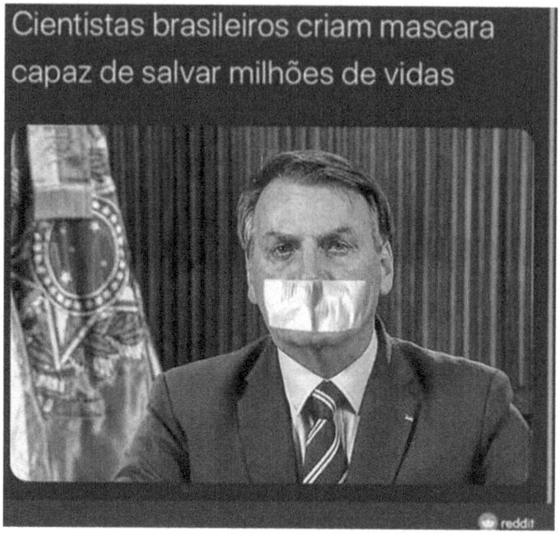

Fig. 3.1 'Brazilian scientists create a mask capable of saving millions of lives.' (All images are taken from the Internet)

kind of routine can be established, a space for humour also becomes possible. Equally, as I have also demonstrated elsewhere (Werneck, 2015, 2016, 2019; Werneck & Loretti, 2018), this deployment of humour is more than just a proof of wit and cleverness: it is usually associated with the circulation of critique—whether using the dynamic of critique to make jokes, or using humour to make critiques. In the image, we see President Jair Bolsonaro become the target of a 'mocking' (a *zoação*: Werneck, 2015) in which his 'mouth' is criticized—that is, his recurrent hapless remarks concerning the health crisis, in a gallery that spans from denial of the risk potential of the virus to prioritization of economic aspects over the need to preserve life, accompanied by his proposal of controversial 'alternative' treatments. In the joke, the protective mask, an essential device in the pandemic discourse—and in some public situations in which the politician proved unable to use them (Alfano, 19/03/2020)—is transformed into stick tape, a form of preventing him from speaking, which in the universe of the joke would be a public health measure.

The argument I have been exploring in the aforementioned previous works is that the *formal matrix* (Werneck & Loretti 2018) of a humorous critique—that is, the composition of its formal elements—plays a role in its *effectuation* (Werneck, 2012),[2] both in private situations or one-off interactions (Werneck, 2015) and in public situations (Werneck & Loretti 2018; Werneck, 2016, 2019, 2020b). Furthermore, this involves the deployment of a specific process, the *ridiculing* (Billig, 2005) of the object of the critique (whether this is a practised action or its practitioner): its worth[3] (Boltanski & Thévenot, 1991) is reduced to a condition of laughable absurdity. When mobilized as a platform for critique, this joking register provides the latter with the construction of a singular observer capable of *effectuating* the critique employing this reduction to the ridiculous, without needing to undergo the rationalist protocol of *testing* (*épreuve*) (ibid), in which proofs and logical arguments are carefully evaluated. As such, the process ratifies the idea of a *transitory truth* (Nielsen, 2019/04/01) to be accepted without any further evaluation. Consequently, the deployment of the *grace* of *inspiration* (Boltanski & Thévenot, ibid) proper of *humour* assumes a prominent role in the operationalization of critiques. Grace is a competence rooted in *inspiration*—on creativity and singularity, in other words—whose evaluation thereby replaces any evaluation of the specific content of the critique.

The point I wish to highlight here is that in situations like that of the pandemic in which there is a vast, monumental transformation of routine, a threefold process becomes established: an *investigation* (Dewey, 1938), *indefinition* (Werneck, 2020a), and *routinization*, which is sustained to a significant extent by critique and benefits remarkably from humour towards this end. This process turns on the same fundamental social phenomenon: the definition of the situation, that is, 'a stage of examination and deliberation [...] preliminary to any self-determined act of behaviour' (Thomas (1966[1923], 42) and that says *what is happening there*, allowing humans to treat these situations as 'real in their consequences' (Thomas & Thomas, 1938[1928], 572), that is, a definition capable of generating effects, effectuating itself (Werneck, 2012). In each of these three stages, a relation with this definition is established with the critique on the horizon, the moral evaluation of things becoming a central element of the equation.

To understand how memes expressed these different regimes for defining the pandemic's general situation in Brazil, I promoted a collection of these circulating signs in the country in the period between March (when our isolation experience began) and August 2020 and proceeded with a semiotic analysis. The observations presented here are based on a sample of around 350 unique memes (in this universe, there exist many versions of the same sign) in a sample space of more than 500. The research showed how different critical investments took place at each stage of the pandemic and how the memes mirrored these phases.

A series of humour formal variables can be identified in the memes circulating during the pandemic.[4] This chapter, though, concentrates on the critical directions chosen by them and their political dimension. In so doing, it dialogues with an expansive area of studies on the use of humour in public protests—in which I include my recent work (T'Hart & Bos, 2008; Beckman, 2014; Yacintas, 2015; Werneck, 2015, 2016, 2019, 2020b; King, 2016; Trnka & Rehak, 2018; Werneck & Loretti, 2018). However, this emphasis on critique seeks to understand this political dimension first and foremost as a morality game: the question is which conceptions of good are deployed to support the critical discourse that encounters a fertile soil in the transition between routines caused by the pandemic and the health measures—made explicit in the critiques in the way in which these goods are disrespected/disregarded. It was possible to observe that these concepts of good took a metonymic form: the critical targets have served as a form of this characterization.

The wave of memes on the pandemic in Brazil seems to have followed three distinct movements (regimes) in four different temporal registers, and the chapter structure follows this movement, each item focused on a different phase or moment in time, with a focus on the critiques produced in each moment/phase. The following table summarizes the matrix:

Moment in time	*Regime*
Emergence(end of 2019–Mar 2020)	Investigative (criticisms motivated by the initial estrangement with the virus)
Isolation(Mar 2020–May 2020)	
Start of the plateau(May 2020–Aug 2020)	Routine (in which the criticisms were consolidated)
Plateau's consolidation (Aug 2020–)	'New normal' (A new routine, new critiques)

The Memes Pandemic and Its Different Phases

The first stage of the 'memes pandemic' could be called, inspired by Dewey (ibid), investigative in which the jokes represent attempts by actors to deal with the upheaval in routine caused by the disease. In the first moment, this regime initially comprehended the infection as something mysterious and distant, 'coming from China' and still yet to be understood, and, mostly, as a future wave to be awaited. A survey published by the Public Policy Analysis Directorate (*Diretoria de Análise de Políticas*

Públicas: DAPP) of the Getulio Vargas Foundation (FGV) on 28 February 2020 (updated on 9 March) showed that, at the end of the second month of the year, around 34% of interactions on social media relating to COVID-19 in Brazil were good-humoured or ironic compared to 17% worried (Camillo 13/03/2020). At that moment, the country had just recorded the first confirmed case of the disease. The memes followed a more or less concentrated trend at the start of the epidemic, their more typical form reflected in the following example:

Figure 3.2 shows a man lying back in a toy float in floodwaters. Another example is a meme showing Zé Gotinha (Joe Droplet), a character created by Brazil's Ministry of Health in the 1980s as a mascot for its child vaccination campaigns, with the caption: 'Joe Droplet says in interview that he'll beat the hell out of Coronavirus.' Coronavirus was considered a far-away danger at the beginning of the year, and the essential information contained in these jokes expresses some indifference to its risk. Nevertheless, they also contained a second layer, self-critical of the country: the disease originating from China is strong, but Brazil already lives with far too many misfortunes on an everyday basis and even has its own diseases—for instance, there are many comparisons with dengue, an endemic consolidated in Brazilian health culture. Coronavirus would be no match, then, for the country's reality. Even the claim that Zé Gotinha would beat up

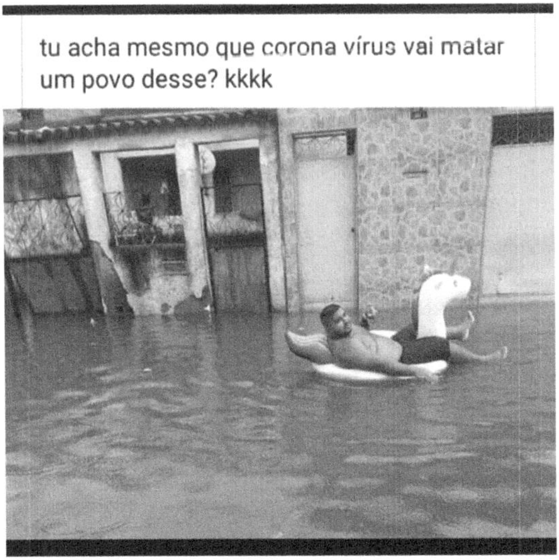

Fig. 3.2 'Do you really think coronavirus will kill a people like this? LOL'

the virus needs to be read in this context marked by ironic speech (Herzfeld, 2001), referring here to Brazil's capacity to deal with the imminent epidemic: the character is repeatedly depicted in the images in a ridiculous form, as a costume worn by an actor pretending to be a superhero at a child's birthday party.

For some analysts, this movement suggested that the disease's closer experience would adjust the proportion between humour and seriousness (Camillo, 13/03/2020). They speculated that people would shift from memes to informative interactions as soon as the situation became clear. No update was made of the figures of web searches on the topic in Brazil, partly because they were undoubtedly affected by the dizzying rise in the total number of mentions of the pandemic on social networks as the year progressed: on March 11 alone, for example, an international consultancy firm reported 19 million references to the pandemic (Enberg, 18/03/2020). After all, the idea that the moment was critical simultaneously swept the ground from beneath people's feet, exposing them to the indeterminacy (Dewey, 1938) and impelling them to become informed and, at the same time, to start an inquiry. That movement helped them understand the world, aware by now that they were facing a pandemic of global dimensions, something easy to comprehend, though still complicated. Then came the government health and economic measures, followed by, in the eye of the hurricane of a massive transformation in people's routines and behaviours, the physical distancing measures, and the consequent home quarantine.[5] This created a *second inquiry movement*, thematically redirecting the humorous speech: while previously it had concentrated on mocking the virus itself, downplaying its potency, as well as other countries and cultures already affected by it (mostly the Chinese and Italians), the start of a strange new routine of a lack of routine imposed by distancing and self-isolation imperatives, situated somewhere between voluntary and government-ordered, enabled a new zone of indeterminacy fed by a new set of critiques.

On the one hand, we find a new kind of image, the apparent antithesis of the (ironic) 'courage' expressed in the previous case. Now the indeterminacy of the future, associated with the hardship of the present, generates memes like the one in which we can see Hannibal Lecter (Anthony Hopkins) from the Oscar-winning film *The Silence of the Lambs* by Jonathan Demme (1991) (and another three films and a series, all based on the books of the writer Thomas Harris featuring the character), with the caption: 'When all the food is gone, we'll still have each other.' Famously, the plot of the films revolves around a psychiatrist who became a cannibalistic killer. Hence the punchline—the part of the joke where the situation set up previously undergoes a twist, revealing its comical nature—is that, when spoken by Lecter, an initially optimistic phrase in fact announces an apocalyptic future. In a second example, we can also observe a high level of what I have previously described in the context of political demonstrations as *mocking the powerful* (Werneck, 2019).

Figure 3.3 involves an international viral joke: the debate on life versus economy—in Brazil, channelled through Jair Bolsonaro's insistence on rejecting the guidelines of the World Health Organization (WHO) on self-isolation, wearing masks and physical distancing—had already become established in various countries and global news reports as a result of the denialism of the US President Donald Trump. In the scene with the dinosaurs watching the giant meteor's approach to cause their extinction, we also see tyrannosaurus, a prehistoric reptile known for its colossal power, saying that it would be bad for the economy. This reveals both the imbecility of the predator (and whoever says the same in real life) and the denialist politician's character: he can only be a *tyrant*osaurus.

Generally speaking, the jokes circulating about the pandemic during this second moment are concentrated on four types of critique, characterized by the following targets: government actions; ourselves' (and others') behaviours; the new routine; and discourses about the pandemic themselves. Below I briefly analyse each type.

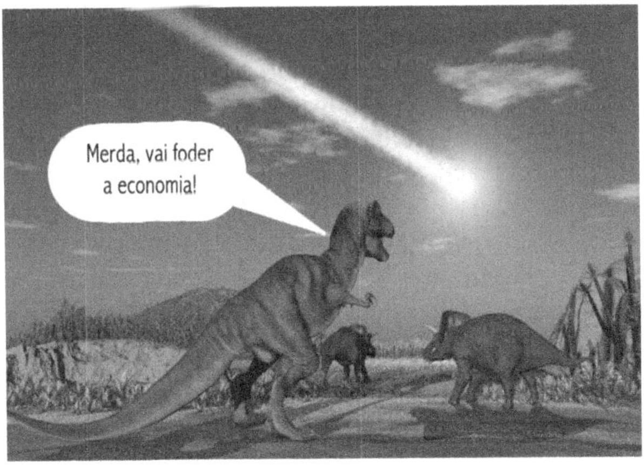

Fig. 3.3 'Shit, that'll fuck up the economy!'

A Government Without Grace and a Disgrace of Government: The Common Good Is State Care

Critiques of governments, especially their executive branch, tend to be based on what Boltanski and Thévenot (1991) call a *civic world*, in which the common good is founded on the representation of many people by a mandated representative (which may be a person, like a president, or a non-human being, like a specialized category or an institution such as the Ministry of Health). The logic of the authors' model is grounded in an 'economy of worth' (ibid) according to which situations are defined with the less worthy (the 'deficient' in terms of worth) depositing their agency in the hands of the more worthy.[6] Thus, the pact that defines what the authors call a *collective polity* (*cité*),[7] characteristic of the functioning of the State and originating from an agreement between the *civic polity* and the *industrial polity* (centred on technical efficiency), is based on the idea that citizens hand over the greater worth to a representative that encompasses them and promotes their well-being. This submission, in turn, is based on the fact that the more worthy in the collective polity is to be a legitimate (civic) representative after having been elected, for example, and, simultaneously, to provide proof of one's executive (industrial) efficiency with, for instance, successful policy initiatives. The joking critiques circulating in the Brazilian memes aimed at political power throw into question precisely these two dimensions. Within the Brazilian government itself, a controversy emerged between technical competence—represented by the Minister of Health[8] and state governors, generally following the WHO guidelines—and political administration, represented primarily by the president and by certain governors and mayors. Bolsonaro was criticized, on the one hand, as egoistic (showing more concern with his re-election than with the health situation, which puts into question the civic legitimacy of his power), and, on the other hand, as lacking policy sensitivity (by showing, as we have seen, more concern with economic issues than health issues, which questions the industrial legitimacy of the mandatary). Thus, we see a large number of memes expressing criticism of the government in the person of President Bolsonaro, as in the following examples (Fig. 3.4):

Both are examples of parodies (when an established sign is imitated, altering its meaning). The first case is a parody of the first verse of the Brazilian national anthem,[9] using a pun to express a convergence between the government and the problem it should be confronting. In the second

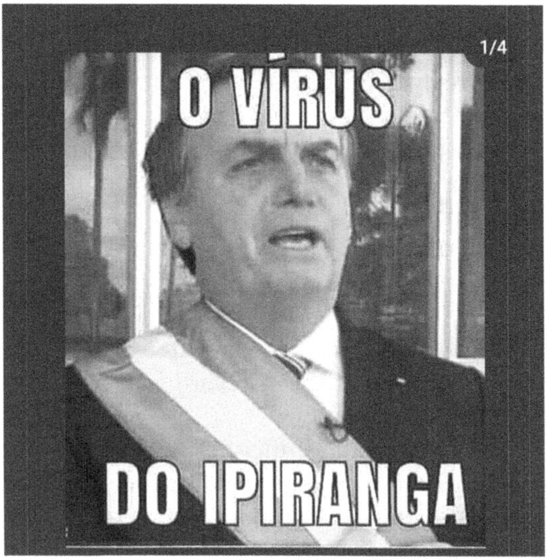

Fig. 3.4 'The virus of Ipiranga'

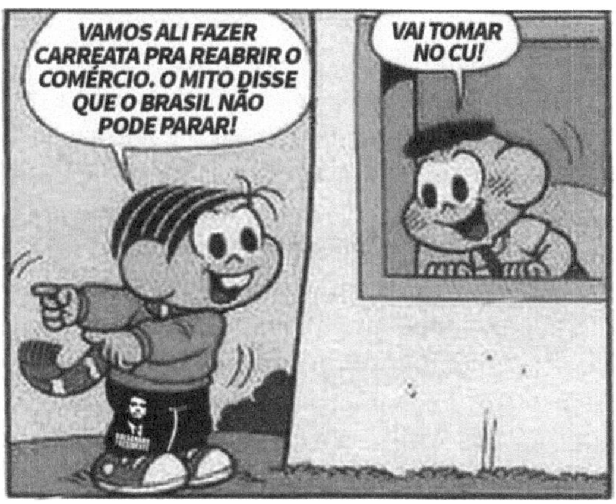
VAMOS ALI FAZER CARREATA PRA REABRIR O COMÉRCIO. O MITO DISSE QUE O BRASIL NÃO PODE PARAR!
VAI TOMAR NO CU!

Fig. 3.5 'Let's hold a rally to reopen the stores. The Myth said that Brazil must not stop!' 'Fuck off!'

(Fig. 3.5), we see the eponymous character from the classic Brazilian cartoon strip Turma da Mônica (Monica's Gang), highly popular in the country. Mônica is standing in front of the window of Cascão (Smudge), her friend, inviting him to go and do something, and he is replying to the invitation. This specific cartoon became a meme for various jokes: as discussed in Note 6, on the formal dimension of the memes, all that is needed to produce the *zoação* (mocking effect) is to change the dialogue. In this case, the structure involves presenting a 'mockable' invitation, followed by a rude reply that conflicts with the two children's lively expressions. In this meme, 'Myth' is how Bolsonaro's followers refer to him, and the joke cites the campaign promoted by his government (under the slogan 'Brazil must not stop') against preventive self-isolation and in favour of a resumption of economic activity.

Leave the Street: The Common Good Is Citizen Care

The most widespread behavioural critique is the neglect of preventive measures, whether the disregard for physical distancing or bad prophylactic habits. For example:

The basis of this criticism is that the common good is founded on a civic division of the fight against the virus—employing the logic of civic-industrial commitment based on a strong engagement of the less worthy, the citizens—focused on two behavioural changes: *personal hygienic habits* (washing hands, sanitization with gel alcohol, use of masks) and *voluntary isolation* (oriented by the government in various cities), along with distancing when it is necessary to leave home. In the first case, the critiques are based on the *isolation-good*, criticizing disbelievers and the disobedient. This is the case of the meme shown in Fig. 3.6, in which we see a photo of Dona Zica and Cartola, classical leading exponents of samba, the Brazilian musical rhythm par excellence, with Cartola sitting in front of his house, 'pronouncing' some of the existential lyrics to 'Quero me encontrar' ['I Want to Find Myself'] by the composer Candeia, one of the singer's biggest hits, and Dona Zica, also his wife, replying to him, already elderly, a member of the risk group, telling him in a rude way to get inside and isolate. The same kind of criticism could be found in another frequent internet hit, which is a critique of those disbelieving the effectiveness of isolation measures. In another meme, no less than Charles Darwin (in a black and white photo) appears to imply that the measures' disobedience exposes humans to natural selection, a central element in his Theory of Evolution: 'Anyone who doesn't want to go into quarantine, fine by me.'

In another set, the critiques take the form of affirming *hygiene-good*, expressed in the accusations against those who fail to follow such procedures. This can be seen in a meme showing Skeletor, the supervillain of the He-Man cartoon universe, an incarnation of evil, appearing at the centre of a moral twist as someone who previously smelt of alcohol (i.e.,

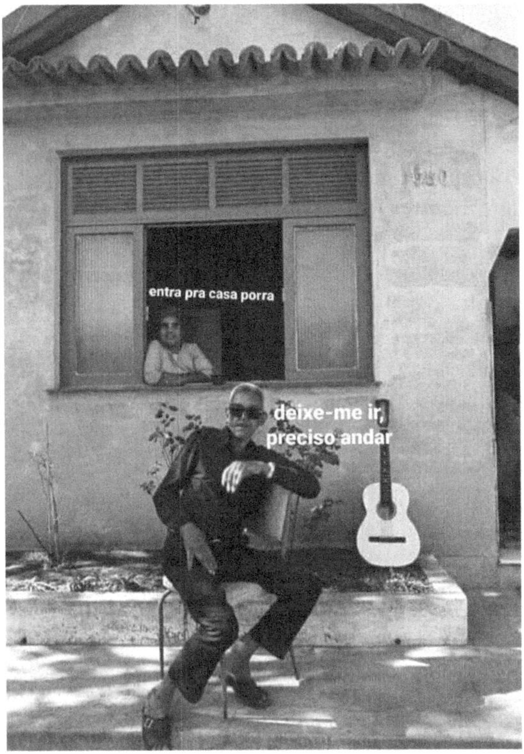

Fig. 3.6 'Get inside, for fuck's sake' 'Let me go, I need to walk'

was an alcoholic) and saying: 'How things change... Now, if you smell of alcohol, people look at you approvingly.' In all these cases, the *sanitary-good* manifests as a core element of the situation and the agency of the actors is made explicit: the critiques hold every citizen responsible for the population's health as a whole, emphasizing the need for civic engagement.

Isolate! The Common Good Is to Resist During the New Routine

In this case, what is ridiculed are precisely the new routine elements, making explicit the absurdity of a situation that messes up everyone's lives. The critique is not of isolation in itself (though it also surfaces) but more especially the *deroutinization* and, in part, people's low resilience at times. This seems to follow the path of accepting inevitable suffering and a logic of 'laughing so as not to cry.' Hence, we see memes emphasizing indeterminacy and the everyday inquiry necessary during this moment. For example:

The meme showed in Fig. 3.7 concentrates on the distinction between people isolating with children and without children—a recurrent theme among the jokes, which always highlight the tremendous suffering of parents and, among this group, the difference between men and women (mothers). Other examples were various. In one case, the reproduction of a Twitter post says: 'I'm trying to maintain my normal routine. For example, I set up a mini-gym here at home and I've never gone there either.' It emphasizes how the routine has changed but not that much. In another, the joke depicts the Dutch painter Vincent van Gogh to ridicule the new habits, altering one of its classical self-portraits to make him try to wear a protective mask forming part of the new routine, but with him saying 'Merde!' (shit, in French), given that he would be unable to use it since he only had one ear. Moreover, the last example I want to present shows a clever pun (which I adapted here to work in English): 'To avoid transmitting Coronavirus, avoid holding parties with more than 20 invitees. You simply CONEED-19.'[10] It mocks those who, during quarantine, insist on holding parties at home.

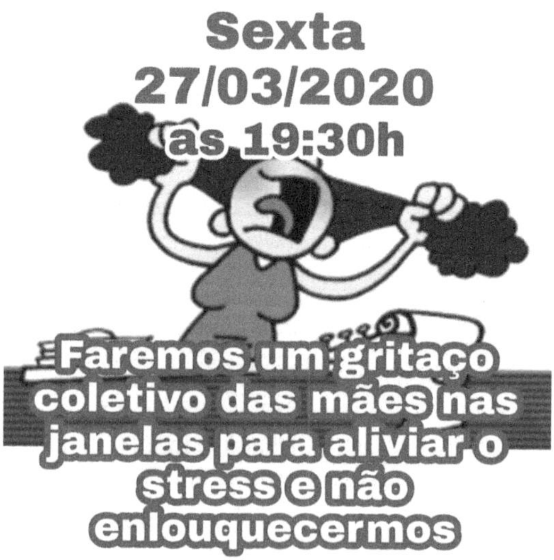

Fig. 3.7 'Friday 27 March 2020 at 7.30pm We'll be holding a collective yelling of mothers at their windows to relieve stress and not go mad'

In each of these cases, like all those presented above, though here it becomes more apparent, the critique exploits the routinization of the debate on the health measures taken as a central element of the humour: as I have shown elsewhere (Werneck, 2015), the *joke*-form, in which the pair of *setup* (definition of the normal situation) and *punchline* (twist of the situation through the revelation of the element of change that makes it comic) works, reveals the presence of grace/inspiration showing how the world changed with the advent of an absurd, unpredictable element.

Humorous Critique Focused on Grace and Inspiration

The final important category of the first routinization is the one that concentrates on the humorous critique of discourses considered to be clichés, banal repetitions, and platitudes, that is, sentences that fail to show themselves as touched by the grace of inspiration. Therefore, ridicule here focuses on those discourses precisely *vis-à-vis* the *inspired worth*. For instance, a pandemic special edition of the regular sketch "Phrases that Deserve a Slap in the Face" from the comedy channel TV Quase, broadcast on YouTube.[11] The sketch has a simple premise: the actor (Daniel Furlan) appears in front of the camera and announces phrases that they deem to be clichés and, after each, is interrupted by a heavy slap to the face. In this special edition, which contained two videos, the sentences are linked to the pandemic and the hand slapping the actor is gloved, as though indicating prevention against COVID-19. Among the phrases, we hear gems like: 'Did you know that in the Mayan Calendar [suggesting some apocalyptical prevision]…?'; 'No, but we're going to learn about humanity with this virus'; 'I'll finally have time to study French'; and the suggestive 'One day, we'll laugh about all this.' They even repeat phrases from Jair Bolsonaro, but within the same continuum of platitudes. The same critique of cliché is contained in memes that reproduce tweets from the social network Twitter, serving as a parody of the clichéd phrases, like the one saying 'A few months from now we'll all sit down and laugh when we remember Coronavirus … In hell.'

A 'New Normal': The Second Routinization and the 'Endemicization' of the Pandemic

The graph below (Graph 1) shows the mortality rate throughout the pandemic in Brazil, from the beginning of quarantine in March to the start of August 2020. It presents the data in absolute figures, represented by the bars, and the *moving average* (i.e., the average of the last seven days, registered day-to-day), shown by the line. This behaviour is almost unparalleled elsewhere in the world with the establishment of a lengthy plateau in the number of deaths (from the last third of May to the end of this sequence, at least, on 8 August, when the country surpassed the mark of 100,000 deaths and 3 million people infected), staying at a very high level of around one thousand deaths per day:[12]

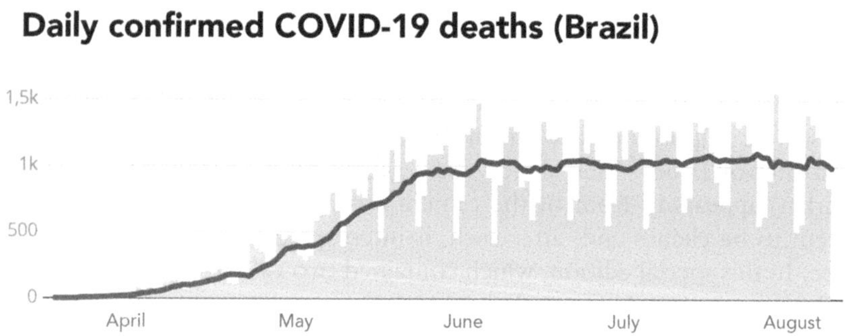

Source: Brazilian news pool, based on data from the states' health departments

I introduce this statistical element into the discussion because it simultaneously reflects and has played a role in forming a new interpretative turn among actors, bringing up a new regime. The new situation is registered in those actors' humour-based critiques, what I call an *endemicization of the pandemic*, a moment in which the epidemic disease is treated as an endemic one:[13] the period during which the plateau became established and consolidated was also when the isolation measures were relaxed and physical distancing became more neglected, registered in numerous news reports during this new stage. The sensation of a new routine seems to have become established, in which the global situation of the epidemic in the country became normalized: the daily number of deaths seems to have generated a feeling that the real 'new normal' was to have this (high) number of deaths every day and that public life would continue oblivious to this figure. It is important to say that Brazil is accustomed to a high number of deaths by homicide at 63,000 per year. At that moment, the country was registering another 'round' number (100,000) of deaths from COVID-19. It was a dramatic landmark. However, it was *another* dramatic landmark as had been the first thousand, then 5000, then 10,000, the tens of thousands, a sequence that, nonetheless, was incapable of reversing the tendency towards anaesthesia and routinization. For all practical purposes, in Brazil, the true 'new normal' seems to have become the death of many from the disease and the life that continues—which in many cities has meant the reopening of commerce and a rush to the beaches and bars (Callegari & Magalhães 02/06/2020).[14,15]

How have the memes registered this weird Brazilian 'new normal'? By shifting to an anecdotal version of evaluating others' behaviour, especially the government: the critiques become concentrated on actions considered bizarre or ridiculous in themselves. This movement follows the dynamic of what I have called 'mocking the powerful' (Werneck, 2019, 642), a form involving 'direct attack on the powerful, concentrated on mocking famous figures and/or those who represent power.' We thus see memes like these:

The first meme (Fig. 3.8) refers to a preposterous declaration of the then Minister of Health, Eduardo Pazuello. Pazuello is a general without any medical training who served as acting minister for an extended period after the second incumbent's sacking in Bolsonaro's government.[16] In a press conference, he stated that the virus' behaviour in the Northeast of Brazil, a region historically famous for its droughts, a vast area of semi-arid climate with tourism centred on its many and beautiful beaches, was closer to those in Northern Hemisphere countries with a cold climate. Hence, the meme factories quickly produced images like the first one of this series, promoting the Winter Olympics in a famous city of the North-eastern Sertão (depicting a landscape entirely different from the reality, filled with snow and alps).

A second example marks one of the most prolific meme sources of this period: after spending months saying that COVID-19 was 'just a little flu' and adopting measures at odds with those recommended as preventive, even encouraging crowds to form at demonstrations in support of his government and demanding the closure of Congress and the Federal Supreme Court, Bolsonaro announced that he had tested positive for the disease on 7 July. Thereafter, an enormous number of memes were directed towards

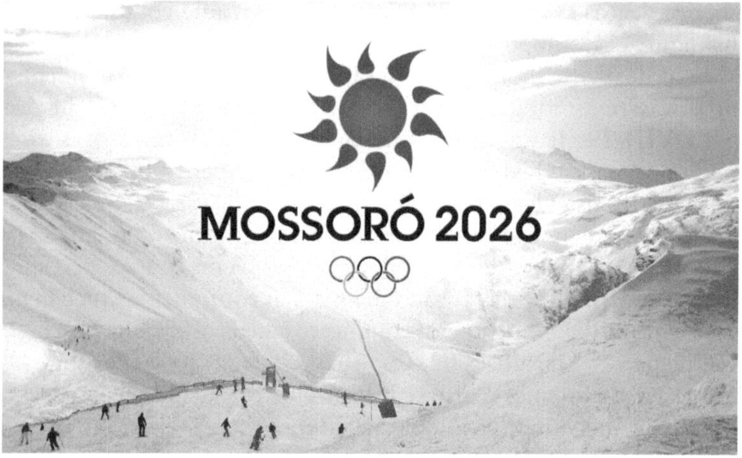

Fig. 3.8 '2026 Mossoro [a city on the Brazilian semi-arid region] Winter Olympic Games'

a kind of retaliation, something like an assertion that the infection was a punishment for his declarations. One meme, therefore, promotes the direct comparison between the president and the disease, indicating that he would make the virus ill: [*over a photo of Bolsonaro quarantined*] 'We need to talk about the three weeks of suffering of Coronavirus in Bolsonaro's body #keepstrongcorona #chloroquine.'

A third example is shown in Fig. 3.9:

The meme refers to an episode known as 'the Antifa Emu': following his positive test, the president had to self-isolate and work from the Alvorada Palace, his official residence whose gardens contain various specimens of the animal (emu). Like Trump, Bolsonaro is also an enthusiast of hydroxychloroquine as a treatment of COVID-19—a medicine that not only lacks any scientific demonstration of effectiveness against the disease but also has proven harmful side effects. He even ordered that Army laboratories should produce pills of the substance on a large scale. This was done, leaving millions of units unused, given that governors and mayors declined to include the medicine in their disease management policies. When he became sick, he claimed that he had been treated with the medicine and it was responsible for his recovery. So, during a walk through the gardens while isolating, he approached an emu and tried to pet it. He was

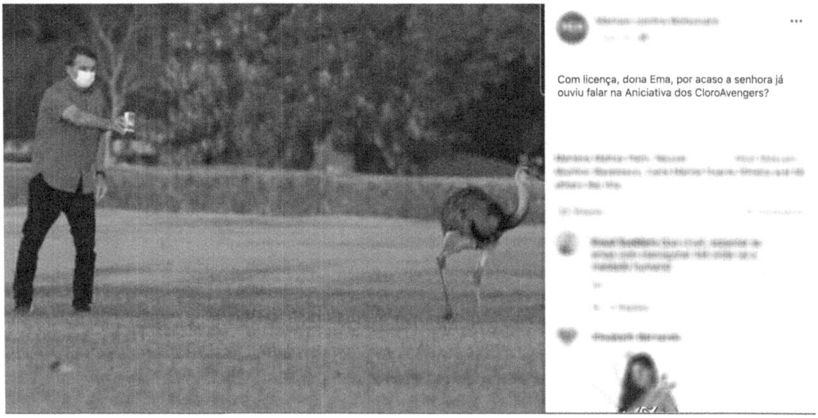
Com licença, dona Ema, por acaso a senhora já ouviu falar na Aniciativa dos CloroAvengers?

Fig. 3.9 'Excuse me, Mrs Emu, by chance have you heard about the [I]niciative of the ChloroAvengers?'

pecked, which generated a wave of memes claiming that the animal was 'politicized,' 'left-wing,' or 'Antifa' (an abbreviation of 'anti-fascist,' a non-party movement against Bolsonaro). Days later, knowing he was being filmed and photographed, Bolsonaro once again approached the bird, this time showing it a box of chloroquine, suggesting to the rhea that it would be protected by the medication.

The last example once again uses the 'peculiar' style (to say the least) of Bolsonaro, combining his anti-preventive behaviour with both his tendency for clumsy actions and rude declarations. In this case, curiously, involving someone else's: at the start of August, the mayor of a mid-sized city in the interior of the country, who is a medic, suggested treating COVID-19 with 'ozone therapy,' the rectal injection of ozone gas, a technique with no proven efficacy against the disease, but which the politician claimed would increase immunity. Of course, the project was a source of enormous controversy and a wave of memes, especially with witty puns and sexual jokes (which the president, himself keen on this kind of anecdote, also ended up making). As an advocate of using chloroquine, Bolsonaro not only ridiculed the plan but declared himself opposed to it. Even so, he permitted for Pazuello to meet the medical mayor in question to discuss the matter. In the meme, a series of references intersect, drawing from the many photos of the president's poor mask use to combine a critique of his neglect with his tendency for measures just as absurd as ozone therapy: it shows a photo of Bolsonaro tapping his own nose, with the caption: 'I think I can smell Ozone coming after our haemorrhoid!'. These combined with referencing his obsession both with projecting a macho image (which had prompted him to say that he would never submit to that kind of medical treatment) and with the idea that the political left persecutes 'our' freedoms and that form part of a conspiracy of world domination—which he expressed in a ministerial meeting as 'What these guys want is our haemorrhoid' (an unexplained expression, but it seems to contain both a meaning similar to 'fuck us' and to use *ass* as a metonym for individual freedom).[17]

This 'new normal' of the pandemic as a simple fact with which the country lives—to some extent a rhetorical victory of Bolsonaro—made the jokes about the country's global situation rarer along with those about people's behaviours in response to the pandemic. Indeed, they even represented a relative acceptance of the critique involving COVID-19.[18]

Conclusion

The observation of the different moments of meme production related to the COVID-19 pandemic in Brazil allows us to map a range of critiques circulating about various *actants* (Callon & Latour, 1981; Latour, 1997[1987]; Boltanski, 1990) related to the health crisis but also about the country's political routine itself. As we have seen, this critique benefits from humour as a form of circulation and operationalization, although it was able to encounter three different moments of routine: an investigative phase, a first routine phase of isolation, and a second routine phase of liberation (here called a 'new normal,' in quote marks, since it involves a normalization amid the ongoing health risk, utterly unrelated to the new normal promised for life after the health crisis). The formal actants observed in this scenario were (a) Brazil with its entrenched ills (which may be extrapolated to the idea of a *big problem* that can never be solved); (b) the government/State; (c) the other as a preventive character (whether by acting correctly or by acting negligently); (d) the routine of isolation; (e) the cliché discourses on the pandemic; and (f) the isolated anecdotal actions of characters who became public.

My interpretation of this scenario led me to the model proposed by Laurent Thévenot (2006) to think about the agential movements of the actors towards social mobilizations—or, as he puts it, towards *actions in common in the plural*: this process involves what he calls *engagements*, that is, the logic through which the actors *coordinate* with each other. My hypothesis here is that the second moment of the wave of memes, marked by voluntary isolation and a new routine, was guided by two types of engagement: the first, called *exploratory* by Auray (2011), founded on the kind of investigative processes outlined by Dewey (1938), seeking what Thomas (1966[1923]) would call a *definition of the situation*. The second is what in another text I referred to as a *circumstantialist* engagement (Werneck, 2020a), founded on what I called, inspired precisely by Thomas, an *indefinition of the situation*, a movement of strategic avoidance, postponing definition, to maintain oneself in a hybrid situation and take advantage of the same. In the ambient of this routine of indefinition—which might be a paradox—the actors experience what Stark (2009) called *dissonance*, a productive friction between what, in principle, are competing logics of action. Critique seems to perform a fundamental role at this moment since it occupies the space produced by the aforementioned friction. During moments like the first two phases of the pandemic, as I argued, the transition between indefinition and the emergence of a new tentative routine to be experienced 'one day at a time,' responding to 'whatever happens,' at the whim of new events and circumstances, offers actors an open-ended universe of meanings to fill with their questionings (and, with them, their critiques). Furthermore, however much actors attempt to find a routine, the memes good-humouredly make explicit how this movement is itself tentative, the circulating critiques still seeking to comprehend the possible good from moment to moment, sometimes benefitting from a definition, sometimes benefitting from indefinition. This *mixed* engagement (Werneck, 2020a) appears to unite everyone in a critical environment based on the fact that we are all immersed in a *big problem* (in which the country and its ills always remain present as a question), something to be experienced through its situated problematizations—that is, something wide open to controversies in which critiques appear as a central element.

Concerning the latest moment, the 'new normal,' my argument sets out from an inversion of the idea of an *engagement on the plan* developed by Thévenot (2006, 113–130): my idea is to approach the concept of the plane in a broader sense, conceiving the future glimpsed by it as a *horizon* rather than an *objective*—and thinking of a plane potentially as a map contemplating a geography rather than simply 'how to arrive'). This means thinking of the plane as a vision of the future, an image of what we expect and how we imagine it will be, and not just how we would wish it to be.

With this interpretation, an engagement on the plane would imply a coordination colonized by this vision. Based on this, I suggest, then, that when they adopt the possibility of contracting COVID-19 as a 'plane,' as a vision of the future, the actors develop a tentative activity through which each moment in which one 'confronts' the world and does not contract the disease, the plane, causes the horizon to gradually adjust, becoming an increasingly failed plane in the eyes of these actors. This in part explains this new 'alternative' normal: the sensation that the pandemic has become absorbed into normality so that even the daily information on another thousand deaths makes little difference to people's routines as they adapt to a critical environment in which only the anecdotal becomes criticizable.

Humour, and the grace that it expresses, therefore, appears in all these moments as an element facilitating these critiques, as I have demonstrated and expressed before: the singular observer who occupies the place of the *humoristic speaker* (just as the poetic speaker in poetry) of the discourses enables the transitory truths circulating in them to ridicule the criticized objects and realize their potency, reducing the worths (and in this sense the agencies) of these objects and making the critique not only more capable of circulating but more potent in a simultaneously subtle and intense form. It is not that the joke is more effective in making a critique potent, but that critique made in a form that suggests presence of grace—littered with elements that enable the humour to be recognized—inserts an *inspired* logic (Boltanski & Thévenot, 1991) into the equation, replacing the rationalist evaluation of the 'serious' critique with a leap over the testing (*épreuve*) of the content that stabilizes the situation as a verification in terms of grace/inspiration. The joke-form is thus converted into a form of making the critique more effective as critique: by demonstrating that it is funny, that is, 'full of grace,' that is, singular, creative, clever, the critique constructs a singularized voice that completes this circle.

Notes

1. As I have already written in Werneck (2019, p. 614), 'a meme is a sign that spreads massively via the internet, originally in a peer-to-peer system, but more recently in a model that we can call peer-to-all, more typical to social networks, through repetitions and/or alterations. The term of everyday use is inspired by the idea of the British biologist Richard Dawkins, who in his book *The Selfish Gene* (Dawkins, 2016[1976]), suggests an explanatory

model for the diffusion of information within a culture […]. For more about memes and their involvement in [critiques], see Mina (2019).'

2. The effectuation to which I refer concerns the effectiveness of the critical collocation and the possibility of presenting a critical discourse (Werneck & Loretti, 2018). Thus, it is not a question of evaluating the effectiveness of the critiques nor humour's role in this effectiveness. Due to its situated character, an analysis of this type would be impossible with the material available. For a discussion of critical effectiveness, see Boltanski (1990) and Hirschman (1972).
3. All citations to this work considered the terminology established by the book's American edition, which was translated by Catherine Porter. I did the Brazilian translation, published in 2020.
4. For instance, visual parodies are commonplace, using images of famous people, especially celebrities, movie scenes, and images from comic strips, changing the dialogues and thus generating a punchline through the semiotic friction between the original scenes and the meaning presented in the meme. This creates a versatile set of signs, which can change the message at the captions' whim, as Barthes (1990[1982]) would say. Logical jokes, puns, and plays of words are equally important, as seen in some of the cases shown here.
5. Unlike in various other countries, a policy of *governmentally oriented voluntary isolation* was adopted in Brazil. Most of its state and local governments did not make home isolation compulsory. Instead, they left each person to decide if they would stay at home or not, issuing guidelines only on the motives for people to go out: they ordered the closure of those activities considered non-essential, a reduction in the circulation of public transport, and so on. Thus, I use the term *governmentality* here in the sense given by Foucault (2007[1978]), as a form of making free people do what one wants, or, in his terms, as 'an administration of things that would think before all else of men's freedom, of what they want to do, of what they have an interest in doing, and of what they think about doing […]. physics of power, or a power thought of as physical action in the element of nature, and a power thought of as regulation that can only be carried out through and by reliance on the freedom of each' (p. 49).
6. The idea of *worth* is opposed to that of *size*, which defines an intrinsic characteristic of the actors. The model does not deal with domination founded on intrinsic traits (e.g., as in class domination), although it does not deny its existence. Instead, it seeks to take the actors' critical capacity seriously and to show how situations are defined through the situated recognition of worths, which can only act if they are justified by them, that is, proven by their capacity to produce the common good, and which exclusively define precedence in decision-making in the situation. These situations only

obtain legitimacy in the justification, effected through the demonstration that the well-being of the more worthy and the less worthy, though different, are read as equivalent, distributing the good in question through a common way.

7. The term *cité* refers to an ordering limited to a determined form of justice, that is, the common good. In their research, Boltanski and Thévenot (1991) initially mapped six polities (*cités*), six forms of justice, privileged in the modern framework of controversies, namely: a *civic* polity; a *domestic* polity (centred on generational hierarchy); a *market* polity (centred on the value of exchange); an *industrial* polity (centred on efficiency); an *inspired* polity (centred on grace, that is, creativity and singularity); and a polity of *fame* (centred on honorific recognition and reputation). Other polities were proposed by themselves and by other authors, but I do not intend to describe or debate them here.
8. From the beginning of the crisis and for a long period during the early phase of the pandemic, a post occupied by the physician and deputy Luiz Henrique Mandetta. In his last weeks of office, Mandetta entered into a series of public clashes with the President, the latter being opposed to horizontal isolation and in favour of treatments not yet fully tested for the disease, while the minister declared himself in favour of following the WHO guidelines, including horizontal isolation. Mandetta was dismissed on 16 April.
9. The section in question is: 'Ouviram do Ipiranga/as margens plácidas/de um povo heroico/o brado retumbante.' The verses of the Brazilian National Anthem, composed in 1831, make frequent phrasal inversions as in this initial section. Here the reference is to the resounding cry of the Brazilian people heard 'by' the shores of the Ipiranga River, the location of the declaration of the country's independence. Note the acoustic overlap between the sections in Portuguese: 'Ouviram do Ipiranga' [They heard from Ipiranga] and 'O vírus do Ipiranga.'
10. The original pun is based on the proximity in spoken Portuguese between the imperative of the verb to invite, *convide*, and pronunciation of the word *COVID*: 'Para evitar a transmissão do Coronavírus, evite fazer festas com mais de 20 convidados. Apenas COVID-19.'
11. Although this case is not a meme, I treat it as a paradigmatic example since it contains all the elements of the viral logic of the former, as well as, at the same time, having itself generated a series of memes, reproducing its screens, especially the opening title.
12. On this last day of this series, the moving average was 990 deaths, 8% lower than the moving average recorded 14 days earlier, a comparison used by epidemiologists to evaluate the behaviour of the pandemic: when the positive or negative variation is higher than 15%, a change is taken to have

taken place (rising or falling), and when the variation is smaller, the trend is considered stable. This fall of 8%, though small, followed a trend that indicated a sequence of reductions, but became diluted amid the news of the global number of dead.

13. An influence that Eugênia Motta and I discussed in another text, due to be published in 2021 (Werneck & Motta, 2020).
14. Faced with the imminence of this landmark figure, Bolsonaro declared: 'We lament all the dead, we're going to reach 100,000, but we're going to get on with life and dodge this problem.' This declaration formed part of a long gallery of declarations of the president on the disease that would merit a text by itself based around the humorous responses. When I finish the draft of this chapter, on 27 October 2020, the confirmed COVID-19 number of deaths in Brazil is around 157,000. After that moment, the number of deaths in Brazil went through a drop until the beginning of November and then a sequence of high, reaching, on April 13, 2021, a peak of 3,808 deaths in one day, with an average of 3,068 deaths in 7 days. With the start of vaccination, the numbers dropped again, but remained for months still at around a thousand daily deaths. From the beginning of the pandemic until mid-August 2021, Covid-19 had claimed around 570,000 lives in Brazil.
15. Another element to be considered in this normalization was the use of masks as a mass preventive measure established by the WHO in June. While this is obviously an essential health policy of already proven effectiveness, it seems to have had a deleterious side effect, contributing to the 'new normal.' I am not suggesting that the use of masks is not a necessary measure. On the contrary, I consider it fundamental. The question was the encouragement to leave home that it gave to those who wanted to disobey isolation guidance.
16. Pazuello was appointed minister on 16 September, remaining as acting minister for almost four months, longer than the period in office of his predecessor, the oncologist Nelson Teich. He remained minister until March 15, 2021, when he was replaced by a physician, Marcelo Queiroga—a measure adpted because Bolsonaro's popularity, high throughout the entire pandemic until taht point, started to drop consistenly. In Pazuello's administration, several crises relating to Covid-19 took place and he became one of the main targets of a parliamentary committee of inquiry investigation for negligence on the federal responsibilities for the mismanagement of the pandemic in the country. By mid August 2021, the disapproval level for Bolsonaro reached 54%.
17. Bolsonaro's discourse as a president has concentrated not only on a denial of the virus's risk potential but also—and more intensely—on a dichotomy between isolation and individual liberty, claiming that the virus is an excuse

for 'the left' to curb 'our freedom.' Much of his presidential campaign was based on intensifying an almost anecdotal association between equality as a degenerative operation promoted by 'communism' and liberty as a supreme value sought by the right, mobilizing a very peculiar mixture of economic neoliberalism and behavioural liberation for 'good people' (the conservatives, who, in Bolsonaro's view, constitute the paradigmatic matrix of the Brazilian). Indeed, the president left no doubt concerning his stance on the matter, stating that for him, 'there is something more important than life: freedom' (Caramuru, 21/05/2020). This tends to be the Bolsonarist activists' slogan, individual freedom for its own sake (Lima, 25/05/2020). Bolsonaro and his followers describe that as a 'good freedom', conceived along the lines of the American 'pursuit of happiness': self-determination to decide one's path and accumulate wealth without interference from the State in one's lives. This is represented by policies such as the incentive towards entrepreneurship and an aversion to the State and its agents and a deregulation policy that involves easing gun control, loosening traffic laws, and valorizing order and security. The left, the 'communists,' for their part, are described as people who advocate not liberty, but 'libertinism,' promoting an agenda of complete liberation only in hedonist behaviours, especially sexual—overthrowing traditional gender roles, promoting 'homosexualism' and 'pedophilia'—and chemical, for instance, demanding the liberation of marijuana use. They would also be against liberty by 'taking our money' (e.g., charging high taxes) to hand over to 'vagrants' (civil servants or socially vulnerable people) and being driven by a project of global cultural domination supposedly inspired by Italian philosopher Antonio Gramsci. However, a more detailed analysis of this conservative agenda and its labelling of opponents would go beyond the scope of this text.

18. The gallery presented in this section has concentrated on Bolsonaro and his minister Pazuello more because of the representativeness of the memes and the cases' anecdotal weight than because of any capacity to synthesize a sample. In fact, at this moment, the critiques were directed at any figures capable of being made public by actions worthy of mocking. Thus, both the medical mayor of ozone therapy and celebrities or even anonymous people who, through the social networks, may have seen their actions reach the general public are included in this selection.

References

Auray, N. (2011). Les technologies de l'information et le régime exploratoire. In P. Van Andel & D. Boursier (Eds.), *La sérendipité: Le hasard heureux* (pp. 329–343). Hermann.

Barthes, R. (1990[1982]). *O óbvio e o obtuso*. Nova Fronteira.

Beckman, J. (2014). *American fun: Four centuries of joyous revolt*. Pantheon.

Billig, M. (2005). *Laughter and ridicule: Towards a social critique of humour*. Sage.

Boltanski, L. (1990). *L'amour et la justice comme compétences*. Métailié.

Boltanski, L., & Thévenot, L. (1991). *De la justification: Les économies de la grandeur*. Gallimard.

Callon, M., & Latour, B. (1981). Unscrewing the big Leviathan: How actors macro-structure reality and how sociologists help them to do so. In K. Knorr-Cetina & A. V. Cicourel (Eds.), *Toward an integration of micro- and macro-sociologies* (pp. 277–303). Routledge/Keegan Paul.

Dawkins, R. (2016[1976]). *The selfish gene*. Oxford University Press.

Dewey, J. (1938). *Logic: The theory of inquiry*. Henry Holt.

Foucault, M. (2008[1978]). Aula de 11 de janeiro de 1978. In *Segurança, território, população: Curso dado no Collège de France (1977–1978)* (pp. 3–38). Martins Fontes.

Herzfeld, M. (2001). Irony and power: Towards a politics of mockery in Greece. In J. W. Fernandez & M. T. Huber (Eds.), *Irony in action: Anthropology, practice, and the moral imagination* (pp. 63–83). The University of Chicago Press.

Hirschman, A. O. (1972). *Exit, voice, and loyalty: Responses to decline in firms, organizations, and states*. Harvard University Press.

King, B. (2016). *Clowning as social performance in Colombia: Ridicule and resistance*. Bloomsbury.

Latour, B. (1987). *Science in action: How to follow scientists and engineers through society*. Harvard University Press.

Mina, N. X. (2019). *Memes to movements: How the world's most viral media is changing social protest and power*. Beacon.

Nielsen, M. (2019, April 1). Comedic lies as transitory truths. *Anthropology News*. http://www.anthropology-news.org/index.php/2019/04/01/comedic-lies-as-transitory-truths. Accessed 28 Sept 2020.

Stark, D. (2009). *The sense of dissonance: Accounts of worth in economic life*. Princeton University Press.

T'Hart, M., & Bos, D. (Eds.). (2008). *Humour and social protest*. Cambridge University Press.

Thévenot, L. (2006). *L'action au pluriel: Sociologie des régimes d'engagement*. La Découverte.

Thomas, W. I. (1966[1923]). *Unadjusted girl: With cases and standpoint for behaviour analysis*. Harper and Row.

Thomas, W. I., & Thomas, D. S. (1938[1928]). *The child in America: Behavior problems and programs*. Alfred A Knopf.

Trnka, S., & Rehak, J. K. (2018). *The politics of joking: Anthropological engagements*. Routledge.

Werneck, A. (2012). *A desculpa: As circunstâncias e a moral das relações sociais*. Civilização Brasileira.

Werneck, A. (2015). 'Dar uma zoada', 'botar a maior marra': Dispositivos morais de jocosidade como formas de efetivação e sua relação com a crítica. *Dados: Revista de Ciências Sociais, 58*(1), 187–221. https://doi.org/10.1590/00115258201542

Werneck, A. (2016). Uma sociologia da compreensão a partir do par crítica e jocosidade. *Civitas: Revista de Ciências Sociais, 16*(3), 482–503. https://doi.org/10.15448/1984-7289.2016.3.21941

Werneck, A. (2019). Política e ridicularização: Uma sociologia pragmática da 'graça' da crítica em cartazes das 'Jornadas de Junho'. *Interseções: Revista de Estudos Interdisciplinares, 21*(3), 611–653. https://doi.org/10.12957/irei.2019.47254

Werneck, A. (2020a). Obstáculos na 'pista livre': Algumas considerações sobre a pragmática dos dispositivos da 'lei do trânsito' no Rio de Janeiro. *Antropolítica: Revista Contemporânea de Antropologia, 50*, 327–355. https://doi.org/10.22409/antropolitica2020.i50

Werneck, A. (2020b). A força da graça, a graça da força: A crítica jocosa aos personagens da 'violência urbana' nas capas de um jornal popular como 'violentização' da fala pública (Working paper, *Necvu*).

Werneck, A., & Loretti, P. (2018). Critique-form, forms of critique: The different dimensions of the discourse of discontent. *Sociologia & Antropologia, 8*(3), 973–1008. https://doi.org/10.1590/2238-38752018v839

Werneck, A., & Motta, E. (2020). Um novo "novo normal" expressado em números: A endemização da pandemia e os usos sociais do "platô" (Working paper, *Necvu*).

Yacintas, A. (Ed.). (2015). *Creativity and humour in occupy movements: Intellectual disobedience in turkey and beyond*. Palgrave Macmillan.

News Reports

Alfano, B. (2020, March 19). Especialistas em epidemias apontam erros de Bolsonaro no uso de máscara em coletiva: Casos confirmados ou sob suspeita devem usar proteção, mas procedimento de presidente em entrevista foi classificado como inadequado. *Época*. https://epoca.globo.com/brasil/especialistas-em-epidemias-apontam-erros-de-bolsonarono-uso-de-mascara-em-coletiva-24314199

Callegari, C., & Magalhães , L. E. (2020. June 2). Com praias cheias e BRT lotado, Rio entra na primeira fase de reabertura gradual durante pandemia de COVID-19: Sufistas movimentam o mar da Zona Sul e da Barra da Tijuca na manhã desta terça-feira; novas regras estão sendo descumpridas, *O Globo*. https://oglobo.globo.com/rio/com-praias-cheias-brt-lotado-rio-entra-na-primeira-fase-de-reabertura-gradual-durante-pandemia-de-COVID-19-24458348

Camillo, M. (2020, March 13). Piada nas redes diminuiu à medida que coronavírus passou de surto para pandemia, *Folha de S. Paulo*, #Hashtag: Mídias Sociais e a Vida em Rede. https://hashtag.blogfolha.uol.com.br/2020/03/13/piada-nas-redes-diminuiu-a-medida-que-coronavirus-passou-de-surto-para-pandemia/

Caramuru, P. (2020, May 21). Bolsonaro: Para mim, tem algo que é mais importante que a vida, a liberdade, *UOL*. https://noticias.uol.com.br/ultimas-noticias/agencia-estado/2020/05/21/bolsonaro-para-mim-tem-algo-que-e-mais-importante-que-a-vida-a-liberdade.htm

Enberg, J. (2020, March 18). How COVID-19 is testing social media's ability to fight misinformation: And what the coordinated effort may mean for their long-term strategies. *eMarketer*. https://www.emarketer.com/content/how-COVID-19-is-testing-social-medias-ability-to-fight-misinformation

Lima, V. (2020, May 25). 'Povo quer liberdade e democracia', afirma Bolsonaro após manifestação: Presidente disse que protesto do último domingo, na Esplanada dos Ministérios, foi 'espontânea' e despistou sobre possível troca na Educação, *R7*. https://noticias.r7.com/brasil/povo-quer-liberdade-e-democracia-afirma-bolsonaro-apos-manifestacao-25052020

CHAPTER 4

'Coromentality': Nigerians' Use of Memetic Humour During the COVID-19 Lockdowns

Aje-Ori Agbese and Edeanya Agbese

Introduction

To prevent or flatten the curve after the coronavirus (COVID-19) pandemic hit, many countries implemented social distancing guidelines and lockdowns. Nigeria was no exception. When the pandemic hit Nigeria on February 27, 2020, the country was unprepared because social media posts claimed Africa's climate was inconducive for its spread, and Black people would not contract COVID-19 (Tangwa & Munug, 2020). Within a month, however, Nigeria had 129 confirmed cases and one death (Toromade, 2020). Therefore, lockdowns and other measures were necessary, considering Nigeria's 206 million population was at high risk of severe effects if the pandemic spread (Wetsman, 2020). Several states

A.-O. Agbese (✉)
Department of Communication, The University of Texas Rio Grande Valley, Edinburg, TX, USA

E. Agbese
Department of Public Health Sciences, Penn State College of Medicine, Hershey, PA, USA

S. Mpofu (ed.), *Digital Humour in the Covid-19 Pandemic*,
https://doi.org/10.1007/978-3-030-79279-4_4

announced lockdowns and stay-at-home orders to curb COVID-19's spread between March 23 and March 27 (Onu et al., 2020). On March 29, President Muhammadu Buhari announced a total lockdown in the hardest-hit areas, Lagos and Ogun states, and the federal capital, Abuja (Adoyi, 2020). He also closed international airports and suspended non-essential services. These actions meant Nigerians had to stay at home, stop businesses and, if possible, work from home. To cope with the change and mitigate COVID-19's psychological impact, Nigerians turned to the internet and social media to cope.

According to Nigeria's National Information Technology Development agency, over 124 million of Nigeria's 206 million population has access to the internet (Dangida, 2021). However, the National Bureau of Statistics (NBS, 2020) determined that Nigeria's more than 136 million mobile subscribers actively use the internet. As of January 2020, 27 million Nigerians were on social media, spending an average of 3 hours and 17 minutes there daily (Tankovska, 2021, Udodiong, 2019). Nigerians belong to multiple social media platforms, with WhatsApp (85%), Facebook (78%) and Instagram (57%) having the highest users (Udodiong, 2019). The highest number of internet users are in the urban areas and mostly in Lagos state (NBS, 2020). In addition, according to Johnson (2021), 75.1% of Nigerians access the internet through mobile phones and three-quarters of them use smartphones. Nigerians go online for a variety of reasons, including seeking information, commentary and entertainment, and the number of internet users grows yearly (Udodiong, 2019).

Despite the growing numbers, however, a digital divide exists in the country that separates those with good internet from those with slow internet, and millions are without internet. Though the federal government met and exceeded its goal of closing the divide with broadband by 30% in 2018, several challenges remain (Olaoluwa, 2019). These include data affordability, providing infrastructures in rural areas to close the urban-rural divide, and encouraging Nigerians to use digital technology (Iteumah, 2019). Nevertheless, that Nigerians are active internet users who are creating content and interacting with people in and outside Nigeria is noteworthy. A widespread tool they use in creating content, which is important to this study, is internet memes.

Internet memes are the most popular way 'to channel humour on the internet and social media' (Taecharungroj & Nueangjamnong, 2015, 289). A meme, according to Patrick Davison (2012, 122), is 'a piece of culture, typically a joke, which gains influence through online transmission.' A meme can be 'written text, a still image, brief animation sequences, or combinations thereof' (Rieger & Klimmt, 2019, 2202). More importantly, memes represent an online participatory culture that encourages discourse interpersonally or with mass audiences on matters of socio-economic and political importance (Rieger & Klimmt, 2019). Memes have allowed Nigerians to 'become more innovative in their patterns of communicating humor' (Chimuanya & Ajiboye, 2016, 255). Consequently, Nigerians' active use of internet memes has garnered scholarly interest (Adegoju & Oyebode, 2015; Alfred, 2019; Tella 2018). Most of these studies have focused on political humour in Nigerian memes. Considering that 'practically every socio-cultural and political event generates internet memes in Nigeria,' there is room to explore how Nigerians use memes and humour in other contexts (Chimuanya & Ajiboye, 2016, 254).

Therefore, this chapter investigated how Nigerians used memes to communicate their positions and concerns during the 2020 COVID-19 pandemic. Specifically, we analysed the humour Nigerians shared through COVID-19 memes. The key questions answered here concerned the types of memes created, the role memes played in the Nigerian context, and how Nigerians made sense of the COVID-19 crisis. We argue that in times of crisis and human suffering, people resort to humour. According to Davis (2003, 19) 'gruesome jokes' have followed major disasters such as famine, earthquakes, terrorist attacks and plane crashes, sometimes within minutes, for decades. The internet, Davis (2003) adds, has accelerated and normalized the spread and popularity of humour in tragic times, despite social mores that forbid people from finding human tragedy funny. Therefore, this chapter theorizes humour will emerge when crisis occurs in Nigeria, and Nigerian memes will channel those feelings. After all, beyond their humorous and discursive abilities, internet memes can 'perform a soothing and uplifting role' in times of tragedy and crises (Dynel, 2020, 2). This is because humour allows people in such situations to reframe 'negative experiences and/or emotions (such as suffering, anxiety and fear)' (Dynel, 2020, 2).

This chapter also contributes to a small but growing body of research that has recognized social media, its actors and shareable content like memes as influential tools in health communication, advocacy and activism (Kostygina et al., 2020). In the following paragraphs, the chapter highlights how humour is used in times of crisis and discusses humour in the Nigerian context. We also detail how Nigerians used memes during the COVID-19 lockdowns in 2020.

Humour in Times of Crisis

Silberman (1987, 102) defined humour as 'the quality that makes something funny, amusing or ludicrous; comicality, also the ability to perceive, appreciate, or express what is funny, amusing or ludicrous.' Humour is socioculturally defined and exists in different forms, including parody, jokes, satire, sarcasm, pun, and ridicule (Cernerud & Olsson, 2004). Humour also has therapeutic value that helps 'maintain, enhance, or improve physical and/or emotional well-being' (Dziegielewski, 2003, 78). However, can people find something to laugh about when a crisis or traumatic event occurs?

According to Sarah Christopher (2015), traumatic events can actually inspire humour and help people cope. Sigmund Freud (1905) theorized that humour can be a defence mechanism that allows people to cope in traumatic times. Telling jokes during trying times, for example, can 'provide for the cathartic release of anxiety or anger while bringing people together and reinforcing the boundaries between in- and out-group' (Hernan, 2016, 58). Research also indicates that humour is an important reason why people turn to social media when crisis or disaster occurs, and also a reason why they ignore social media when disaster occurs (Liu et al., 2011). Crises and disasters create black, dark, disaster or gallows humour, 'a type of humour that arises from stressful, traumatic or life-threatening situations' (Christopher, 2015, 611). Dark humour is incongruous, meaning it is out of place or inappropriate. According to Kuipers (2005, 71), 'this incongruity can be between real and unreal (absurd humor), between taboo and nontaboo (sexual humour, toilet humour, aggressive humour), or between the gruesome and the innocent, the banal, or even the cheerful (sick humour).' The incident is humorously connected to an incompatible topic. According to Davis (2003), dark humour connects with people's need to defy a system that sees such expressions as taboo. Dark humour is simply 'a way of playing with the forbidden for the sake of amusement' (Davis, 2003, 32). When disaster strikes, dark humour could also be 'a symptom or litmus test of a general population's feelings and anxieties' (Sheftel, 2012, 147).

Scholars have examined tragedies and discovered that dark humour played integral roles in how people responded to such events (Christopher,

2015). For example, Steve Lipman (1991) studied humour and laughter's importance during the Jewish Holocaust. He found that Jews used humour during the Holocaust to stay hopeful. Humour was also a 'psychological weapon and a defense mechanism. It was a social bond among trusted friends...a diversion, a shield, a morale booster, an equalizer, a drop of truth in a world full of lies' (Lipman, 1991, 10). In her work on survivors of the Bosnia-Herzegovina war, Sheftel (2012, 147) also discovered funny stories were a 'way of expressing memories that otherwise seem dangerous' during and after the war. In a study on South African prisoners of war (POWs), Karen Horn (2011) found that humour helped POWs cope, recall and reconstruct memories, and acted as a defence mechanism during captivity.

In another study, Smyth (1986) found Americans circulated jokes five weeks after the Challenger space shuttle exploded during takeoff, killing everyone on board in 1986. Smyth (1986, 260) contends that joking probably helped people deal with anxiety about death and attacked societal 'taboos on talking about and describing death or disaster.' Bill Ellis (2003) also found people posted dark humour online immediately after the September 11, 2001 attacks on the World Trade Center. Though many people reacted 'within seconds, with angry, violent, and obscene attacks on the contributor' of these jokes, six days later, others perceived the jokes as 'an inevitable, healthy response to disaster' (Ellis, 2003, 44).

Apart from wars and attacks, scholars have examined the use of humour in health crises. Marcus and Singer (2017) found that people spread digital humour using a female anime character called Ebola-chan during the Ebola epidemic from 2014 to 2015. Users of 4chan, a message board, also used the anime to spread misinformation, racial stereotypes and fear about Ebola as pranks. In contrast, Chimuanya and Ajiboye (2016) examined the semiotic patterns Nigerians used in Facebook memes when the Ebola pandemic spread in West Africa in 2014. They found the memes raised awareness on the disease and offered solutions. To date, studies indicate that digital humour, especially memes, were also important tools for coping, reducing stress and commenting on COVID-19-related issues, such as wearing face masks, social distancing and hoarding supplies (Ambrose & Idegbekwe, 2020; Dynel, 2020).

Overall, these studies suggest humour plays a function in times of crisis. However, Kuipers (2005, 72) warns that because traumatic events have become more mass mediated, meaning the media cover these events, dark humour may no longer be about coping with tragedy or venting about it.

She argues that media images of disasters evoke not only shock and grief, 'but also less empathic emotions: fascination, gloating, or even outright triumph. Explaining the appreciation of such disaster jokes with one specific emotion, such as coping with grief, seems unhelpful for such global genres' (Kuipers, 2005, 72). In addition, humour is 'a system of rules and expectations that every human being acquires simply by being a member of a particular sociocultural system' (Farb, 1981, 763). People interpret humour negatively or positively depending on their 'environment and the people therein' (Sprowl, 1987, 50). Therefore, to understand the humour Nigerians reflected in COVID-19 memes, it is important to understand what humour means in the Nigerian context.

Context

Humour appears in different forms in Africa and allows people to express themselves. Africans largely express humour interpersonally, in groups, through mass media, and live shows like stand-up comedy. Whatever the form, a common thread in African humour is that it is 'one of the most important means by which the majority define, "get even with," and "resist" the power elite and the dominant power relations' (Obadare, 2009, 244). Contemporary African humour, Obadare (2016, 63) explains, 'allows the put-upon postcolonial subject to imagine a place and reality that is radically different from the current one of widespread abjection, constant humiliation and desperation.' In postcolonial Africa, where one may wonder what there is to laugh about, Africans continuously find something to laugh about (Obadare, 2009). In the African context, humour and laughter serve 'a variety of functions for the oppressed African subject – as vengeance, coping mechanism, a means of escape, subversion, not to mention as a means of resistance' (Obadare, 2009, 243–244). Yet, African humour 'remains relatively under-investigated and is still far from seriously regarded' (Obadare, 2009, 244). In response, several scholars have studied African humour in different contexts. As this study's focus is Nigeria, this chapter discusses humour in the Nigerian context.

Nigerian humour could be defined as anything that causes laughter, including jokes, puns, satire, caricature, mockery and ridicule, but also expresses 'cultural beliefs, attitudes and ideological dispositions' (Filani, 2018, 1). Nigerians often use humour to:

> express their expectations of and disappointments in the socio-political leadership of the country. Common Nigerian jokes indicate the country's travails with ethnicity and failed political leadership. They also enunciate populist perspectives on nationhood, identity and the challenges of everyday living. (Filani, 2018, 1)

Scholars have studied Nigerian humour in three categories—precolonial/traditional humour, stand-up comedy (SUC), and online/digital humour. According to Filani (2018, 3), the last two areas have 'brought about an increase in the sourcing and use of humour in Nigeria, and have generated more sociocultural awareness, socio-political activism, and self-consciousness among the country's citizens.' Nigerian humour predates colonial times. Adeleke (2005) found that among the Yorubas in precolonial times, humour was a communal discursive act for social and political reform. The Yorubas also ridiculed or mocked antisocial behaviour using comic songs. Likewise, the court jester (Wawan Sariki) performed for the king and people in Hausa-Fulani societies and used puns, songs, satire and jokes to 'communicate serious messages…without creating any form of embarrassment' (Kofoworola, 2007, 105). Among the Igbos, jesting and exchanging insults were common strategies for building relationships (Nwankwo, 2019). These precolonial strategies are still used in Nigerian societies. In the 1970s and 1980s, comedy became a popular genre on Nigerian television, with shows such as *The New Masquerade*, *Samanja* and *Bassey and Company* entertaining Nigerians and addressing 'the social, religious, cultural and political realities' facing the country (Ajayi, 2020, 1). Then in the 1990s, the rebirth of the Nigerian movie industry provided new spaces for performing comedy. One of these spaces was SUC (Adetunji, 2013). Much of the literature on Nigerian humour has focused on SUC humour (Filani, 2020).

For example, Adetunji (2013) examined the pragmatic strategies in Nigerian SUC and found it used pidgin English, 'stereotyping, call-and-response, formulaic response, self-deprecation and shared experiences' to reach audiences. Sesan's (2018, 14) study of SUC also found performers created humour with 'topical issues such as politics and corruption to lampoon the system and the "culprits."' Filani (2020, 335) adds that Nigerian SUC uses humour to 'actively perpetuate and create a social consciousness' about Nigeria. Nwankwo (2019) also examined Nigerian SUC and found it addressed poverty, bad leadership, religion, tribalism, ethnic stereotypes and heterosexual relationships. Filani and Ajayi (2019, 142) sum up Nigerian SUC as humour that provides 'a comic dimension to the country's socio-political situation' and helps people 'strategically cope with the sociocultural realities of Nigeria.'

The final area of scholarship on Nigerian humour is digital humour. Social media's emergence in the 2000s revolutionized Nigerian humour because it offered 'more opportunities for the audience to access comedic entertainment' and provided new 'avenues for comedians to propagate their crafts' (Filani, 2018, 6). Social media, unlike traditional media (television, radio and newspapers), also provided an environment free of government censorship and control. This is a 'carnival-like environment in which laughter constitutes another kind of catharsis' for Nigerians, one that 'occasions a collapsing of the barriers between writers and readers, and through endless remixability, erases the distinctions between producers and consumers of data' (Yékú, 2016, 248). Therefore, Nigerians who were passive audiences on traditional media became active participants and content creators on social media and the internet overall. According to Awa-Kalu (2016), social media sites like Instagram, YouTube and Twitter also created a 'second wave of Nigerians comedians' who 'talk about anything and laugh about everything, sparing no topic the caustic end of the tongue.' Examples of these new comedians include Falz the Bahd Guy, Mr. Macaroni, K10, Taaooma and Maraji. Furthermore, social media created a 'laughing space' where Nigerians 'disillusioned with abuse of state power, and the consequences of political hierarchies', can laugh at themselves and people in power (Yékú, 2016, 249).

Nigerian online humour largely consists of short video skits, graphics/animation, and texts that employ satire, jokes, music, exaggeration, mockery, and ridicule as humour strategies. Scholars have examined digital humour in the Nigerian context from different angles, with most focusing on the pragmatic and linguistic strategies online humour contains (Ajayi, 2020).

For example, Filani (2017) examined readers' responses to Akpos narrative jokes (jokes created about an imaginary character called Akpos) on Facebook and found that an audience's response to online jokes is still dependent on knowing the language in which jokes are expressed and its context. Otherwise, audiences may contest a joke's funniness. Yékú (2016) also studied Akpos jokes and determined that the jokes reinvented the trickster hero found in traditional Nigerian folklore and mythologies. Akpos, through jokes, also reflected, among many things, Nigerians' coping strategies, Nigerian youths' pessimism about the future and the failure of the political class. Scholars have also examined Nigerians' use of internet memes. Besides humour, memes can 'raise very serious socio-political issues, critique social ills and communicate messages' (Taiwo, 2018, 320). Alfred (2019) contends that for Nigerians, using memes is a 'subtle and more convenient way of expressing political ideologies, possibly because it guarantees anonymity of the source of the meme.' Memes can also shape and reflect the 'collective actions and mindsets' of specific cultures at a given time (Shifman 2007, 189). Davis et al. (2018, 3900) found that memes are tools of 'silly citizenship' that allow people to humorously participate and comment on political events and politicians. To Milner (2012, iii), the internet's participatory nature also allows people to change any meme they receive and share it with others. Recipients can create or alter a meme with a meme-generating site and share with others through the internet or social media. Each time a meme is shared and/or remixed, it is 're-appropriated in order to produce new iterations and variations of broader ideas, mostly without signature or citation' (Milner, 2012,12).

To determine the patterns of humour that exist in political discourse online, Adegoju and Oyebode (2015) studied memes Nigerians shared on Facebook, WhatsApp and Twitter regarding the 2015 presidential election. The study found Nigerians discussed the elections and the candidates with several humour strategies, including puns, satire, parody, hyperbole and ironic sarcasm. In 2018, Akin Tella (2018) also examined memes about the 2015 presidential election but focused on how Nigerians used humour to frame the candidates. He found that the memes provided humour and framed the candidates negatively and positively. Surprisingly, he also found that though the internet 'widened the scope' of discourse on the election, it had not 'significantly transformed the quality of campaign discourses in Nigeria' because the frames were very negative and maintained that elections were fights over scarce resources (Tella, 2018, 114). Bukola Alfred (2019) also found Nigerians criticized the ruling political party and discussed Nigerians' sufferings through memes.

Beyond politics, Ajayi (2020) examined humour-evoking memes to determine the social realities they revealed about Nigerian society. He found that through memes, Nigerians discussed several social realities and ideologies, such as marital infidelity, electricity and un/employment problems, religiosity, and exorbitant spending during festive seasons like Christmas. Recently, Ambrose and Idegbekwe (2020) investigated the deeper meanings available in COVID-19 memes from a Nigerian perspective. They found that Nigerians used memes to echo their concerns and fears about the pandemic. However, the study focused on the echoic and pragmatic relevance of the COVID-19 memes and did not examine the humour angle. This chapter closes that gap. Considering the COVID-19 pandemic was a traumatic event that killed millions of people globally, created fear and confusion, this chapter adds to a growing literature on digital humour's role in the COVID-19 pandemic. The study argues that the pandemic, like other traumatic events examined so far, produced a dark humour that co-existed 'with daily reports on the death toll and infection numbers' (Dynel, 2020, 2). That such humour was prevalent at a tragic time suggests its significance in society. Therefore, this study is important because it presents an opportunity to understand how Nigerians use humour in times of crisis. An understanding of how Nigerians used memes during the country's COVID-19 lockdown is crucial to our understanding of people's coping mechanisms during a pandemic that required isolation and social distancing to prevent/control transmission.

Theoretical and Conceptual Framework

Humour is difficult to define because it is personal and differs from culture to culture. This, according to Meyer (2000), makes humour a seemingly difficult subject to investigate. Still, scholars have studied humour because it is a prevalent 'social phenomenon' that is popular and persuasive (Meyer, 2000, 311). Scholars want to know what makes people laugh, explain humour's roles and causes and have created theories for these reasons. According to Cernerud and Olsson (2004), more than 100 humour theories exist. The dominant ones are classified as incongruity, superiority and release/relief theories (Billig, 2005).

The incongruity theory of humour states that laughter can occur when a joke violates expectations or uses a mishap or surprise. A play on words like a pun is an example of incongruity humour because people do not expect others to spell or pronounce words wrongly. Incongruity can appear as 'contradiction, understatement, exaggeration, surprise, reversal, ludicrous, or the totally unreal' (Shade, 1996,11). The superiority theory suggests laughter results when people belittle others because they feel superior to them in some way. For example, when someone makes a mistake or wears something unfit for the context. It also means making fun of people's woes and incompetence. The release/relief theory proposes humour can relieve people's stress from 'everyday reality, boredom or even oppression' (Plester, 2015, 22). In his overview of the theories,

Meyer also (2000) argued that humour plays four basic functions: identification, clarification, enforcement, and differentiation. Identification means people use humour to connect and identify with others. Clarification means a person uses a short humorous line or memorable phrase to clarify a stand or to persuade (Meyer, 2000). Next is enforcement, whereby a person can 'enforce norms delicately by leveling criticism while maintaining some degree of identification with an audience' (Meyer, 2000, 320). The enforcement function typically occurs when people are ridiculed because they violated social norms or expectations. Humour's fourth function is differentiation and occurs when people use humour to differentiate themselves from others.

Though studies have applied these theories individually, Meyer (2000) argues that all three theories can appear in a joke because release jokes can be used in incongruous or superiority situations. Robbins and Vandree (2009, 58) add that 'humor and laughter are also modulated by underlying hostility or a sense of superiority over the target.' As internet memes are a popular form of humour online, scholars have applied these theories to their study of memes.

In their work, Shifman and Blondheim (2010) found that people used incongruity, superiority and relief to tell jokes about computers, its users and creators. In another study, Shifman (2007) found that internet memes used jokes that fit in these theories and created six types of humour online. These were 'interactive humor, funny photos, maniphotos, phanimation, celebrity soundboards and PowerPoint humor' (Shifman, 2007, 196). Interactive humour involves participating in a fun activity. A maniphoto is a digitally manipulated picture, and a phanimation is an animated version of a maniphoto. Celebrity soundboards are 'digitized celebrity sound bites taken from movies, radio and TV, which are presented on the Internet to facilitate prank calls' (Shifman, 2007, 198).

Meyer's (2000) functions of humour suggest that communicative messages like memes do not only make people laugh. Rather, people can use memes to comment on, criticize, question, dispute or acknowledge issues and events in society. This way, they can share important information and opinions indirectly. However, for readers to interpret humorous memes correctly, they must have knowledge of current events or the culture in which the memes originate (Grundlingh, 2018). Memes are therefore a good source for examining people's thoughts about issues like COVID-19 because humour is often 'used to mask a more serious issue or problem or to express a negative opinion about an individual in power (politicians, religious figures, etc.)' (Grundlingh, 2018, 163). This study applied the three humour theories and asked:

RQ1: What types of internet memes did Nigerians create and/or share during the COVID-19 lockdowns in Nigeria?
RQ2: What role did COVID-19 memes perform during the lockdowns in Nigeria?
RQ3: How did Nigerians make sense of the virus and share their fears through memes?

Methodology

To answer the research questions, we searched for user-generated memes created and/or shared between March 23 (the start of the lockdown) and June 30 (when most of it was lifted) in Nigeria on WhatsApp. WhatsApp is a Facebook-owned messaging application that allows people to send text and voice messages, make voice and video calls and share a variety of content, including images, videos and documents. Our rationale for using WhatsApp to collect memes is that it is the most popular social medium and messaging system in Nigeria (Udodiong, 2019). We also observed that as a cross-platform application, people can download and share content gleaned from other social media networks on WhatsApp and were more likely to save those they liked (pictures and videos are also automatically saved in people's phone galleries in a WhatsApp folder). Taylor (2020) also reported that WhatsApp saw 'the greatest gains in usage' of all social media when lockdowns began. Therefore, we asked 20 friends and family members in Nigeria's six geographical regions to send us any memes they received during the lockdowns and assessed them for those on COVID-19. We received 60 memes and 47 were on COVID-19. To avoid researcher bias because humour is personal, all 47 memes on COVID-19 were analysed. The 47 memes were also only in English or Pidgin English.

The memes were analysed using quantitative content analysis. Quantitative content analysis is a systematic method for describing a text's contents (Ahuvia, 2001). It involves putting data into categories and counting the frequency with which each category occurs in the data. This method suited this study because it is a popular methodology in communication research. As there was no codebook we could replicate, we selected 10% of the memes and examined them to find common characteristics we could use to create a codebook. Each meme was considered a unit of analysis because internet memes use 'textual and visual elements simultaneously in order to create humour, and as such, any attempt to separate these properties would be unwise' (Drakett et al., 2018, 115).

To address the research questions, we categorized the memes into type of meme and type of humour used. Using Reiger and Klimmt's (2019) meme categories, the memes were classified as written text only (memes that used only text to address the subject), still image (memes that used only still images to address the subject), combination (memes that combined text and images/animations to address the subject) and video. Using Billig's (2005) humour categories, the types of humour used in the memes were grouped into three types: incongruity (e.g., memes that employed puns or surprise elements), release/relief (e.g., memes that elicited laughs or eased tensions) and superiority (e.g., memes that made fun of others or elevated oneself). Once the categories and subcategories were created, we independently assessed intercoder reliability using 10% of the sample.

We compared our coding afterwards and any disagreements were discussed and resolved. Cohen Kappas on the categories ranged from 0.85 for type of humour to 0.98 for type of meme. According to Landis and Koch (1977), a kappa above 0.80 indicates almost perfect agreement. Following the pretest, we coded all 47 memes. For both categories, memes were counted in each sub type once. We also took notes regarding observations we made about the memes as quantitative content analysis examines mostly manifest information. Taking notes helped us determine the latent content, which allows researchers to make 'inferences about people' because, presumably, the 'behaviors, attitudes, meanings, and values found in the text reflect the behaviors, attitudes, and values of the people who create the material' (Keyton, 2011, 245).

Data Presentation and Analysis

Results from the content analysis revealed that Nigerians shared different types of memes during the lockdowns from March 23 to June 27, 2020. Fifty-seven per cent of the 47 memes combined text and still image/animation and 34% used text only (Fig. 4.1). We found one video meme and three that used only still images. These findings answered RQ1. The analysis also determined that the memes employed three types of humour—incongruity (46.8%), relief/release (29.8%) and superiority (23.4%). The memes provided important insight into how Nigerians use memes to

Meme Types	Frequency (N=47)	Percent
Written Text Only	16	34.0
Still Image	3	6.4
Combination	27	57.5
Video	1	2.1
Total	47	100

Fig. 4.1 Types of internet memes shared by Nigerians during the COVID-19 lockdown

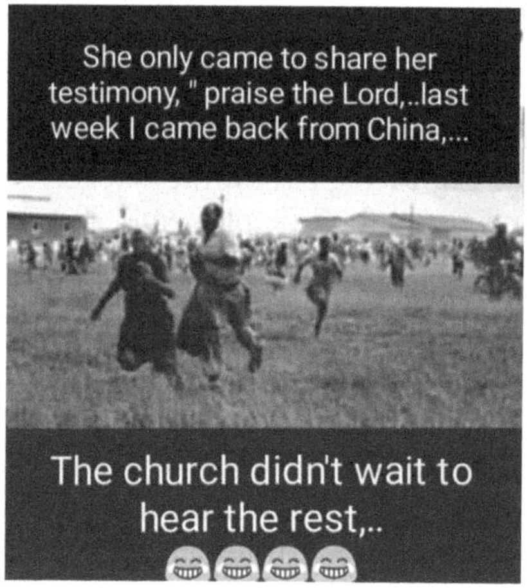
She only came to share her testimony, " praise the Lord,..last week I came back from China,...
The church didn't wait to hear the rest,..

Fig. 4.2 Combination meme

depict social realities and indirectly express the challenges people are facing at the time. In addition, the results supported Sprowl's (1987) argument that humour is successful if the context is known. However, our findings suggest that some still image-only memes could be unfunny or misunderstood without text and context.

For example, Fig. 4.2 is a combination meme that needs text to interpret the photo/still image. It shows people running and one would not know why without the text. The text says they are running from church after a woman testified that she just returned from China. Considering COVID-19 began in China, the meme implies the woman must be avoided because she may have contracted coronavirus in China, causing people to flee the church service. The laughing emojis at the bottom also prime the reader to see the meme as funny. In contrast, Fig. 4.3 is an example of a written text-only meme that does not need a picture. Yet, context is required to understand the humour.

Money is essential in all societies and the meme incongruously twists the social distancing rule to say what is safe and unsafe. The lockdowns caused Nigerians financial difficulties. Therefore, the writer wants money to know it can violate the distancing rule. In fact, it should come closer because it is needed. The meme in Fig. 4.4 is a picture of a fridge filled with food during the lockdown. Unlike Fig. 4.2, this meme has no text. But someone who does not know about Nigeria's electricity problems could miss the joke or need text to prime him/her. Following years of corruption and inefficiency, Nigeria has epileptic power supply. Yet, someone filled a fridge with food that could spoil quickly (the freezer has no frost).

Nevertheless, one can conclude from these examples that humour is successful when one knows the social realities that produce it (Obadare, 2009). The analysis also identified three thematic issues in the memes that explained the roles the memes played during the lockdowns and how Nigerians used memes to make sense of COVID-19 and share their fears about it.

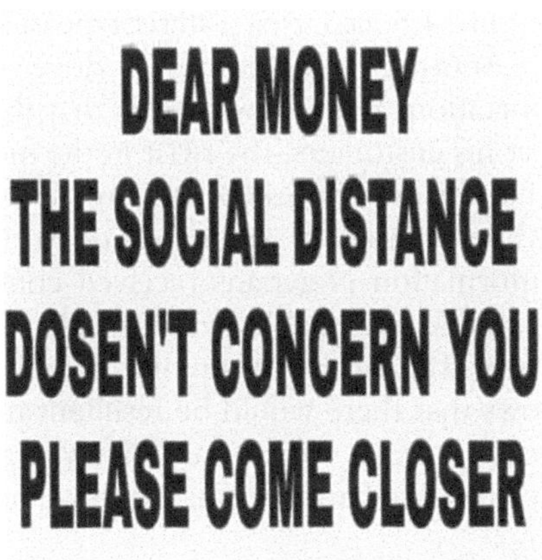
DEAR MONEY
THE SOCIAL DISTANCE
DOSEN'T CONCERN YOU
PLEASE COME CLOSER

Fig. 4.3 Written text meme

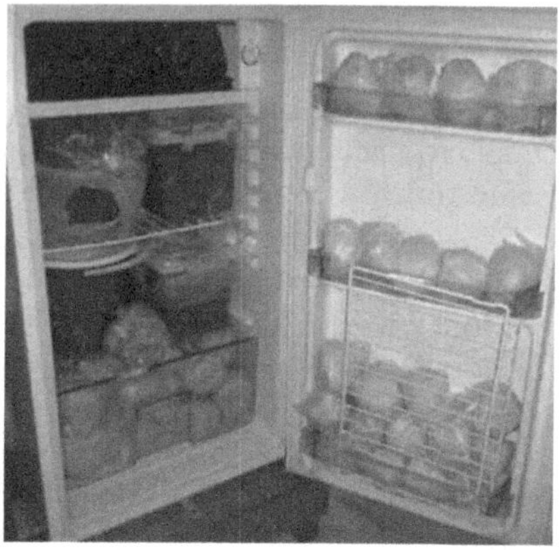

Fig. 4.4 Still image/animation example

Need to Practise Safety Habits and Have Information

A majority of the memes addressed the new safety habits implemented nationwide to curb the spread of the coronavirus with an undertone of incorrect and wrong implementation. Wearing face masks and constantly using hand sanitizers are not normal habits in Nigeria. Implementing such new habits required time and understanding. Therefore, some memes highlighted these changes and raised awareness about what was happening by mocking people who wore masks incorrectly or used items like soap dishes and lettuce leaves for masks. Such memes used a superiority approach to differentiate and ridicule those they believed were doing something wrong. Two examples are offered in Figs. 4.5 and 4.6. Figure 4.5 also used a stereotype of Ibadan people as backward.

Another meme addressed driver-provided face masks in public transportation. While it was great that the driver in the meme had face masks for his customers, the twist in the meme comes when we learn at the end that the driver uses the same mask for different passengers. These memes, while humorous, also raised questions about the amount and quality of information Nigerians received concerning masks; whether masks were available, affordable, what people could use as masks, and how to wear them. If people were uninformed or the messages were ambiguous, it follows that there would be resultant misuse. Memes also drew attention to handwashing, which was portrayed as excessive (e.g., a meme said a man washed his hands so many times, he found answers to his eighth-grade

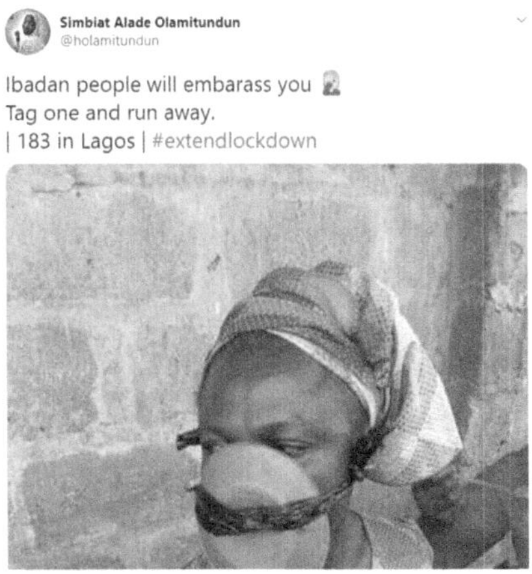
Simbiat Alade Olamitundun
@holamitundun
Ibadan people will embarass you
Tag one and run away.
| 183 in Lagos | #extendlockdown

Fig. 4.5 Woman using bowl for mask

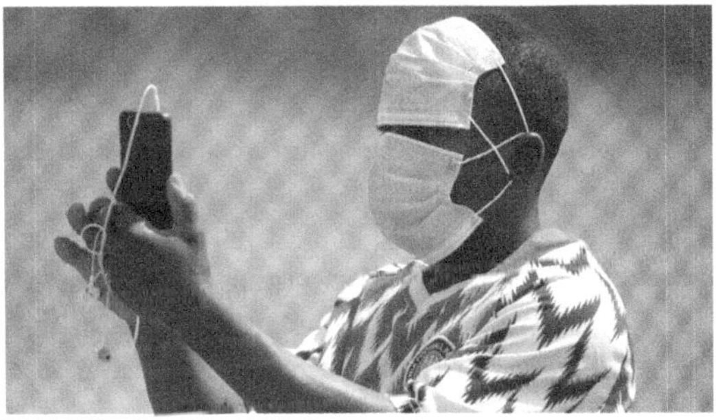

Fig. 4.6 Man wearing mask covering forehead

social studies test), and using hand sanitizers, which was framed as hands drinking alcohol.

Two memes also addressed discrepancies in the information states like Kano provided on confirmed COVID cases. After the news reported the number of confirmed and recovered cases, the memes highlighted the discrepancies in what was reported. According to one meme, Kano reported 840 confirmed COVID-19 cases, but then reported 970 recovered COVID-19 cases. This 'means COVID-19 is owing them extra 130 cases.' These memes sarcastically suggested government/leaders in the state exaggerated their numbers and hinted at corruption in the system. The memes also hinted at the lack of good information and record keeping on the virus in the country. If states could not provide accurate numbers, how would people know the virus' true effect?

Overall, while these memes talked about the need to be safe and practise new safety habits, they made fun of the changes. This way, the memes also served as release because they allowed people to laugh at the situation. The memes also indirectly raised questions about the problems following these practices caused in Nigeria and highlighted people's concerns with how the disease could spread if people were uninformed or using masks wrongly. This supports Grundlingh's (2018) and Taiwo's (2018) view that humour can express serious problems.

Consequences of a Protracted Stay at Home

A second theme found in the data concerned the effects of staying at home. Apart from the once-a-month environmental cleaning that required Nigerians to remain home for three hours in the early 1980s, 2020 was the first time Nigeria implemented daily stay-at-home orders (Olowoporoku, 2017). As a social country, Nigerians struggled with the new normal. Some of the memes addressed people's inability to go on holidays. Instead, people were 'travelling' within their homes (one meme was a passport that was stamped at the bathroom, bedroom, living room and kitchen). Memes also addressed the impact staying at home for an extended period could have on families, marriages and/or relationships. These memes addressed the lack of privacy, extramarital affairs and how spouses, being forced to stay at home together, would learn new and troublesome information about each other. Oguntayo et al. (2020) found that the lockdown caused 'unprecedented stress' that disrupted marriages and increased rates of intimate partner violence. Understanding that this was an issue, memes proffered suggestions for what spouses could do to survive the lockdown.

Figure 4.7 provides an example of such a solution. The meme offers husbands a 'rescue' from their wives to a location of their choice. As people could not go out, the meme creatively suggests husbands can hire people disguised as members of the Nigerian Centre for Disease Control's COVID-19 taskforce. They would pretend the man had the virus and use that excuse to take him away. Aside from providing entertainment on how one could escape a spouse, the meme also points out Nigeria's patriarchal culture. Only men need rescuing, not women. Secondly, the meme creatively presents Nigerians' creative tendencies to make money and use opportunities to their advantage. This meme features incongruity, release and superiority humour because it used violations of social expectations

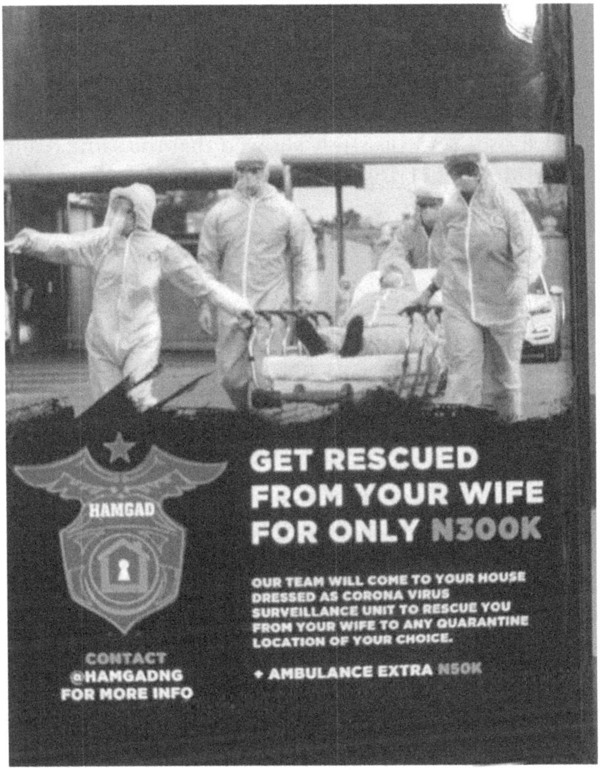
GET RESCUED
FROM YOUR WIFE
FOR ONLY N300K
OUR TEAM WILL COME TO YOUR HOUSE DRESSED AS CORONA VIRUS SURVEILLANCE UNIT TO RESCUE YOU FROM YOUR WIFE TO ANY QUARANTINE LOCATION OF YOUR CHOICE.
+ AMBULANCE EXTRA N50K
HAMGAD
CONTACT
@HAMGADNG
FOR MORE INFO

Fig. 4.7 Husband rescue meme

(obey the law, fidelity and family time), provokes laughter to relieve stress, and ridicules men's superiority (they need help to leave home).

In addition, five memes featured the lockdown's financial impact. Some businesses could not operate, and people were unable to work during the lockdown. Therefore, lost income was a source of anxiety, especially as Nigeria did not provide adequate relief for Nigerians. Palliatives that the federal government created to help 'vulnerable' citizens, including food and cash, were not distributed (Eranga, 2020, 222). To make money some people started new businesses that fit the context. One was handwashing stations. Figure 4.8 uses a photo of one such handwashing station for a meme. The meme emphasizes that Igbo women, who are considered industrious, thought of the new business. However, it is telling that though socially distanced, none of the women in the picture are wearing masks. It also highlights how no facilities for washing hands exist outside homes and restaurants in Nigeria. Thematically, these memes also matched Ajayi's (2020) findings about the social realities that humour-evoking memes can expose. Yet, this study showed that the same realities he identified can occur during a crisis.

Need for Entertainment

The final theme the analysis revealed was Nigerians' need for entertainment. The confusion and uncertainty COVID-19 created and the resulting lockdown meant Nigerians needed distractions. According to Tom McTague (2020), COVID-19 was the 'worst global health crisis,' and the resulting lockdowns created a 'mass outpouring of gags, memes, funny videos and general silliness.' COVID-19 created what we called a 'coromentality' in Nigeria; a mental state focused on COVID-19 because it impacted people psychologically. Nigerian memes probably tapped into people's need for entertainment to deal with the lockdown's psychological impact. All 47 memes evoked humour to help people find release and remove their minds from the public health crisis and its present and future impacts. For example, in the meme the creator makes fun and suggests that wearing masks for extensive periods would alter ear shapes. People would need to normalize their ears after the pandemic. Therefore, they will wear masks in reverse to return ears to their original positions.

Another example is provided in a meme, through a superiority frame, that gives Nigerians hope. The creator purports that Nigeria is going to beat the coronavirus just as it did Ebola. The meme takes a superior tone asking coronavirus if Ebola did not tell it about Nigeria. This suggests Nigeria was the 'wrong nation' for COVID-19 to come to. The caption of the meme, which features a child holding her chin reads, 'corona, you mean Ebola did not gist you? This is Nigeria oh! corona just landed in the wrong nation, ask Ebola what eternal life and prayers did to it. I have seen you crushed already.' The creator is also insinuating that as a highly religious country, Nigerians will be definitely praying against the virus, another source of superiority.

The seriousness of the pandemic also did not stop Nigerians from making jokes about the safety practices they encouraged in the memes. For example, a meme on social distancing said a man was asked what he would do for his community if he won 80 million Naira. He replied that he would 'practice social distancing.' A temperature meme also addressed how COVID-19 was the great equalizer because it empowered people of a lower class. It asked, 'Did you ever think a time will come when a security man will check the temperature of a doctor at a bank?' A doctor is of a higher social class than a security man (who mans the door or gate). But in this scenario, because the security man determines who enters a bank and who cannot, he has more power than the doctor. Two memes also made fun of the irony that a disease discovered in China had such a lasting effect. For example, one meme showed a sad looking chimpanzee and the text points out that this is the longest something made in China has ever lasted. It plays on the stereotype that things made in China do not last.

Overall, our findings supported Kostygina et al.'s (2020) research that memes can be used for activism to address issues in society. These memes were also timely because they addressed issues Nigerians were experiencing at the time. Our findings further cement Moreno-Almeida's (2020, 2) position that no matter 'how serious or humorous they are, all memes are political because they speak to the ways people see themselves in terms of race, class, gender, sexuality, ability and so forth.'

Conclusion

This study explored the memes Nigerians created and shared during the COVID-19 lockdowns that began on March 23, 2020. The study found that during the lockdowns, Nigerians created and shared 47 memes with a COVID-19 theme. The analysis also determined that the memes were primarily created to entertain but also comment on issues COVID-19 caused. Although this study used a small sample of internet memes, it sheds light on how Nigerians use memes in times of crisis. Unlike previous studies on dark humour that found humorous material when people died, none of the Nigerian memes in this study talked about or made light of death. This was probably because only four deaths were recorded during the period of study. One could say these memes show Nigerians use dark humour to laugh at themselves and the country, and not others' suffering.

Overall, the study's findings are important for understanding how Nigerians used humour during a global pandemic because these memes were created in a period when people were forced to isolate and rely on social media for information, companionship and entertainment. Further studies on Nigerian memes could explore the other communicative acts that Nigerian user-generated memes can perform. Though it was challenging to find Nigerian created memes for this study, future studies could explore other social media networking sites for user-generated content from Nigeria on the coronavirus. The entertainment-themed memes also raise questions about the emotions the memes raised and why they were made. According to Kuipers (2005), dark humour in a mediated society raises less empathic emotions beyond coping. Future studies could explore why Nigerians make memes in times of crisis.

References

Adegoju, O., & Oyebode, O. (2015). Humour as discursive practice in Nigeria's 2015 presidential election online campaign. *Discourse Studies, 17*(60), 643–662.

Adeleke, D. (2005). Ethos of laughter among the Yoruba. *Ihafa: A Journal of African Studies, 5*(2), 43–62.

Adetunji, A. (2013). The interactional context of humour in Nigerian stand-up comedy. *Pragmatics, 23*(1), 1–22.

Adoyi, A. (2020, March 29). COVID-19: President Buhari announces total lockdown in Lagos, Abuja. *Daily Post.* https://dailypost.ng/2020/03/29/breaking-COVID-19-president-buhari-announces-total-lockdown-in-lagos-abuja-full-statement/. Accessed 1 June 2020.

Ahuvia, A. (2001). Traditional, interpretive, and reception-based content analyses: Improving the ability to address issues of pragmatic and theoretical concern. *Social Indicators Research, 54*, 139–172.

Ajayi, T. M. (2020). Beyond joking: A pragmatic (de)construction of "Nigerian realities" in selected humour-evoking Facebook memes. *Israeli Journal for Humour Research, 9*(1), 47–71.

Alfred, R. (2019). Analysing verbal and visual indexes in internet memes on the APC-led administration and "change" slogan in Nigeria. *Covenant Journal of Language Studies, 7*(1), 1–20.

Ambrose, C. L., & Idegbekwe, D. (2020). Echoic communication and pragmatic relevance of COVID-19 memes in Nigeria's social media space. *Indian Journal of Language and Linguistics, 1*(1), 1–1.2.

Awa-Kalu, N. (2016, May 11). The new funny: How social media is disrupting comedy in Nigeria. *Ventures Africa.* https://venturesafrica.com/features/the-new-funny-how-social-media-is-disrupting-comedy-in-nigeria/. Accessed 26 Jan 2021.

Billig, M. (2005). *Laughter and ridicule. Towards a social critique of humour.* Sage.

Cernerud, L., & Olsson, H. (2004). Humour seen from a public health perspective. *Scandinavian Journal of Public Health, 32*, 396–398.

Chimuanya, L., & Ajiboye, E. (2016). Socio-semiotics of humour in Ebola awareness discourse on Facebook. In R. Taiwo, A. Odebunmi, & A. Adetunji (Eds.),

Analyzing language and humour in online communication (pp. 252–273). IGI Global.

Christopher, S. (2015). An introduction to black humour as a coping mechanism for student paramedic. *Journal of Paramedic Practice, 7*(12), 610–615.

Dangida, A. (2021, January 28). Over 124 million Nigerians are using internet – NITDA. *Vanguard.* https://www.vanguardngr.com/2021/01/over-124million-nigerians-are-using-internet-nitda/. Accessed 29 Jan 2021.

Davis, C. (2003). Jokes that follow mass-mediated disasters in a global electronic age. In P. Naverez (Ed.), *Of corpse: Death and humour in in folklore and popular culture* (pp. 15–34). Utah University Press.

Davis, J. L., Love, T. P., & Killen, G. (2018). Seriously funny: The political work of humour on social media. *New Media & Society, 20*(10), 3898–3916.

Davison, P. (2012). The language of Internet memes. In M. Mandiberg (Ed.), *The social media reader* (pp. 120–134). NYU Press.

Drakett, J., Rickett, B., Day, K., & Milnes, K. (2018). Old jokes, new media – Online sexism and construction of gender in internet memes. *Feminism & Psychology, 28*(1), 109–127.

Dynel, M. (2020). COVID-19 memes going viral: On the multiple multimodal voices behind face masks. *Discourse & Society, 32*(2), 1–21.

Dziegielewski, S. F. (2003). Humor: An essential communication tool in therapy. *International Journal of Mental Health, 32*(3), 74–90.

Ellis, B. (2003). Making a Big Apple crumble: The role of humour in constructing a global response to disaster. In P. Navarez (Ed.), *Of corpse: Death and humour in in folklore and popular culture* (pp. 35–79). Utah University Press.

Eranga, I. O. (2020). COVID-19 pandemic in Nigeria: Palliative measures and the politics of vulnerability. *International Journal of Maternal and Child Health and AIDS, 9*(2), 220–222.

Farb, P. (1981). Speaking seriously about humour. *The Massachusetts Review, 22*(4), 760–776.

Filani, I. (2017). "Laf wan kill me die" (I almost died laughing): An analysis of Akpos jokes and the readers' responses. *European Journal of Humour Research, 4*(4), 5–25.

Filani, I. (2018). Editorial: Dis laf fit kill person: An overview of Nigerian humour. *European Journal of Humour Research, 694*, 1–9.

Filani, I. (2020). A discourse analysis of national identity in Nigerian stand-up humour. *Discourse Studies, 22*(3), 319–338.

Filani, I., & Ajayi, T. M. (2019). Ideologies of Nigerian stand-up comedy. *Linguistik Online, 100*(7), 141–158.

Freud, S. (1905). *Jokes and their relation to the unconscious.* Norton.

Grundlingh, L. (2018). Memes as speech acts. *Social Semiotics, 28*(2), 147–168.

Hernan, A. (2016). Joking through hardship: Humour and truth-telling among displaced Timbuktutians. *African Studies Review, 59*(1), 57–76.

Horn, K. (2011). 'Stalag Happy': South African prisoners of war during World War Two (1939–1945) and their experience and use of humour. *South African Historical Journal, 63*(4), 537–552.

Iteumah, O. (2019, November 29). Uneven playing fields: Nigeria and the digital divide. *The Republic*. https://republic.com.ng/october-november-2019/nigeria-and-the-digital-divide/. Accessed 30 Jan 2021.

Johnson, J. (2021). Number of internet users in Nigeria from 2015 to 2025. https://www.statista.com/statistics/183849/internet-users-nigeria. Accessed 13 Jan 2021.

Keyton, J. (2011). *Communication research: Asking questions, finding answers* (3rd ed.). McGraw-Hill.

Kofoworola, K. G. (2007). The court jester in Nigerian drama. In D. Robb (Ed.), *Clowns, fools and picaros: Popular forms in theatre, fiction and film* (pp. 101–114). Rodopi.

Kostygina, G., Tran, H., Binns, S., Szczypka, G., Emery, S., Vallone, D., & Hair, E. (2020). Boosting health campaign reach and engagement through use of social media influencers and memes. *Social Media + Society, 6*(2), 1–12.

Kuipers, G. (2005). "Where was King Kong when we needed him?" Public discourse, digital disaster jokes, and the functions of laughter after 9/11. *The Journal of American Culture, 28*(1), 70–84.

Landis, J. R., & Koch, G. G. (1977). The measurement of observer agreement for categorical data. *Biometrics, 33*(1), 159–174.

Lipman, S. (1991). *Laughter in hell: The use of humour during the Holocaust*. Jason Aronson.

Liu, B. F., Austin, L., & Jin, Y. (2011). How publics respond to crisis communication strategies: The interplay of information form and source. *Public Relations Review, 37*, 345–353.

Marcus, O. R., & Singer, M. (2017). Loving Ebola-chan: Internet memes in an epidemic. *Media, Culture & Society, 39*(3), 341–356.

McTague, T. (2020, April 3). Yes, make coronavirus jokes. *The Atlantic*. https://www.theatlantic.com/international/archive/2020/04/humor-laughter-coronavirus-covid19/609184/. Accessed 27 Jan 2021.

Meyer, J. C. (2000). Humour as a double-Edged sword: Four functions of humour in communication. *Communication Theory, 10*(3), 310–331.

Milner, R. M. (2012). *The world made meme: Discourse and identity in participatory media*. PhD dissertation. University of Kansas. https://kuscholarworks.ku.edu/handle/1808/10256. Accessed 10 June 2020.

Moreno-Almeida, C. (2020). Memes as snapshots of participation: The role of digital amateur activists in authoritarian regimes. *New Media & Society*, 1–22.

National Bureau of Statistics. (2020). *Telecoms data: Active voice and internet per state, porting and tariff information* (Q1 July 2020).

Nwankwo, I. E. (2019). Incongruous liaisons: Routes of humour, insult and political (in) correctness in Nigerian stand-up jokes. *European Journal of Humour Research, 7*(2), 100–115.

Obadare, E. (2009). The uses of ridicule: Humour, infrapolitics and civil society in Nigeria. *African Affairs, 108*, 241–261.

Obadare, E. (2016). *Humour, silence and civil society in Nigeria*. University of Rochester Press.

Oguntayo, R., Oyeleke, J., John-Oguntayo, O., & Aajayi-Hutchful, F. (2020). Personality traits, emotional intelligence, socio-contextual factors and spousal violence: The trajectory of COVID-19 pandemic lockdown. *International Journal of Behavioral Sciences, 14*(2), 101–107.

Olaoluwa, J. (2019, August 28). Broadband penetration: Nigeria exceeds 30% target. *Nairametrics*. Broadband penetration: Nigeria exceeds 30% target | Nairametrics|Broadband penetration: Nigeria exceeds 30% target | Nairametrics. Accessed 29 Jan 2021.

Olowoporoku, O. (2017). A recipe for diaster: An assessment of environmental sanitation situation in Nigeria. *Journal of Environmental Science, 1*, 1–5.

Onu, N., Aiwerie, O., Adeyemi, K., Anthony, B., Anioke, O., Alabelewe, A., & Omokhunu, G. (2020, March 27). Nigeria in lockdown. *The Nation*. https://thenationonlineng.net/nigeria-in-lockdown/. Accessed 1 June 2020.

Plester, B. (2015). *The complexity of workplace humour: Laughter, jokers and the dark side of humour*. Springer.

Rieger, D., & Klimmt, C. (2019). The daily dose of digital inspiration 2: Themes and affective user responses to meaningful memes in social media. *New Media & Society, 21*(10), 2201–2221.

Robbins, B. D., & Vandree, K. (2009). The self-regulation of humour expression: A mixed method, phenomenological investigation of suppressed laughter. *The Humanistic Psychologist, 37*, 49–78.

Sesan, A. A. (2018). Narrating self and topicality in AY and Elenu's stand-up comedy. *European Journal of Humour Research, 6*(4), 10–23.

Shade, R. A. (1996). *License to laugh: Humour in the classroom*. Libraries Unlimited.

Sheftel, A. (2012). Monument to the international community, from the grateful citizens of Sarajevo: Dark humour as counter-memory in post-conflict Bosnia-Herzegovina. *Memory Studies, 5*(2), 145–164.

Shifman, L. (2007). Humor in the age of digital reproduction: Continuity and change in internet-based comic texts. *International Journal of Communication, 1*, 187–209.

Shifman, L., & Blondheim, M. (2010). The medium is the joke: Online humour about and by networked computers. *New Media & Society, 12*(8), 1348–1367.

Silberman, I. N. (1987). Humor and health: An epidemiological study. *American Behavioral Scientist, 30*, 100–112.

Smyth, W. (1986). Challenger jokes and the humor of disaster. *Western Folklore, 45*(4), 243–260.

Sprowl, J. (1987). Humor theory and communication research. *World Communication, 16*, 47–65.

Taecharungroj, V., & Nueangjamnong, P. (2015). Humour 2.0: Styles and types of humour and virality of memes on Facebook. *Journal of Creative Communications, 10*(3), 288–302.

Tangwa, G. B., & Munung, N.S. (2020). COVID-19: Africa's relation with epidemics and some imperative ethics considerations of the moment. *Research Ethics, 16*(3–4), 1–11.

Tankovska, H. (2021). Global social networks ranked by number of users. https://www.statista.com/statistics/272014/global-social-networks-ranked-bynumber-of-users/. Accessed 13 Jan 2021.

Taiwo, R. (2018). *Beyond the text: Critical discourse analysis and the quest for meaning in cyberspace interactions.* OAU Press.

Taylor, D. (2020, March 31). COVID-19: Social media use goes up as country stays indoors. *Victoria News.* https://www.vicnews.com/news/COVID-19-social-media-use-goes-up-as-country-stays-indoors/. Accessed 1 June 2020.

Tella, A. (2018). Humour generation and multimodal framing of political actor in the 2015 Nigerian presidential campaign memes. *European Journal of Humour Research, 6*(4), 95–117.

Toromade, S. (2020, March 20). Timeline of coronavirus cases in Nigeria. *Pulse.ng.* https://www.pulse.ng/news/local/coronavirus-timeline-and-profile-of-cases-in-nigeria/k9p6lbk. Accessed 1 June 2020.

Udodiong, I. (2019, February 8). Here is how Nigerians are using the internet in 2019. *Pulse.ng.* https://www.pulse.ng/bi/tech/how-nigerians-are-using-the-internet-in-2019/kz097rg. Accessed 1 June 2020.

Wetsman, N. (2020, February 20). Some African countries at risk for the new coronavirus aren't prepared. *The Verge.* https://www.theverge.com/2020/2/20/21145378/coronavirus-africa-egypt-algeria-nigeria-travel-vulnerability. Accessed 1 June 2020.

Yékú, J. (2016). Akpos don come again: Nigerian cyberpop hero as trickster. *Journal of African Cultural Studies, 28*(3), 245–261.

CHAPTER 5

An Analysis of Internet Memes and Discourses on Traditional Medicines as Remedies for COVID-19 in Zimbabwe

Mbongeni Jonny Msimanga, Lungile Augustine Tshuma, and Mphathisi Ndlovu

Introduction and Context

The outbreak of the novel coronavirus disease (COVID-19) resulted in an unprecedented global crisis. Given this public health crisis of multifaceted dimensions, this chapter examines how memes produced and circulated by Zimbabweans on social media demonstrated citizens' sense of agency to comment on the treatment for this pandemic. With the Zimbabwean government yet to avail plans for vaccination, traditional herbs such as *umsuzwane/zumbani* became sought after. Traditional means of curing flu such as steaming became popular during this pandemic. However, in the wake of the second wave of infections, some members of the public turned to traditional remedies and medicinal plants. However, this indigenous

M. J. Msimanga (✉) • L. A. Tshuma
University of Johannesburg, Auckland Park, South Africa

M. Ndlovu
Stellenbosch University, Stellenbosch, South Africa

S. Mpofu (ed.), *Digital Humour in the Covid-19 Pandemic*,
https://doi.org/10.1007/978-3-030-79279-4_5

knowledge system is hotly contested as health experts warned the public against the use of traditional herbs. Against the backdrop of the search for COVID-19 cure, this study examines how social media memes reflected on people's lived experiences and knowledge contestations.

Since the virus broke out in Wuhan (China) in December 2019, COVID-19 has continued to wreak havoc across the globe. In March 2020, it was declared a pandemic by the World Health Organization (WHO). More than 175 million people have contracted this virus across the globe, with nearly four million fatalities recorded. The symptoms of COVID-19 include dry cough, fever and shortness of breath. Prominent debates have been centred on epidemiological responses to this global disaster. Countries across the globe adopted sweeping measures such as lockdowns, sealing of national borders and imposing other travel restrictions to curb the spread of this infectious disease. Health experts recommended hand hygiene, social distancing and mask wearing as some of the measures for mitigating and preventing the spread of the virus. With the non-existence of a cure, measures such as "hand hygiene, social distancing and quarantine" were said to help people to "protect themselves and others" (Teti et al., 2020, 2).

Although countries are implementing measures such as social distancing, there was an urgent need for the development of a vaccine to curb the spread of COVID-19. Thus, there is a race to "develop and deploy safe and effective vaccines" (WHO, 2021). However, there are concerns about the lack of equitable access to vaccines, or what the United Nations regards as the problem of "vaccine nationalism" (EWN, 2021). Wealthy countries are hogging COVID-19 vaccine doses, a situation that may lead to what the WHO director-general Tedros Adhanom Ghebreyesus terming a "catastrophic moral failure" (EWN, 2021). Given these structural inequalities and the hoarding of COVID-19 vaccines by powerful nations, African countries are being left behind in obtaining the vaccines. Besides the challenge of vaccine nationalism, there are myths about COVID-19 vaccines that are circulating on social media, and some of the rumours include a claim that the vaccines will alter people's DNA. In March 2020, Zimbabwe's Minister of Defense claimed that COVID-19 was God's punishment on the Western countries for imposing sanctions on Zimbabwe. In Zimbabwe, COVID-19 fears were compounded by the lack of emergency preparedness, poor healthcare system and the deepening economic crisis. Given the fragile health system in the country and uncertainty surrounding the COVID-19 pandemic, some Zimbabweans resorted to the use of herbal remedies such as *umsuzwane/zumbani*, concoctions and steaming as preventive measures (CITE, 2021). At the time of writing this chapter, the country was yet to receive doses of COVID-19 vaccines. Health experts in the country have been warning citizens against the use of steam inhalation and local herbs as COVID-19 remedies. Our chapter considers how Internet memes gave citizens a voice and agency to comment on prescribed treatments for the COVID-19 pandemic.

In January 2021, South Africa became one of the first African countries to receive doses of COVID-19 vaccine. Seychelles was the first country in sub-Saharan Africa to vaccinate its citizens against COVID-19 (McSweeney & Chingono, 2021). As of February 3, 2021, Egypt, Algeria, Seychelles and Morocco were the only African states that had begun vaccinating their populations (McSweeney & Chingono, 2021). Tanzania's head of state, on the other hand, declared that his country will not accept COVID-19 vaccines (BBC, 2021). President Mugufuli had been urging Tanzanians to use steam inhalation and herbal medicines to cure COVID-19. Earlier in June 2020, he declared Tanzania "COVID-19 free" (BBC, 2021). Almost a year later, in March 2021, he was killed by the virus. Social media reports abound that a herbal concoction was launched and promoted in Madagascar to cure COVID-19, despite warnings by the WHO against the use of traditional herbal remedies (Ndlovu-Gatsheni, 2020). Against the backdrop of the myths, complexities and politics surrounding COVID-19 vaccines, this chapter examines the memes that circulated on social media platforms such as Facebook, Twitter and WhatsApp as citizens attempted to cope and make sense of the cure for COVID-19 pandemic. In the next section, we review literature on humour and health communication.

Literature Review

Humour, since time immemorial, has been dedicated to exposing human folly with its goal to inspire critical thinking and reasoned social engagement (McClennen & Maisel, 2014, 108). It is mostly accompanied by irony, parody and word play. It is critical in nature and has a didactic meaning on issues expressed. By possessing such qualities, humour is sometimes a critical mode of addressing those in power as the press is viewed too timid and does not convey political and social events the way it does (Gray et al., 2009). Highet (1962, 5) further suggests that humour is "topical; It claims to be realistic (although it is usually exaggerated or distorted); It is shocking; It is informal; (and although often in a grotesque and painful manner) it is funny". Thus, satire ought not to be funny per se, although it maintains its characteristic of scorning those who wield power. In the process, humour is a means of speaking back to power, laws or institutional policies in a given context or scenario (Critchley, 2002; Neale & Krutnick, 2006; Gray et al., 2009). The attack of power by the genre also enables deliberative discussions permitting unconscious reflections amongst audiences on socio-political and socio-economic issues. In this way, satire has the power to "energize civic culture, engaging citizen-audiences…inspiring public political discussions, and drawing citizens enthusiastically into the realm of the political with deft and dazzling ease" (Gray et al., 2009, 4). The genre's calling card is the ability to produce social scorn or damning indictments through playful means transforming the aggressive act of ridicule into a more socially acceptable act of rendering something ridiculous.

However, most studies in the Global South have assessed how satire, memes and humour are avenues for challenging and critiquing the ruling elite (Willems, 2011; Siziba & Ncube, 2015; Mpofu, 2019). These studies are in relation to how humour is oppositional and transgressive in nature and is used as political weapons. Moreover, humour are weapons of the weak used to expose self-aggrandisement, ineptness and nepotism of political leaders, mishaps and inability to serve in positions of power (see Nyamnjoh, 2009, 99). Thus, humour is a means of political communication that plays the role of an alternative public sphere and gives space for postcolonial subjects to deliberate and think about issues presented to them that affect them on a day-to-day basis (see Mbembe, 2001). In this way, humour is a social and political construct arising from the society in which we are embedded. Mbembe (2001, 142), drawing his examples from Togo and Cameroon, comments on the significance of humour and aesthetised art in postcolonial Africa alluding that "as a figure of speech, the image is always a conventional comment, the transcription of a reality, a word, a vision, or an idea into a visible code that becomes, in turn, a manner of speaking of the world and inhabiting it". In the process, humour is significant in the *deterritorialisation* of political leaders and is an attempt to *delegitimise* a particular person, idea or position circulating within the wider social sphere or community (Eko, 2015). A recurring theme amongst this corpus of literature shows how satire and humour provides a space for communicating and venting out displeasure towards government officials and policies.

However, in this study we consider how memes were a means to comment on indigenous herbs and as COVID-19 treatments. We consider how memes then act as counter-hegemonic and countercultural weapons regarded as significant political actions (see Mina, 2014; Pearce & Hajizada, 2014). As Goriunova (2012, 223) further states, memes are forms of "aesthetic expression" created and circulated through social media platforms. They are a means of silent resistance, take on forms of manipulated videos, phrases images and words (see Siziba & Ncube, 2015, 517–518). They can be used to advertise or commercialise products on social media platforms (Siziba & Ncube, 2015). This performance and playfulness online, particularly through the creation of memes and viral videos, gives individuals the capacity to create and express political and cultural discontent. They also create subcultures that oppose dominant discourses. The strong visual language embedded in Internet memes and their culture, which consists of creative remixing and fosters communal participation, provides a platform which allows for new forms of public debate and community building to take place.

There is, however, a dearth of literature on the intersection of humour and health communication in the Global South. Studies have shown how humour has been used during health campaigns as a way of persuading people to accept aversive information (see Hendricks & Jansen, 2017, 595). Some however examine people's response to humour with findings showing that people including patients respond positively to life-threatening information when communicated with humour (see Lee et al., 2015). Referring to Malawi, Tavory (2014, 287) observes how people make fun of HIV/AIDS stating, "where AIDS constantly hovers over social life, it becomes both constant resource-for and the butt-of humour". There is a growing interest on the intersection of humour and health communication on the COVID-19 pandemic because of citizens' access to social media and their inclination to debate issues online. Wasserman (2020) contends that during the COVID-19 pandemic, humour has been used as a coping mechanism that speaks to socio-cultural, political and psychological reasons. Taking a leaf from this study, we argue that humour plays an important role in communicating health-related information by analysing memes that circulated on social media platforms during the COVID-19 pandemic. Particularly, this chapter will assess how audiences communicated information on indigenous ways of treating the COVID-19 pandemic. Thus, this chapter acts as a springboard for further research on the intersection of health communication and humour as the effects will be felt for years to come. In the next section, we provide an outline of the theoretical perspectives that the study will adopt.

Theoretical and Conceptual Framework

The chapter adopts a Bakhtin's theoretical lens so as to understand memes that circulated on social media platforms. The carnivalesque is developed from the term carnival, and these were common cultural activities in medieval Europe and elsewhere. It is through an analysis of these that Bakhtin developed a theory of the carnivalesque (Ngoshi, 2013, 54). The carnivalesque denotes a rebellion of the social order against hierarchic authority. This traditional institute or body legitimises specific rules and regulations that are meant to be abided to by society. Stam (1989, 95) further notes that the carnivalesque atmosphere "is more than a party or a festival; it is the oppositional culture…a counter-model of cultural production and desire". Thus, a carnivalesque atmosphere suspends rules, laws and any form of hierarchical institutions and rules that attempt to hunker down society and its participants. In the process, "second life" is imagined as a "world" where everyone on free and familiar contact is established. We consider these aspects as social media platforms in Zimbabwe were used to challenge the COVID-19 vaccines approved by the World Health Organization (WHO) and the Zimbabwean government. Instead, people preferred the traditional means of treating the virus. We also consider how the new relationship espoused by a carnivalesque atmosphere enables a "new mode of interrelationship between individuals, counterpoised to the all-powerful socio-hierarchical relationships of non-carnival life" (Stevens, 2009, 1).

Within this space, ordinary people have an opportunity to interact with the "untouchables", that is, those who wield institutional, political and economic power in the non-carnival life. Stam (1989, 87) supports this view stating that within a carnivalesque atmosphere, all hierarchical distinctions, all barriers, all norms and prohibitions are temporarily suspended, while a qualitatively different kind of communication, based on "free and familiar contact", is established. The space enables the breaking down of barriers, overcoming of power inequalities and hierarchies through free interactions (see Rayner, 2010, 6). It challenges dominant discourses, conquering power inequalities and societal hierarchies through humour and mockery. Deveau (2012) submits the carnival is a form of political weapon that seeks to undermine hierarchy and authority bringing together people in a "common discursive" body, this manifesting in the form of social media platforms. Thus, Hess, for example, argue that social media provides a platform for "parody and pastiche [which] are vital forms of speaking out and resistance" (2009, 429). In the same vein, Burgess and Green (2009, 103) state that social media platforms are characterised by a "sense of playfulness and affect". Papacharissi further states that social media "provide irreverence, humour, unpredictability necessary for rejuvenating political conversation trapped in conventional formulas" (2010, 151). She further advances this view stating that social media platforms elicit "sarcasm, humour or satire which are equally important forms of political thought and expression" (Papacharissi, 2010, 151). Drawing on social media platforms Twitter, Facebook and WhatsApp where these humorous conversations are circulated, we consider how audiences appropriated social media platforms to communicate indigenous ways of boosting the immune system and treating COVID-19. In the next section, we outline the methodological premise underpinning this study.

Methodology

This qualitative study uses data drawn from three social media sites—Twitter, Facebook and WhatsApp. The choice for selecting these sites is based on our observation of many of memes on these platforms. Selected social media memes were in various forms which include images, videos, words and phrases. For this study we focus on images and words because they were dominant. From the selected social media platforms, researchers monitored memes from December to February and used thematic analysis to derive thematic issues that arose from the memes. Thematic analysis is a process of identifying and analysing various themes within a given data set. Braun and Clarke (2006) note that themes are captured aspects about data in relation to the research questions and objectives and represent a certain level of patterned response or meaning within the data set. There are two types of thematic levels explained by Braun and Clarke (2006) and fall under semantic and latent themes. Semantic themes "exist within the explicit or surface meanings of the data and the analyst is not looking for anything beyond what a participant has said or what has been written" (Braun & Clarke, 2006, 84). The latent level focuses on the deeper meanings of the data and "examines the underlying ideas, assumptions, and conceptualizations – and ideologies – that are theorized as shaping or informing the semantic content of the data" (Braun & Clarke, 2006, 84).

The research adopts the latter. As such, key themes identified for the study showed how humour became a means to prescribe alternative treatment for the COVID-19 vaccine prescribed by the World Health Organization, the commercialisation of traditional medicines and how social media platforms were used for social commentary during the COVID-19 indigenous treatment. Resultantly, 17 memes were analysed as they directly spoke to COVID-19-related memes and indigenous treatment that circulated on social media platforms. These memes were circulated between March 2020 (when COVID-19 was declared a pandemic) and January 2021. For further analysis, semiotic analysis was used for image-based memes. Major issues accessed how meaning is layered: and the two layers are denotation and connotation. The former looks at the descriptive features of an image, while the latter responds to issues such as ideas and values that are expressed through what is represented and the ways in which issues are reported (Van Leeuwen, 2005).

Data Presentation and Analysis

COVID-19, Traditional Herbal Medicines and Epistemic Struggles

In his decolonial reading of COVID-19, Ndlovu-Gatsheni (2020, 368) regards this pandemic as multifaceted, with "ecological, existential, and epistemic dimensions". Although Africa has a "long history and experience of grappling with epidemics and pandemics", Ndlovu-Gatsheni (2020, 370) bemoans that there is a reluctance to "tap into this history, experience, and knowledge about responding to the COVID-19 pandemic". Ndlovu-Gatsheni (2020, 370) further posits that COVID-19 provides an opportunity for:

> Africa in particular and the Global South in general not to look up to the Global North for salvation but to shift the geopolitics of knowledge by using African endogenous knowledge and the epistemologies of the Global South.

Rather than "copy and paste" responses from the Global North, there is need for Africans to draw on their rich history, experiences and knowledge systems (Ndlovu-Gatsheni, 2020, 372). A herbal remedy called "COVID Organics" was developed in Madagascar as an endogenous mitigation strategy (Ndlovu-Gatsheni, 2020, 373). WHO responded by warning the public against using unproven medication. Whilst the point of caution is "well taken", the challenge, as noted by Ndlovu-Gatsheni (2020, 373), is that the "geopolitics of power and knowledge are still titled toward the Global North as the only site of credible science and only space to look to as the world waits for the vaccine". The initiative taken in the Global North on the development of a vaccine are "not subjected to the same dismissal as those being carried out by the African scientists" (Ndlovu-Gatsheni, 2020, 273).

There are social media memes that constitute rallying calls for the use of indigenous knowledge systems as mitigation strategies and alternative remedies against COVID-19. Steam inhalation, or steam therapy, is popularised in these memes that are reproduced and circulated in cyberspace. In countries such as Zimbabwe, steam therapy is one of the common home remedies for flu. As such, one of the memes is a visual depiction of three toddlers undergoing a steam therapy. A message, written in Zimbabwe's chiShona language, accompanies this image and reads: *Pamberi neku natira!!! Vanoseka hameno henyu #staysafe* (translated: Forward with steaming!!! It does not matter even if they laugh at you). This meme depicts partially naked toddlers in a humorous manner as they endure steam inhalation. Through this use of humour, this meme seeks to promote African traditional medicine and endogenous knowledge by reifying *kunatira* (steam inhalation). Although *kunatira* does not cure or prevent COVID-19, this meme constructs and celebrates steaming as an alternative episteme. Ndlovu-Gatsheni (2020, 366) examines the geopolitics of power and knowledge and develops an argument that seeks solutions to COVID-19 "based on the African knowledge and epistemologies from the Global South". We consider how, from a carnivalesque point of view, memes from Zimbabwe and the Global South then became an oppositional culture and counter-model of production. This oppositional culture, as evidenced by the memes, undermines official and legitimate discourses (Bakhtin, 1984).

In addition, there are memes that celebrate local knowledge. For example, in Fig. 5.1, a visual text projects lemons, garlic and ginger as preventive measures against COVID-19 in a humorous manner. Although these do not prevent or cure COVID-19, there is an additional message that reads: "Dear COVID 19, you are in a wrong country". Given the crumbling healthcare system in countries such as Zimbabwe, some members of the public have resorted to traditional medicine. Other memes celebrate

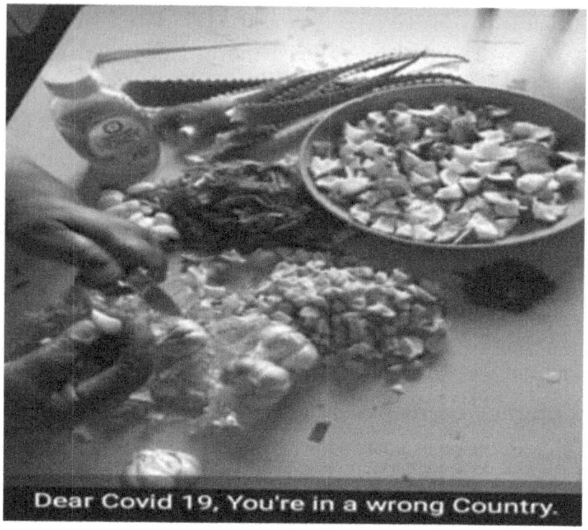

Fig. 5.1 Illustration of ginger, garlic, honey and aloe vera that are seen as immune boasters to counteract against COVID-19

herbal medicine as a remedy for COVID-19. One meme depicts a man wearing a mask and having a face covered with *umsuzwane/zumbani*. The message attached to the image is a declaration against COVID-19: "Corona for what! No chance here". In this regard, traditional herbal medicines are celebrated as a remedy for the pandemic. Through humour, an image of traditional herbal medicine serves to invoke and reclaim subjugated local knowledge. The dominant Western science that is associated with pharmaceutical drugs and vaccines is being challenged and resisted by endogenous knowledge systems. However, this reclaiming of indigenous knowledge systems by virtue of the memes shows how humour suspends already known rules or knowledge, and any form of hierarchies that attempt to filter alternative viewpoints (Thompson 2009). Thus, a "second life" is imagined as a "world" where everyone is imagined to be "equal" recapturing the public sphere and "reopening the discussion of 'serious' affairs…that signals that anyone can participate in it" (Thompson, 2009, 223).

In celebrating traditional herbs, some memes project vaccines as poisonous. There are various anti-vaccine assumptions and myths that focus on the toxic nature of immunisation. COVID-19 vaccines are denounced as having adverse effects on the physical and mental wellbeing of the users. There are claims that COVID-19 vaccines will supposedly alter DNA (Goodman & Carmichael, 2020). Others add that tracking microchips will supposedly be implanted in individuals who receive the coronavirus vaccines (Goodman & Carmichael, 2020). In Fig. 5.2, a meme with a message: "Dear black people. Your Minister will not tell you to steam with *umhlonyane*, *umsuzwane* and gum tree coz it will collapse his poison project. Wake up guys". An image of eucalyptus leaves serves to reinforce this notion that traditional medicines are safer and effective as compared to what is deemed as "poisonous" vaccines. In addition, another meme explicitly represents a particular herb as a cure for COVID-19. The message reads: "umuthi wokuvikela I Corona uyahlikihlela emhlane" (a medicine to protect you from COVID-19. Rub it on your back"). As such, there is an assumption that traditional herbal medicine is a treatment of COVID-19 (Fig. 5.3).

Another meme depicts a man in a bushy area seemingly full of umsuzwane. The avowal: "We still have umsuzwane, *insangu*,[1] gumtree and other. You won't finish us. And we will never stop using those" constitutes a resistance against the taking of COVID-19 vaccines. Evidently, steam inhalation and traditional herbal medicines are celebrated as an African endogenous knowledge that challenges the hegemony of Western science. Thus, in the context of Zimbabwe, one would note the way social media

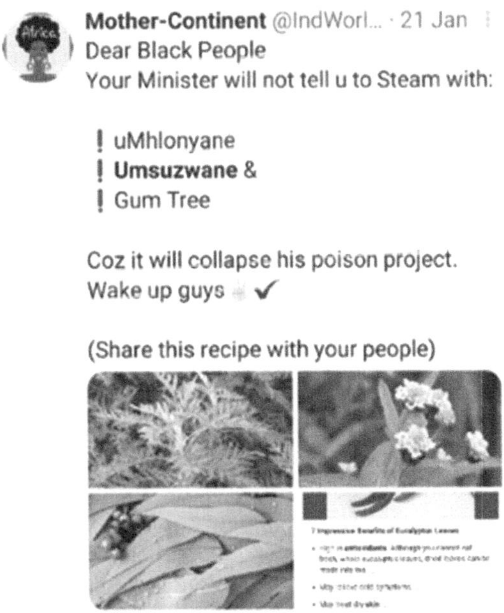

Fig. 5.2 Traditional herbs such as umsuzwane that are regarded as preventative measures against COVID-19

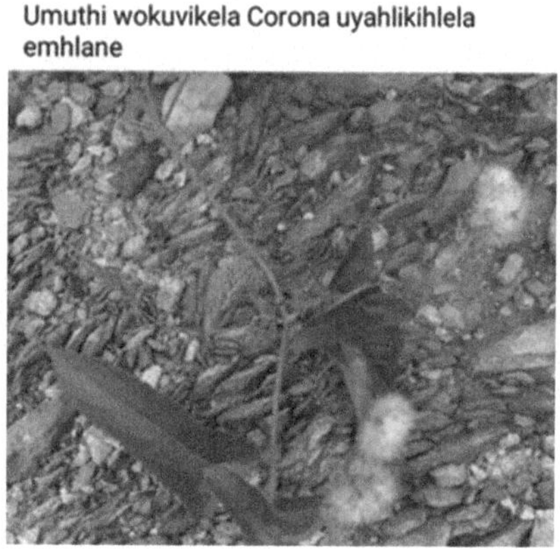

Fig. 5.3 A shrub that is seen as a cure for COVID-19

platforms are characterised by a "carnivalesque mode of expression" (Karekwaivanane, 2018, 56) that then go on to challenge institutionalised knowledge on topics with health-related issues. In the next theme, we discuss how memes were used to comment on indigenous knowledge systems on COVID-19.

COVID-19 Vaccines and the Social Commentary

Humour comes in various formats and these include irony, satire, parody and also sarcasm. Given that memes are easily created and manipulated by audiences "they provide an ideal social media tool for responding to current events through humour" (Ross & Rivers, 2018, 289). Debates that centred on COVID-19 addressed the need to use indigenous knowledge systems, although they were laced with social and everyday life commentary offering comic relief. These everyday issues mostly touched on how old people and the political elite should could use indigenous systems as an alternative to the cure for COVID-19. Thus, humour serves as a key for the understanding of social and cultural issues (see Shifman, 2014, 187). It is, however, through various memes that one is able to understand how memes reflected on indigenous medicines and how audiences commented on them. In Fig. 5.5, the meme reads *kana wakambopfeka maZico, gara mumba, idya mafruits akawandisa, natira 4 times a day and usatendere vayenzi pamba pako* which when translated means (if you once had Zico sandals, you should steam 4 times a day and don't allow visitors at your house). Zico are sandals that were once popular in the early 1990s. As such, the background of the meme suggests that people who wore the sandals are now old and likely to be infected by the virus as statistics have shown the majority of people who succumbed to COVID-19 are old people. The meme captures discourse on the pandemic as humour is used to comment and advise elderly people, likely to have ailments to use indigenous medicines as an alternative immune booster or treatment for COVID-19. Therefore, memes play an important role in communicating health information as humour, a component of Internet memes, "is easier to relate to for most people" (Ross & Rivers, 2018, 288).

In Fig. 5.4, the meme comments on the pandemic by highlighting a collage of five different images—Mazoe orange crush, Farino juice, Chibuku opaque beer, green boxers commonly used for playing soccer

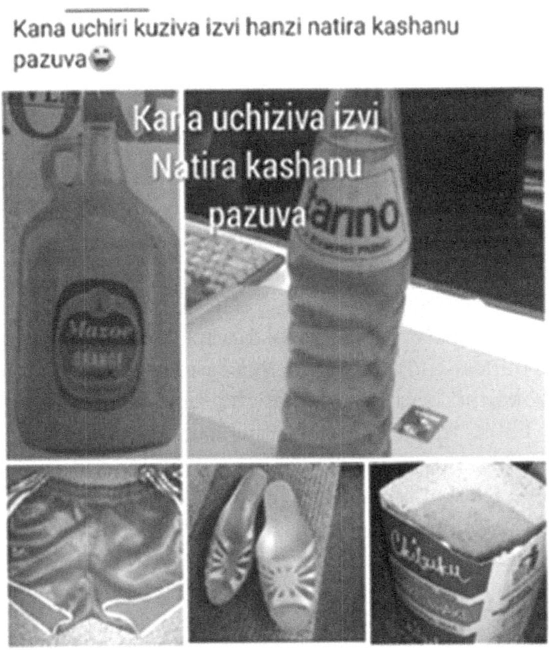
Kana uchiri kuziva izvi hanzi natira kashanu pazuva
Kana uchiziva izvi
Natira kashanu
pazuva
farino
Chibuku

Fig. 5.4 is a collection of items that are supposedly known only by the elderly. Such people are being encouraged to steam as they are deemed more vulnerable to COVID-19

and a pair of sandals for women. These were common in Zimbabwe's early years of independence in 1980. The message inscribed, in Zimbabwe's chiShona language, juxtaposed with the images reads; ***kana uchiri kuziva izvi natira kashanu pazuva*** (if you still know these steam five times a day).

Therefore, the meme suggests that people of the old age should take measures that will protect them from the COVID-19 virus—preferably using indigenous ways of treating a flu such as steaming. In this case, the meme serves as a way of reflecting the views of audiences on how to combat the COVID-19 virus. Furthermore, social media platforms play an important role in sharing information in the wake of applications that give audiences the power of autonomy to create messages that reflect how society understands issues related to treatment of COVID-19. They, however, reflect audiences' opinions on important or topical issues, in this case COVID-19 treatment.

However, another meme reads; ***umuntu wesifazane imbali, kodwa mayenesishwapha*** umsuzwane (beautiful woman deserves roses but unattractive ones should get umsuzwane). The message is accompanied by a rose which supposedly should be given to a beautiful lady and umsuzwane for less attractive women. The meme is derogatory in two ways; first, it constitutes body shaming as certain women are being devalued. Second, it constructs umsuzwane as less appealing than roses. As such, this meme undermines indigenous knowledge systems. The meme circulates at a time when people have discovered that umsuzwane has long been used to cure flu-like diseases and can play a part in reducing the risk of being infected by the COVID-19 virus. Such memes relate with what Burgess and Green (2009, 103) view on social media platforms that are characterised by a "sense of playfulness and affect". In this case, memes give people avenue where they poke fun at each other at the same time discussing issues of importance. Thus, this brings out the carnivalesque atmosphere that enables a "'free'discussion…second life, a second world… a 'world inside out'" (Bakhtin, 1984, 11). In this "second life", the "world" is imagined where everyone is subjected to being "equal" despite their societal ranking.

Social commentary also extends to sexual-related issues where memes are used to show infidelity that people in society are involved in. Another meme captures a conversation between a man and his wife. The message, written in Shona language, reads: wife: *ukuitei, its now 9 send pic repauri* when translated means: "what are you doing, it's now 9 send a picture of where you are", hubby: *ndichangopedza kunatira* (I have just finished steaming). The message is inscribed with a male individual sweating purporting to have finished steaming. The underlying message is that the husband is having sex with someone, hence the sweat (steam) in the picture. The image captured in the meme attracts people's attention, and this shows the "secondary layer of language" imbedded in the meme which constitute shared spheres of cultural knowledge allowing individuals to convey ideas through the creation of images, symbols or short phrases (Shifman, 2014). Furthermore, through social commentary, one is able to understand that steaming (*ukufutha/natira*) is one of the ways that society adopts to treat the virus. Memes, however, reveal the dominant discourses or issues circulating in society to raise more awareness of the pandemic that has changed people's way of life. Thus, memes just like other forms of communication are effective in communicating health-related discourses because of their power in influencing the general public as well as opinion leaders on issues of public health (Evans & Ulasevich, 2005). Resultantly, memes have played a crucial role in educating, informing people on health and medical conditions.

Memes as a Critique of the Commercialisation of Indigenous Medicines

Traditional medicines have always been used to address common illnesses in the Global South. It is a common heritage that most African countries share and have been used to since time immemorial. However, their value is not recognised as practitioners are not placed at the centre of policy formulation and implementation. Traditional medicines thus speak to the practice of cultures. In this section, we consider how a vast number of memes that circulated on social media platforms showed how traditional medicines such as *umsuzwane/zumbani* were promoted and commercialised on social media as an alternative treatment for COVID-19. We identified four memes that critiqued the commercialisation of traditional medicines in Zimbabwe. One of the memes that circulated pokes fun at individuals with medical aid subscriptions (see Fig. 5.5). The meme, accompanied by laughing emojis, reads: *Nghlekiswa ukuth nalabo abanama medical aid sikha nabo* umsuzwane which means: "I find it funny that those on medical aid are the very same people who are going to use Zumbani as well". However, there are many possible meanings to this meme. Its playfulness could be a way of rejecting medical aid subscriptions—especially in a dire economic and a healthcare system that has been described as a "silent genocide".[2] Subscribing to a medical aid is

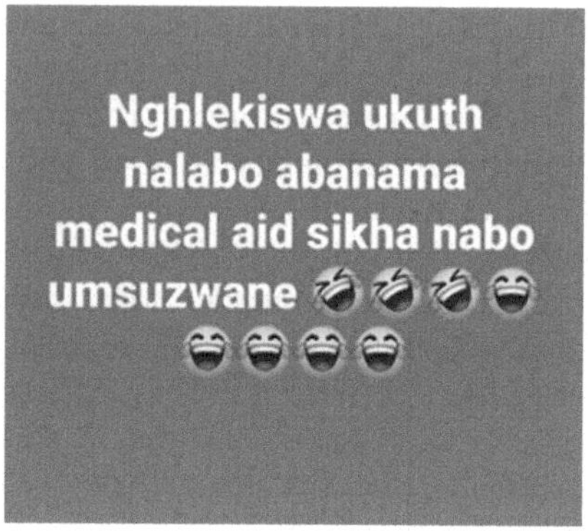

Fig. 5.5 People on medical aid who are using Zumbani

somewhat costly, considering how hospitals in Zimbabwe are facing drug shortages or have poor medical facilities. Instead of using medical aid, the meme is promoting and urging people to use traditional medicines that are readily available as indigenous shrubs. In part, the meme could also be "laughing" at elitists who can afford medical aid subscriptions especially during a pandemic. It somehow shows how the powerful and untouchable in society who can afford medical aid payments in developed countries also resort to using traditional medicines in the face of an irresolvable global pandemic. In relation to the Zimbabwean case, memes empower citizens to contribute and critique the elite on important issues that they are often excluded from. Social media platforms are characterised by laughter that then becomes an arena for free expression and engagement. The elite and those with institutional, economic power are mocked and reduced to ordinary people, stripped of institutional or political control they possess in the non-carnivalesque life.

Another meme (Fig. 5.6) pokes fun at how commercial supermarkets are now selling umsuzwane in Zimbabwe. The meme shows *umsuzwane/zumbani* placed at a vegetable section with price tag. The meme questions how a common plant is now sold in shops and being commercialised as an alternative to treat and boost immune systems. Similarly, another one (Fig. 5.7) shows an individual pushing a trolley full of umsuzwane selling the plant for 10 South African rands. Another meme (Fig. 5.8), with the Nigerian actor Osita Iheme also questions the boom of umsuzwane sales in Zimbabwe. The meme written in isiNdebele language reads: *Kanti* umsuzwane *is now commercialised wona ugcwele egangeni?..sokusele ukuthi sithengise iaki kuphela komgodoyi* which means: "Zumbani is now

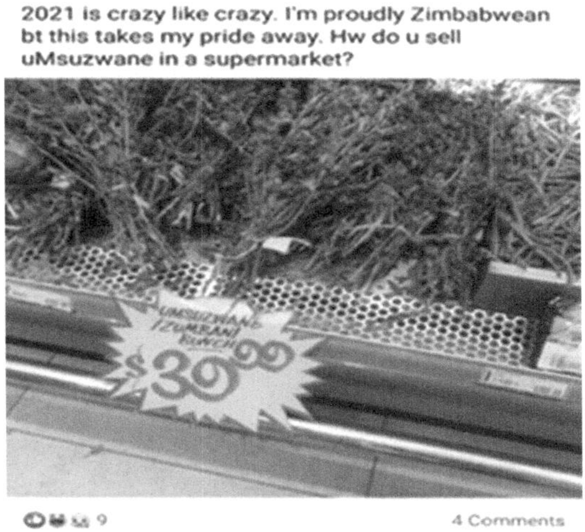

Fig. 5.6 A critique of the commercialisation of plants such as Zumbani

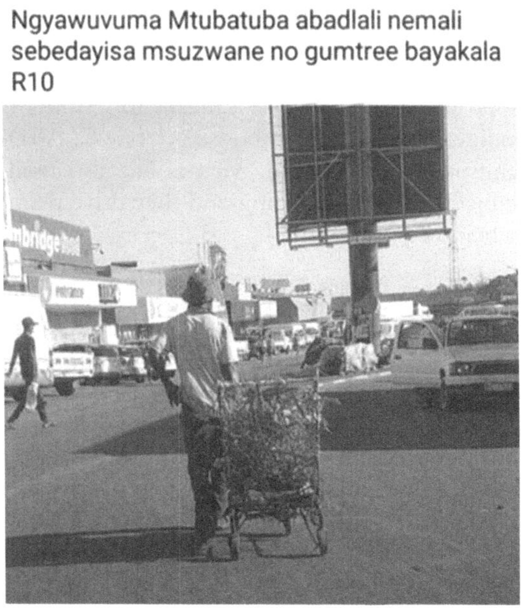

Fig. 5.7 A man pushing a trolley with umsuzwane which is being sold for 10 South African rands

Fig. 5.8 The boom of umsuzwane sales in Zimbabwe

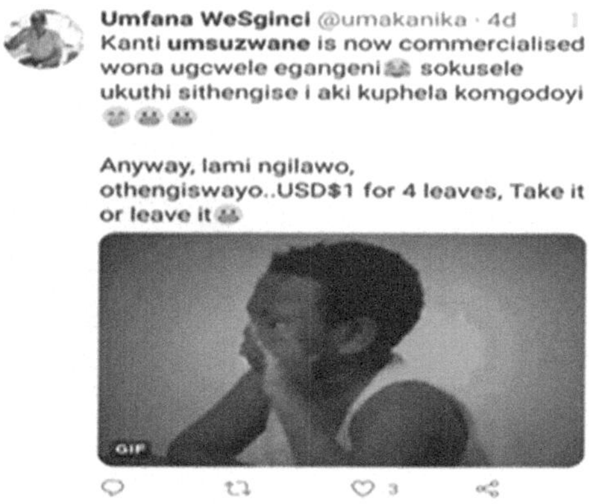
Umfana WeSginci @umakanika · 4d
Kanti umsuzwane is now commercialised wona ugcwele egangeni sokusele ukuthi sithengise i aki kuphela komgodoyi
Anyway, lami ngilawo, othengiswayo..USD$1 for 4 leaves, Take it or leave it
GIF

commercialised yet it's a common plant in the bush? The only thing left is for us to sell our buttocks". In part, the meme reflects how people now make a living in society by selling the indigenous herb. Overall perspective, as shown by these memes, humour is used by audiences to communicate and educate people about alternative immune boosters and COVID-19 treatments such as Umsuzwane/Zumbani. Social media users appropriated humour as a means for critiquing the commercialisation of indigenous immune boosters or COVID-19 treatments such as Umsuzwane/Zumbani. Memes are also used to communicate about a subject that is frightening and they drive people to pay attention to what is being communicated.

Conclusion

This study concludes by arguing that humour plays an integral part in health communication. The findings demonstrated that memes are used to promote the use of indigenous knowledge to help fight the virus. Such knowledge comes on the backdrop of scepticism on the use of WHO-approved vaccines. Citizens are appropriating and utilising the Internet as a means of voicing their opinions on prevention and treatment of COVID-19. These memes constitute counter-hegemonic forms and practices as they challenge the dominant Western scientific knowledge systems.

Notes

1. Insangu or Insango is Cannabis, also known as marijuana, among other names, and is a psychoactive drug from the Cannabis plant used primarily for medical or recreational purposes.
2. https://www.dailymaverick.co.za/article/2019-10-22-zimbabwean-healthcare-system-a-silent-genocide/

References

Bakhtin, M.M. (1984). *Rabelais and his world* (H. Iswolsky, Trans.). Indiana University Press.

BBC. (2021, February 6). Coronavirus in Tanzania: The country that's rejecting the vaccine. *BBC*. https://www.bbc.com/news/world-africa-55900680. Last accessed 19 Feb 2021.

Braun, V., & Clarke, V. (2006). Using thematic analysis in psychology. *Qualitative Research in Psychology, 3*(2), 77–101.

Burgess, J. E., & Green, J. B. (2009). *Video and participatory culture*. Polity Press.

CITE. (2021). Herbalists cashing in on coronavirus panic. *CITE*. https://cite.org.zw/herbalists-cashing-in-on-coronavirus-panic/. Last accessed 10 Feb 2021.

Critchley, S. (2002). *On humour*. Routledge.

Deveau, D. J. (2012). The Aristocrats! Comedy, grotesqueries and political inversions of the masculine code. *Humor, 25*(4), 401–415.

Eko, L. (2015). The art of satirical deterritorialization: Shifting cartoons from real space to cyberspace in Sub-Saharan Africa. *International Communication Gazette, 77*(3), 248–266.

Evans, W. D., & Ulasevich, A. (2005). News media tracking of tobacco control: A review of sampling methodologies. *Journal of Health Communication, 10*(5), 403–417.

EWN. (2021, January). World facing 'catastrophic' moral failure on vaccines: WHO chief. *Eye Witness News*. https://ewn.co.za/2021/01/18/world-facing-catastrophic-moral-failure-on-vaccines-who-chief?fbclid=IwAR0ljj9BJfsRPR18q-wjOBiqOqFzkds6WuDy6UsIISLXdxls2Miuy7Cfi8A. Last accessed 10 Feb 2021.

Goodman, J., & Carmichael, F. (2020). Coronavirus: Bill Gates 'microchip' conspiracy theory and other vaccine claims fact-checked. *BBC*. Available at https://www.bbc.com/news/52847648

Goriunova, O. (2012). New media idiocy. Convergence. *The International Journal of Research into New Media Technologies, 19*(2), 223–235.

Gray, J., Jones, J. P., & Thompson, E. (2009). The state of satire, the satire of state. In J. Gray, J. P. Jones, & E. Thompson (Eds.), *Satire TV: Politics and comedy in the post network era* (pp. 3–36). New York University Press.

Hendricks, H., & Jansen, L. (2017). Frightfully funny: Combining threat and humour in health messages for men and women. *Psychology and Health, 33*(5), 594–613.

Hess, A. (2009). Resistance up in smoke: Analyzing the limitations of deliberation on YouTube. *Critical Studies in Media Communication, 26*(5), 411–434.

Highet, G. (1962). *The anatomy of satire.* Prince Town University Press.

Karekwaivanane, G. H. (2018). 'Tapanduka Zvamuchese': Facebook, 'unruly publics', and Zimbabwean politics. *Journal of East African Studies, 13*(1), 54–71.

Lee, J. Y., Slater, M. D., & Tchernev, J. (2015). Self-deprecating humour versus other-deprecating humour in health messages. *Journal of Health Communication, 20*(10), 1–11.

Mbembe, A. (2001). *On the postcolony.* University of California Press.

McClennen, S. A., & Maisel, R. M. (2014). *Is satire saving our nation? Mockery and American politics.* Palgrave Macmillan.

McSweeney, E., & Chingono, N. (2021, February 5). Western countries have 'hoarded' Covid vaccines. Africa is being left behind as cases surge. *CNN.* https://edition.cnn.com/2021/02/05/africa/vaccine-race-africa-intl/index.html. Last accessed 10 Feb 2021.

Mina, A. X. (2014). Batman, pandaman and the blind man: A case study in social change memes and Internet censorship in China. *Journal of Visual Culture, 13*(3), 359–375.

Mpofu, S. (2019). Pornographic intersections: Race and genitalia in South African political art in the age of digital media. *Critical African Studies, 11*(2), 230–261.

Ndlovu-Gatsheni, S. (2020). Geopolitics of power and knowledge in the COVID-19 pandemic: Decolonial reflections on a global. *Journal of Developing Societies, 36*(4), 366–389.

Neale, S., & Krutnick, F. (2006). *Popular film and television comedy.* Routledge.

Ngoshi, H. (2013). Carnivalising postcolonial Zimbabwe: The vulgar and grotesque logic of postcolonial protest in NoViolet Bulawayo's we need new names. *Journal of Literary Studies, 32*(1), 53–69.

Nyamnjoh, F. B. (2009). *Press cartoons and politics: The case of cameroon.* In J. A. Lent (Ed.), *Cartooning in Africa.* Hampton Press.

Papacharissi, Z. (2010). *A private sphere: Democracy in a digital age.* Polity Press.

Pearce, K., & Hajizada, A. (2014). No laughing matter: Humour as a means of dissent in the digital era: The case of authoritarian Azerbaijan. *Demokratizatsiya, 22*(1), 67–85.

Rayner, L. (2010). *Bakhtinian thought and the picturing of a vulgar African identity* (pp. 1–14). In Research report submitted to the Department of Fine Arts, University of Witwatersrand.

Ross, A. S., & Rivers, D. J. (2018). Internet memes as polyvocal political participation: Discourse, disruption, and digital democracy in the 2016 presidential election. In D. Schill & J. H. Allen (Eds.), *The presidency and social media discourse, disruption, and digital democracy in the 2016 presidential election* (pp. 285–308). Routledge.

Shifman, L. (2014). *Memes in digital culture*. MIT Press.

Siziba, G., & Ncube, G. (2015). Mugabe's fall from grace: Satire and fictional narratives as silent forms of resistance in/on Zimbabwe. *Social Dynamics: A Journal of African Studies, 41*(3), 516–539.

Stam, R. (1989). *Subversive pleasures: Bakhtin, cultural criticism and film*. John Hopkins University Press.

Stevens, A. (2009). Carnival and comedy: On Bakthin's misreading of Boccaccio. *Opticon, 1826*(3), 1–5.

Tavory, I. (2014). The situations of culture: Humour and the limits of measurability. *Theory and Society, 43*(3), 275–289.

Teti, M., Schatz, E., & Liebenberg, L. (2020). Methods in the time of COVID-19: The vital role of qualitative inquiries. *International Journal of Qualitative Methods, 19*, 1–5.

Thompson, E. (2009). Good demo, bad taste: South Park as carnivalesque satire. In J. Gray, J. P. Jones, & E. P. Thompson (Eds.), *Satire TV: Politics and comedy in the post network era*. New York Press.

Van Leeuwen, T. (2005). *Introducing social semiotics*. Routledge.

Wasserman, H. (2020, March 15). Laughter in the time of a pandemic: Why South Africans are joking about Corona virus. *The Conversation*. https://theconversation.com/laughter-in-the-time-of-a-pandemic-why-south-africans-are-joking-about-coronavirus-133528. Accessed 20 Jan 2021.

WHO. (2021). Accelerating a safe and effective Covid-19 vaccine. Available at: https://www.who.int/emergencies/diseases/novel-coronavirus-2019/global-research-on-novel-coronavirus-2019-ncov/accelerating-a-safe-and-effective-covid-19-vaccine. Accessed 27 Sept 2021.

Willems, W. (2011). Comic strips and 'the crisis': Postcolonial laughter and coping with everyday life in Zimbabwe. *Popular Communication, 9*(2), 126–145.

CHAPTER 6

"Can we Uninstall 2020 and Install It Again? This Version Has a Virus!": Humourous Pundemic and Misinforming Infodemic about COVID-19 Pandemic on Social Media

Adamkolo Mohammed Ibrahim, Nassir Mohammed Abba-Aji, and Phuong Thi Vi

Introduction

Exponential development in the internet and social media have tremendously influenced online memes. A meme is a way of expressing one person's ideas, thoughts or behaviour to others. Whether in the form of

A. M. Ibrahim (✉) • N. M. Abba-Aji
Department of Mass Communication, University of Maiduguri, Maiduguri, Nigeria
e-mail: adamkolo@unimaid.edu.ng; click2nass@unimaid.edu.ng

P. T. Vi
Faculty of Journalism, Communications, and Literature, TNUS - Thai Nguyen University of Science, Thai Nguyen, Vietnam
e-mail: phuong_vt@tnus.edu.vn

S. Mpofu (ed.), *Digital Humour in the Covid-19 Pandemic*,
https://doi.org/10.1007/978-3-030-79279-4_6

images, hyperlinks, videos, websites or hashtags, memes are shared on the internet. Online memes are popular because they can be accessed by users as jokes, satires and expression of feelings. The development of memes on social media is influenced by universal language (Juditha, 2015). To reinforce some social media arguments, mass media often become references and "weapons". Social media memes are backgrounded by individual or group business and people's "understanding of meme definition based on the subject of the meme, patterns or components, forms of discourse, and language" (Fadly, 2020, 2; Hartini, 2017, 23; Msughter, 2020).

Virtual society has massively consumed the presence of this visual phenomenon. Besides the case of COVID-19 is being discussed on social media. In social media, many visualisations of images or memes associated with COVID-19 are increasing. In general, COVID-19 memes contain images or sentences informing society of quotations and satires. To prevent the spread of the COVID-19 virus, these memes are aimed at educating society. As everyone knows, they are trying to stop the spread of the COVID-19 virus all over the world, including Indonesia. The creators, with all their creativity, try to create funny memes as a preventive step. Hopefully, the community will understand the WFH (Work and Worship from Home) policy and the government's go-home ban (Msughter, 2020).

To be understood by society, the creators combine creativities, arts, messages and humour intentionally. But, sometimes, the phrases do not follow the standards. They use sarcastic language freely; they satirise a certain group, without thinking about the effect. Most memes about COVID-19 satirise societies that disobey the rules of the government. It is not possible to change the cultures of society, such as going home, disobeying physical distance, gathering at restaurants and inviting many people to the party, immediately. The existence of COVID-19 memes could draw the attention of social media users with satires to these problems. In many social media, especially Facebook, Instagram and web blogs, it can be shown from the numerous uses of COVID-19 memes that everyone can read them, especially millennials. We should know, however, that the COVID-19 memes tent with hyperbolic language to concentrate on parodist aspects, so it needs to understand deep thinking. The languages used in memes also vary from traditional languages to Indonesian. The chosen construction of language has symbolic power. Intentionally, the creators wrapped it in such a way that it can be criticised, not taken for granted (Msughter, 2020). A meme is a cultural transmission that constructs certain cultural patterns in the form of thought, idea, inspiration, habit, song or fashion (Dawkins, 2006, 215 in Isnaniah & Augustina, 2020; Msughter, 2020).

Within several disciplines, such as communication, linguistics, psychology, sociology, philosophy and even medicine, the past few decades have seen intensive development in humour research. Therefore, using a review of relevant literature, this chapter explores how social media users use humour about the COVID-19 pandemic and its related issues, say one thing and mean another, and the pivotal role that context plays in explaining the intended meaning. Several coronavirus-motivated humour, jokes, memes (otherwise called "pundemic") and fake news, misinformation and hoaxes (otherwise known as "infodemic" (Richtel, 2020)) on social media are pragmatically discussed in this chapter. Using Mey's theory of pragmatic acts as its theoretical framework, the chapter highlights the strategies and practises used in the projection of reality by the memes and humour in a period of, as Ogungbe and Omolobi (2020) and Pauliks (2020) describe it, "sociological consensus among individuals".

Communication in a Humour

Communication is a tool for a targeted audience to convey specific intentions. In conversations, such intentions can range from idle conversations to injecting humour, to serious issues such as the coronavirus pandemic, reports on certain issues, as well as to share compassion as shown in obituaries. According to Ross (1998), humour is influential and has a high profile in our society; Ross further defines humour as "something that makes a person laugh or smile" (p. 3). While humour is "a universal phenomenon", Andrew (2012) argues that "it is also culturally dependent on a particular time and place for its specific content". Humour is also seen as "a way for both the young and the old to exercise some control over our anxieties about ageing and death" (Andrew, 2012, 11, 14; Williams, 2020).

The literature shows that humour can be used through satirisation, depending on the context (especially academic). It can be viewed as a comedy on television, constructed in play or before a live audience (e.g. sitcom). Humour can be evoked in family, interpersonal or group interactions through jokes and sometimes puns, and so on. It can be inferred in all the identified environments that humour is potentially an effective instrument for maintaining any person or society's peace, stability and general well-being. Therefore, humour can be seen as a means of social interaction (Chapman, 1983). Andrew identified the fundamental functions of humour by stating that "humour uses situations, characters, speech, writing or images to create fun in the form of entertainment. He added that it entertains the audience by making them "less pretentious, make them politically and medically conscious, reduce stress hormone levels, provide physical exercise, promote solidarity and serves as a coping strategy from a pandemic" (p. 13). Therefore, over the years, humour has attracted scholarly attention as an established means of releasing stress and tension and has been identified as an effective means of interaction. It is an effective way to arouse and stimulate the interest of learners in teaching and learning (Aboudan, 2009 cited in Akinola, 2018). "Humour is capable of creating an atmosphere of relief from anxiety (Williams, 2020), anger and pain; its profile in society is high", according to Ross (1998, p. 2). In human society, humour plays many roles. Katayama (2009) argues that "humour brings people together through shared laughter" (p. 25). This indicates that humour is a collective phenomenon as opposed to being an individualised phenomenon. This implies that it functions as a means to unite individuals.

Humour also has some sociological roles besides this (Campisano, 2016). Friedman and Kuipers (2013) argue that there is no complete sociological consensus on the role of humour in sociology. Be that as it may, humour performs the role of promoting social inclusion and exclusion (p. 181). As Alatalo and Poutiainen (2016) noted, humour also decreases and strengthens differences in status and enhances the sense of connectedness. The problem of the coronavirus pandemic ravaging the world could aptly be seen in these aforementioned functions. Despite the severity of the pandemic, to douse the tension, people still tend to make humour flavour out of it, and maybe make people laugh consciously or unconsciously. Furthermore, humour is caused by specific mechanisms that can be grouped into three main categories: cognitive theory, the theory of superiority and the theory of relief (Roux 2008, 89 cited in Ogungbe & Omolobi, 2020). Campisano (2016) also defines cognitive theories of humour, superiority and relief, similar to Roux's assertion. The difference is that Campisano calls them the main sociological theories of humour, while Roux refers to them as mechanisms that trigger humour. The subject has been conceived as a complex multi-faceted phenomenon (Marin-Arrese, 2005). Therefore, it is important to take from communications and language and the function they perform in humour motivated by the coronavirus situation. This is because communication and language are an avenue for individuals, in a particular context, to perform several acts aimed at having intended perlocutionary effects on the audience, readers or listeners (Ogungbe & Omolobi, 2020).

Pragmatics is a communication linguistic branch that focuses on how words are used to perform different acts, how meaning is negotiated between speaker and listener, and how the context plays a pivotal role in interpreting an utterance, as well as explaining aspects of meaning that cannot be found in the plain sense of words or structures. According to Mey (2001, 6), "Pragmatics studies the use of language in human communication as determined by the conditions of society". It is generally concerned with the way people convey meaning through the communication medium of language in any given social context. This meaning includes both verbal and non-verbal meanings, and depending on the context, the interlocutor relationship and many other social factors, it varies. This means that what someone communicates may differ from what will be interpreted by the other party. Therefore, before significance is adequately conveyed pragmatically, both the speaker (and writer) and the listener (or reader) must have a meeting point. Hence, before humour can be successfully created, some components of pragmatics must be present. This explains why it has been claimed that a speaker can only say a joke when he or she knows that the addressees are conscious of the underlying assumptions that are required for the joke's interpretation. These background assumptions include the "belief that the addressees are not going to take the joke at face value, and the belief that the interaction situation allows them to tell a joke" (Filani, 2016, 8; Ogungbe & Omolobi, 2020).

The Bases of Memes

Usually, we think of funny images and videos on the internet, not evolutionary biology, if we hear the term "meme". But this is where the term originated, precisely. In 1976, decades before the World Wide Web, the well-known atheist and evolutionary biologist Richard Dawkins introduced the term "meme" in his book *The Selfish Gene*. What Dawkins means by a meme is a cultural unit which is transmitted via imitation from person to person. The evolutionary biologist uses "meme" by analogy with genes to describe a new, cultural replicator driving human evolution. Ideas, ideologies, religions, sayings, melodies, clothing styles and so on, which evolve in the course of cultural history, are examples of such memes (Dawkins 2006 in Pauliks, 2020). The title of one of his often-quoted essays, Dawkins (2006), conceives memes as "viruses of the mind". On one hand, what he means by this is that memes take on their own lives, and on the other, memes are as infectious as real viruses. Thus, Dawkins (2006, 192) understands memes as "living structures, not only metaphorically, but technically". In his view, to survive in the meme pool, memes replicate spontaneously. Humans act solely as vehicles for memes to be transported and spread. There is a competition between various memes in the logic of evolutionary theory (e.g. between scientific theories, political ideologies or religious dogmas). The meme that will survive, that is, human needs and social circumstances, is the one that is best adapted to its environment. The more infectious memes are, the greater their chances of survival are, and the better they can stay in the human brain and be transmitted to other individuals (Ogungbe & Omolobi, 2020; Pauliks, 2020).

Online Memes

Is it the same thing with memes and internet memes? The original concept of the meme provides a very good description of what can be found on the internet today, as far as Dawkins is concerned. Not that far away from the original is the meaning, "It is anything that goes viral" (Dawkins 2006 cited in Solon, 2013). Memes, as he sees it, are viral content that spreads on the internet by its own accord. This is not an unproblematic view. Virality gives a false impression of how content circulates on the internet, according to Jenkins, Ford and Green (2013, 16-23). The idea that users are infected and then passively spread by viral content is, they argue, a marketing myth. They see users as actively engaged in the process of deciding what content they are going to share with other users instead. No doubt the truth lies between these two arguments. Jenkins et al. (2013, 195-228) acknowledge that content for better dissemination is "designed". Nevertheless, it must be emphasised that content such as internet memes does not spread on its own, but depends on user creativity and participation, which is incompatible with Dawkins' original "self-copying memes" concept (2006, 194; Pauliks, 2020). Another incompatibility with the theory of Dawkins comes from the fact that the terms "meme" and "viral" on the internet do not mean the same thing. A viral is "a single cultural unit" (e.g. a music video, a political image or an advertising slogan), according to the communication studies scholar Shifman (2014, 56), whereas memes are "always a collection of texts" (e.g. image macros with various captions). So, when content is copied and changed, a meme on the internet only becomes a meme. In contrast, virals consist only of a single version, although this can form the basis for internet memes (Pauliks, 2020).

Internet memes are not viruses, but they make it possible to communicate about viruses, particularly if the virus is an omnipresent topic due to a global pandemic. Memes are often used on the internet to comment on current issues. Memes facilitate discursive exchanges about events within society as a means of communication and a critique of these events. The use of humour involves the latter, allowing critical distance from the subject. Thus, humorous memes allow users to address sensitive topics and express criticism, which without an ironic undertone would not be possible. How internet memes critically comment on the coronavirus pandemic.

Crisis-Motivated Humour

In addition to the fact that informal humour has been under-researched, there is a shortage of literature on one aspect of informal humour, particularly public health related. Crisis-motivated humour refers to socio-economic or political jokes built to express the experience of the composers of challenging situations in their environments (Arning, 2020). In other words, a crisis motivated humour is any joke created as a coping strategy for a person's difficult social or health experiences (Williams, 2020). Such problems include any problem that brings about some psychological crisis in the individuals, and as a means of cushioning the effects, the individuals experiencing the difficulties resort to building humour (Arning, 2020; Attardo, 2017). Alongside the various subjects that convey the experiences, how this is carried out will be examined (Dawkins 2006 in Ogungbe & Omolobi, 2020). Traditionally, the study of humour has been seen as a sub-part of the study of aesthetics and has, therefore, been of primary interest to philosophers. According to Jones (2005) and Shelley (2003), humour has been studied since the times of Plato and Aristotle. Plato was the first of the two Greek philosophers to consider the nature of humour and laughter. He believed that the absurd was based on an unfortunate lack of self-knowledge, claiming in Philebus that people experience a combination of both delight and envy when they laugh at what is ridiculous in others, that is, when people mix both pain and pleasure (Jones, 2005; Shelley, 2003). In the second part of Poetics, Aristotle also considered the character of Ludicrous. It is believed that he also considered the ridiculous to be rather ugly and distorted. The studies of humour range from psychology, sociology, anthropology, literature, medicine, mathematics and linguistics across academic disciplines (Ferrar, 1992; Attardo, 2017; Ogungbe & Omolobi, 2020).

Humour studies are in harmony with the fact that jokes are generated from incongruous social experiences, with many humour studies focusing primarily on the first two of the three possible humour variants: formal, non-formal and informal humour. In a situation where the occasion is strictly formal, humour is perceived as formal and the primary purpose of the event is not just to evoke laughter. Examples include audiences, business forums, political meetings, corporate meetings and many others at national day celebrations. Any gathering organised for the main purpose of being entertained can refer to non-formal humour. These include weddings, birthdays, home movies, reality shows, comedy shows, TV drama series and many others (Akinola, 2018; Ogungbe & Omolobi, 2020).

The person evoking such humour is aware of the audience here, and he/she does this to fulfil the overt objective of entertaining the audience. Here, in terms of space and time, the performer and the viewer are limited. The motivation for this kind of humour is the entertainer's compensation or reward. For the sake of banter, the third form, informal humour, is often spontaneously evoked (Ogungbe & Omolobi, 2020). This will include jokes between friends, husband and wife, parents with their kids, teachers in a classroom with students, just to name a few. There is no direct incentive for the individual to evoke anything other than the satisfying feeling of having lightened the mood of others by evoking smiles or laughter. In some other cases, as a result of unwanted social and environmental experiences, it can be evoked to just release built-up emotions (Holmes & Marra, 2002).

To survive tough times, humour is an essential coping tool. Shared laughter gives us strength in adversity and, when the future looks uncertain, can help us feel a little more in control. And laughter literally strengthens us (Williams, 2020). Recent research has found that a good laugh can increase our levels of dopamine and even shore up our immune systems. Most importantly, funny jokes bring us together and help us feel linked, including coronavirus and quarantine jokes, one pandemic quarantine pod to another (Kelleher, 2021). So, while we obviously need to take COVID-19 very seriously and follow the CDC and WHO recommendations, we have to laugh as well. We could all use a few moments that feel lighter in the day, and a well-timed pandemic joke could just take your mind off the world's apocalypse-adjacent state and serve as a reminder that there is always something to smile about, however small. Here are some of the funniest quarantine, COVID-19, pandemic and virus jokes on the internet, from convos with pets to lockdown spins on classic knock-knocks (Kelleher, 2021).

Most of the humour and memes about COVID-19 that go viral on social media and the internet sound like a comedy, which is described as "a tragedy plus time", according to an adage. This has been true for many awful events, when humour and laughter are eventually restored after periods of shock and sadness (Allen, 1957). However, it seems the current pandemic (COVID-19) is different. People have not stopped joking. Even as an increasing number of people around the world get sick and die, memes and funny videos are everywhere on social media. Why is this occurring? Why is there no gap between the catastrophe and the humour that has been created around it?

One thing that makes the current situation of the coronavirus unique is that, in a particular place and time, it is not a single event. It is a rolling and ongoing crisis, endlessly spreading across continents with no end in sight. Therefore, the shock factor is reduced compared with, for instance, a single terror attack. This allows individuals to adapt to what is happening more easily, and humour may be one of the best ways to do just that. In these dire times, of course, many individuals will feel uncomfortable laughing, particularly if they know someone who has been directly affected. However, for others, in the face of the pandemic, it is not only acceptable to use humour, but it may also even be a necessity (Greengross, 2020). Of course, people do not laugh at the tragedy itself, at the victims of the virus, or at the people who suffer from it. Rather people can aim at the seemingly absurd situation in which we all find ourselves. This is because humour is a great defence mechanism from a psychological point of view, which helps us deal with emotionally challenging situations, especially those that are overwhelming and unpredictable. In an attempt to cope and distract themselves from the serious situation, many cancer patients and their doctors, for instance, routinely tell jokes and laugh about the disease (Beach & Erin, 2017).

Humour as a Strategy of Coping the Pandemic

On top of that, humour may become more prevalent, not less, in the unique conditions surrounding the pandemic (see Fig. 6.1). First, many individuals now have an unusual amount of time on their hands. Being

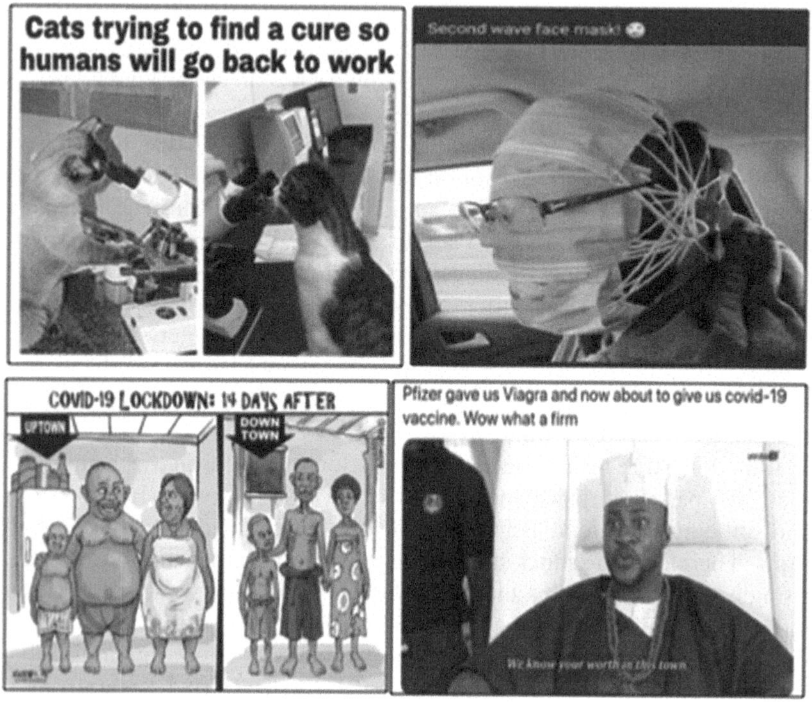

Fig. 6.1 A collage of memes shared in Nigerian social media platforms

stuck with not much to do at home forces individuals to find ways to be more creative, and, while the situation is serious, we are mostly concerned with more mundane tasks in our daily activities such as what to do all day, how to entertain kids, how not to eat too much, and how to stay sane in general. Second, being a little frightened, tense and in a state of alert is actually a good thing to develop humour. In creating and enjoying humour, these physiological and emotional arousal states serve as driving forces. Usually, intermediate arousal levels are best. You are bored with too little, and with too much—you are too excited to enjoy humour. Perfect is right in the middle. After hearing a good joke, the laughter serves as a release of all the physiological and emotional energy built-up, and that is what makes us feel good about it (Roberts, 2017, 2019; Greengross, 2020).

Another important element of humour that is prominent during the pandemic is what is termed "incongruity" by humour researchers. There needs to be something odd or surprising in the situation for something to be funny. There are many such oddities revealed in the current situation. Here is a joke that illustrates the point: "I thought the tumble dryer was shrinking my clothes all this time. It turns out it was the refrigerator, actually". The joke is built on the unusual conditions in which people live, of being stuck at home. The setup is the common understanding that clothes can shrink from the heat of a tumble dryer, but then, there is a surprise. It is not a faulty dryer, but the fridge where we store our food. By realising we are getting fatter from eating too much when we are at home, we resolve this incongruity. This resolution provides for the "Aha!...", which makes the joke funny. And yes, analysing a joke ruins it, too (Greengross, 2020; Morreall, 2020).

Therefore, while humour might not get us out of this terrible crisis, it can help us cope with it. We cannot alter the reality or the economic impact of the disease, but we can try to change how we feel about it. We can cope better and ease some of the tension due to the pandemic by creating and sharing humour. We can have at least some control of the situation in that way (Williams, 2020). And what better way than having a good laugh to do that—especially on social media?

Nigerian Comedians, COVID-19 and Social Media Humour

Nigerian comedian Maryam Apaokagi has a sure-fire way of getting people to listen to her coronavirus health advice—she delivers it with a hard slap in the face. The 21-year-old has joined a line-up of the nation's top performers working health tips into their routines to spread the word about COVID 19. In one of her online videos, she plays the role on an all-knowing, all-controlling Nigerian mother who watches in horror as a young man sneezes into his hands. Within seconds, she grabs a bottle of sanitiser from her bra (the bosom of her dress, typical of African women), slathers it over her palms, then hits him hard in the face. "Ah, a sanitised slap", her companion gasps in mock horror, as the young man learns his lesson the hard way. Apaokagi, who goes by the stage name Taaooma, says she puts out the meme video to reach out to people who would usually ignore or dismiss advice from official sources about the risks of the virus—people like her own mother, as she puts it, "The main reason why I did the coronavirus skit was because of my mom, because you cannot tell her not to go and worship" (Ukomadu, 2020).

Authorities in Nigeria like in all parts of the world have issued a policy on avoiding large gatherings and the importance of washing hands. However, people's trust in the government is low; hence conspiracies and bogus health tips spread fast on social media. The comedian laments that parents "are the ones that are ... the most difficult people to tell not to do things… So, when they watch it and laugh, they will also remember the message that they said we should not go to the mosque, they said we should not go to the church for now". In the skit, she advises anyone who is about to cough to "do the dab" as she puts it (Ukomadu, 2020). The dab is a dance movement involving raising and stretching one arm and bending the other as if one is shooting with a rifle, with one's face getting covered in the elbow of the bent arm.

Furthermore, a Nigerian male comic artiste, Osarenkhoe Lawrence, conjures up a world where diseases have their own governing committee. In the video, performers are made to act Ebola and cancer and lay official complaints to the government that the new kid in the block (i.e. COVID-19) is stealing the show. The solution, the head of the government rules, is to put COVID-19 in its place by maintaining personal hygiene and social distance. "We are no longer joking, we are actually affecting lives, and I think, this period we need more videos, we need more funny content", said the performer from Benin City, South-south of Nigeria and who goes by the stage name MC Casino (Ukomadu, 2020). Nigeria's health ministry has spotted the trend and enlisted popular comedian Bright Okpocha, alias Basketmouth, to appear in a public service video about the dangers and of spreading misinformation. The messages are getting through, said Cyril Oto-Obong, a comedy fan who works as an accountant in Lagos. "It is not everyone who understands the safety measures when it is spoken in English, but once a comedian makes it a laughing matter, one [sur]e thing is [that,] it will make people pay attention", says Mr. Oto-Obong.

Fake News as Humour on Social Media

Fake news can be interesting, and understanding it is increasingly becoming imperative. This chapter's focus on this phenomenon is, therefore, crucial because it presents some of the features of the environment in which the Nigerian social media space is regarding rumours and conspiracy theories about COVID-19 which "have significant consequences for journalism" and news media (Siapera, 2018, 157). To understand these, it is necessary to start with the quest to identify fake news and its varieties. Cited in Ibrahim (2019: 62), Ojebode (2018: 3) defines fake news (which includes misinformation and disinformation) as "the product of a person's imagination for the purposes that may or may not be mischievous", "an oxymoron since news is supposed to be factual (rather than based on imagination or opinion)" and "any story presented as news, but which does not reflect what happened, or which reports what did not happen". Ojebode's second definition focuses on the whimsical definition of what constitutes misinformation, which the researcher describes as "the Trumpian definition of fake news".

From the media and journalism institutional/organisational perspective, Ethical Journalism Network (EJN) and the BBC have both defined what constitutes fake news. According to EJN cited in Pate, Gambo and Ibrahim (2019, 22), fake news is information deliberately fabricated and published to deceive and mislead others into believing falsehood or doubtful messages (EJN, 2017). Whereas the BBC defines fake news as "completely false information, photos or videos purposefully created and spread to confuse or disinform; information, photos or videos manipulated to deceive, or old photographs shared as new; satire or parody which means no harm but can fool people" (BBC News, 2018). Moreover, as used in this chapter, fake news is interchangeably used as disinformation, a term that refers to "deliberately spreading [of] false or inaccurate information", as opposed to misinformation, which "is the spreading of inaccurate or false information while mistakenly thinking one is sharing accurate information (in reality, the person or organisation spreading it is misinformed)" (Bunger et al., 2017; Harsin, 2018).

Furthermore, Wardle (2017), cited in Siapera (2018, 157), has formulated a typology of fake news based on three main dimensions as follows: (i) the type of content created and shared, (ii) the intentions of those behind it and (iii) forms of publication. Wardle also offered seven different categories of fake news, "which she places on a continuum": satire/parody, misleading content, imposter content, fabricated content, false connection, false context, and manipulated content (Fig. 6.2). However, she argues that "The intentions of the communicators are crucial as satire has no intention to deceive, while manipulated content has been developed to manipulate and deceive" (157).

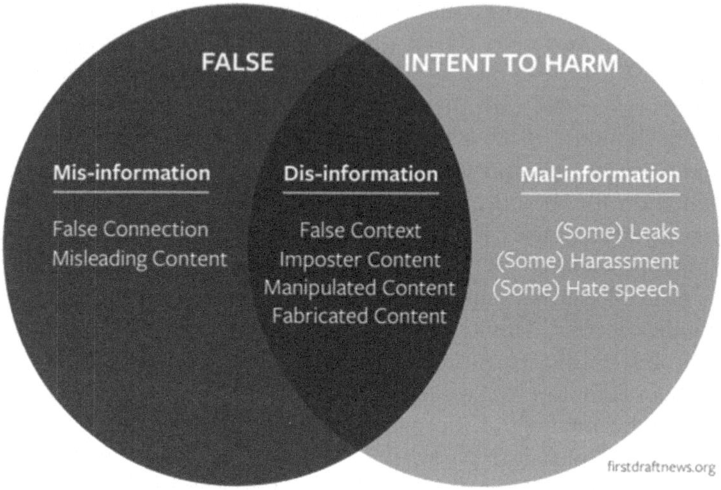

Fig. 6.2 Themes of fake news. (Source: Wardle and Derakhshan (2018, 46))

Furthermore, fake news and disinformation about COVID-19 are rife in the Nigerian social media space. In addition to creating confusion about what is true and what is not regarding the virus, how it is contracted and how to practise preventive measures, fake news and misinformation also are capable of creating the worst scenario—that of deceiving individuals into adopting harmful practices, attitudes, beliefs and behaviours especially when it involves false medication or preventive substances that could lead to loss of lives or impairment. The factors that drive manipulated information dissemination may vary, but the effect is the same—taking advantage of the goal of the message. However, the remedy to this manipulation is clear: "increasing the capacity of readers or audience to separate the wheat from the chaff through exposure to media literacy, critical thinking, and fact-checking". While humour could be useful health wise, misinformation and fake news can worsen the situation. The internet especially social media is a double-edged sword, with good and bad effects. Some health-related humour spread on social media may be useful, but misinformation, which equally spread on social media, is rather harmful. The culture industry should seize this opportunity to enlighten people about disease prevention measures using memes, jokes and humour. Since the

COVID-19 pandemic is a global health crisis so is misinformation about it. Given that in the reviewed literature in the preceding sections a lot has been discussed about the pandemic in a global perspective, now it is worth taking an inward view at the Nigerian context and examining how Nigerians defy health crises (Fig. 6.3).

The challenge to misinformation is that it can come from other credible sources. For example, on March 20, 2020, the (then) US President, Donald Trump, was televised saying that chloroquine showed very encouraging results in the treatment for COVID-19 infection. Since then, Nigeria has seen an increase in the demand for chloroquine despite the US Food and Drug Administration has quickly clarified Trump's statement that the effects of the drug were still being tested. The popularity of chloroquine as a treatment for COVID-19 may have been the result of many factors, not confined to the knowledge of the treatment for Nigerians who had previously used it as medication for malaria. The factors include the need

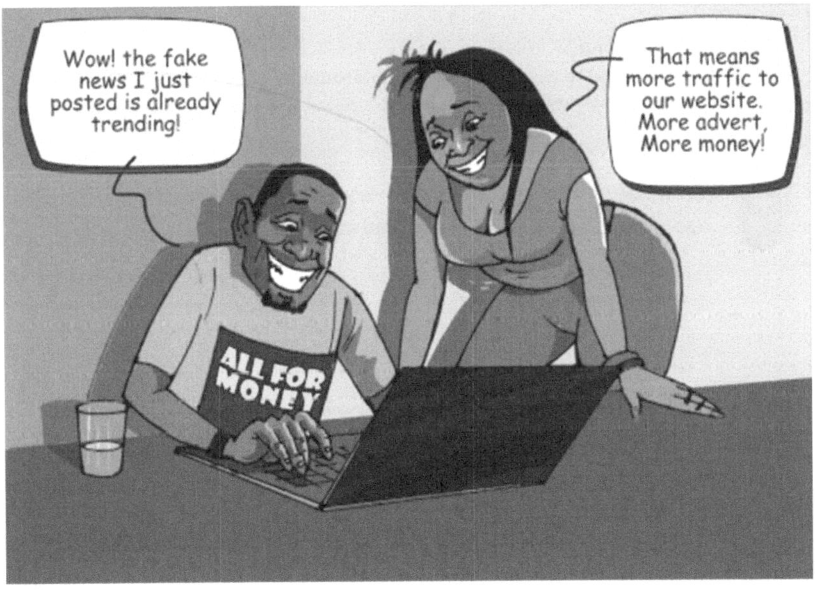
Wow! the fake news I just posted is already trending!
That means more traffic to our website. More advert, More money!
ALL FOR MONEY

Fig. 6.3 A comical illustration of young internet users sharing fake news online. Their conversation (shown in the bubbles) indicates the reasons they (and many of their like) share false information. (Source: PTCIJ Dubawa (2020))

to share an alleged life-saving treatment and the impact of the (then) President Trump's endorsement of the drug on television. One Twitter user (see Fig. 6.4) says, "Chloroquine that was banned in Nigeria has proved to be an anti-viral drug for Corona Virus after showing promising results in trials across 10 hospitals. Who would've thought chloroquine…?" (PTCIJ Dubawa, 2020). An overview of the most popular false stories on COVID-19 is outlined below with fact-checking comments. Moreover, as the virus spreads and tests intensify, Nigeria will need to address health misinformation (Cinelli et al., 2020).

The above memes demonstrate how Nigerians engaged with fake news in a humorous manner. In some cases, some people, unaware that the information being shared online was fake, fell victim. It seems those who joked about fake news either they were knowledgeable enough to fact check or simply knew what is true and false, hence witty and humorous reactions to these instances of fake news.

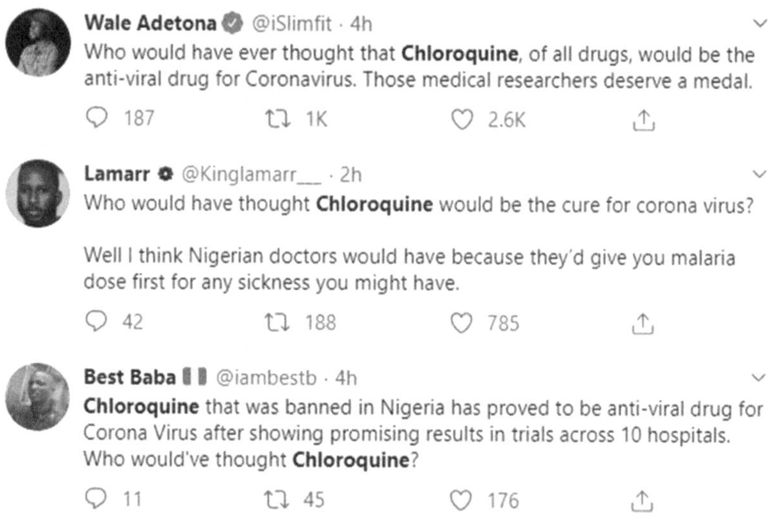

Fig. 6.4 A Twitter hoax on the use of chloroquine as a medication for COVID-19. (Source: David, 2020)

Conclusion

The internet especially social media has been, for the most part, a liberating force during this prolonged time of confinement for many people worldwide. The fact is that apart from our immediate families or loved ones, in the absence of our usual face-to-face interactions, from whom we may now sometimes feel we need a break, online humour, absurdity and wit, along with cartoons or memes revealing the nonsense and grotesque on the part of our beloved leaders act as a source of minor, temporary, salvation. We laugh when authoritarian bureaucrats and self-admiring politicians put themselves above us because, in their handling of this deadly pandemic, they also put themselves above common sense. In terms of the most important humour styles that are at play during the COVID-19 era (success is measured by the degree to which any humorous discourse that distracts us from the downside of the pandemic has an upside), this chapter shows that the different psychological explanations of humour, relief, release and catharsis, spliced on existential humour and the theory of incongruity. The best coronavirus humour provides people with light-hearted fun, brief interludes in otherwise virtually indistinguishable days.

This chapter captures and highlights how social networking sites serve as an avenue that contributes to citizen engagement and the use of unhindered freedom of expression through the use of images, as well as the disappearance of authorship over the creation, distribution and consumption of internet memes to raise awareness and lighten the tense mood of people on COVID 19. As a measure to curb the spread of the virus, internet memes can be used as a tool to transmit messages to the general public. To attack, share sensitive information, pull a prank and derail a topic, internet memes are used. Internet memes serve as an avenue for direct communication that not only contributes to raising awareness of the coronavirus infection but also encourages individuals to adhere to non-clinical preventive measures such as face mask-wearing, social distancing, hand washing, testing and ultimately vaccination. Finally, a couple of research questions have generated for future research to consider finding empirical solution to. The questions are: People have not stopped joking. Despite increasingly more people around the world are getting infected with COVID-19 and dying, memes and funny videos are everywhere on social media. Why is this occurring? Why is there no gap between the catastrophe and the humour that has been created around it?

References

Akinola, A. J. (2018). Pragmatics of crisis motivated humour in computer mediated platforms in Nigeria. *Journal of Language and Education, 4*(3), 6–17.

Alatalo, S., & Poutiainen, A. (2016). Use of humour in multicultural classroom. The Israeli *Journal of Humour Research*, 5(1), 65–79. 7

Allen, S. (1957, February). Steve Allen's Almanac. In *Cosmopolitan* (Vol. 142). Hearst Corp.

Andrew, P. (2012). Laughter is the best medicine: The construction of old age in ageist humour. In J. Chovanec & I. Ermida (Eds.), *Language and humour in the media* (pp. 11–24). Cambridge Scholars Publishing.

Arning, C. (2020, May 29). The risks and rewards of humour in COVID-19. *WARC* blog. https://www.warc.com/newsandopinion/opinion/the-risks-and-rewards-of-humour-in-COVID-19/3640. Accessed 8 Feb 2021.

Attardo, S. (2017). *Humour in language: Linguistics.* Retrieved from https://linguistics.oxfordre.com/view/10.1093/acrefore/9780199384655.001.0001/acrefore-9780199384655-e-342

BBC News. (2018). *World – Africa: What we've learnt about fake news in Africa.* http://bbc.com/news/world-africa-46138284

Beach, W. A., & Erin, P. (2017). Laughter, humour and cancer: Delicate moments and poignant interactional circumstances. *Health Communication, 32*(7), 791–802.

Bunger, L., Gary, J., Venturinirini, T., & Mauri, M. (2017). *A field guide to fake news and other information disorders: A collection of recipes for those who love to cook with digital methods.* Public Data Lab.

Campisano, F. (2016). A case study of comedian Hannibal Buress and humour as an agent for change. *Elon. Journal of Undergraduate Research in Communications, 12*(2), 25–35.

Chapman, A. J. (1983). Humour and laughter in social interaction and some implications for humour research. In P. E. McGhee & J. H. Goldstein (Eds.), *Handbook of humour research.* Springer.

Cinelli, M., Quattrociocchi, W., Galeazzi, A., Valensise, C. M., Brugnoli, E., Schmidt, A. L., Zola, P., Zollo, F., & Scala, A. (2020). *The COVID-19 social media infodemic.* arXiv:2003.05004. https://arxiv.org/abs/2003.05004. Accessed 21 Mar 2020.

David, T. (2020). *Chloroquine does not cure Coronavirus!* https://dubawa.org/chloroquine-does-not-cure-coronavirus/. Accessed 23 June 2020.

Dawkins, R. (2006). *The selfish gene* (30th ed.). Oxford University Press.

EJN. (2017). *Ethics in the news: EJN report on challenges for journalism in the post-truth era.* Ethical Journalism Network.

Fadly, A. (2020). Evaluative language in the discourse of Cebong Vs Kampret ("Tadpole Vs Microbats") on Twitter. *Bahtera: Jurnal Pendidikan Bahasa Dan Sastra, 19*(1), 1–14.

Ferrar, M. 1992. *The Logic of the Ludicrous: A pragmatic study of humour* (unpublished PhD. Thesis). University College, London.

Filani, I. (2016). Humorous meaning strategies in Nigerian stand-up comedy: An example of 'I go dye' performance. *Papers in English and Linguistics, 17*, 193–220.

Friedman, S., & Kuipers, G. (2013). The divisive power of humour: Comedy, taste and 20 symbolic boundaries. *Cultural Sociology, 7*(2), 179–195.

Greengross, G. (2020, May 11). Coronavirus: When life gives you a pandemic, it's okay to laugh about it. Humour can be a great stress buster, especially during this trying time. *Scroll.in* blog. https://scroll.in/article/961546/coronavirus-when-life-gives-you-a-pandemic-its-okay-to-laugh-about-it. Accessed 10 Feb 2021.

Harsin, J. (2018). Post-truth and critical communication. In *Oxford Research Encyclopedia of Communication.* Oxford University Press.

Hartini, S. (2017). Analisis Discourse pada Meme Gamers Mario Teguh di Facebook. *Jurnal Kinesik, 4*(2), 111–126.

Holmes, J., & Marra, M. (2002). Having a laugh at work: How humour contributes to workplace culture. *Journal of Pragmatics, 34*(12), 1683–1710.

Ibrahim, A. M. (2019). Theorizing the journalism model of disinformation and hate speech propagation in a Nigerian democratic context. *International Journal of E-Politics, 10*(2), 60–73.

Isnaniah, S., & Augustina, T. (2020). "COVID-19" meme in social media: Study of Roland Barthes semiology. *Bahtera: Jurnal Pendidikan Bahasa dan Sastra, 19*(2), 351–378.

Jenkins, H., Ford, S., & Green, J. (2013). *Spreadable media: Creating value and meaning in a networked culture.* New York University Press.

Jones, J. D. (2005). *A complete analysis of Plato's philosophy of humour.* Jonathonjones.

Juditha, C. (2015). Meme di social media: Analisis semiotik meme Haji Lulung. *Jurnal Pekomnas, 18*(2), 105–116. https://doi.org/10.30818/jpkm.2015.1180204

Katayama, H. (2009). A cross-cultural analysis of humour in stand-up comedy in the United States and Japan. *JoLIE, 2*(2), 11–19.

Kelleher, E. (2021). 53 Coronavirus and quarantine jokes to retrain your face to smile: It's a pandemic. *Fatherly* blog. https://www.fatherly.com/play/best-coronavirus-jokes/. Accessed 8 Feb 2021.

Marin-Arrese, J. I. (2005). Humour as subversion in political cartooning. In M. L. Postigo (Ed.), *Approaches to critical discourse analysis* (pp. 1–22). McGraw-Hill.

Mey, J. (2001). *An introduction to pragmatics*. Blackwell Publishing.

Morreall, J. (2020). Philosophy of humour. In E. N. Zalta (ed.), *The Stanford encyclopedia of philosophy*. https://plato.stanford.edu/archives/fall2020/entries/humor/

Msughter, A. E. (2020). Internet meme as a campaign tool to the fight against COVID-19 in Nigeria. *Global Journal of Human-Social Science (A), 20*(6), 27–39.

Ogungbe, E. L., & Omolobi, I. (2020). The pragmatics of coronavirus motivated humour on the social media. *All Nations University Journal of Applied Thought, 8*(1), 1–20.

Ojebode, A. (2018). *Fake news, hate speech and the 2019 general elections: The redemptive role of the Nigerian media*. Paper presented at the 13th Annual Federal Radio Corporation of Nigeria (FRCN) lecture, November 29, NICON Luxury Hotel, Abuja, Nigeria. Retrieved from https://www.researchgate.net/publication/329307521

Pate, U. A., Gambo, D., & Ibrahim, A. M. (2019). The impact of fake news and the emerging post-truth political era on Nigerian polity: A review of literature. *Studies in Media and Communication, 7*(1), 21–29.

Pauliks, K. (2020). Memes of the virus: Social criticism of the corona pandemic on the internet. *Televizion, 33*(E), 46–49.

PTCIJ Dubawa. (2020, June 22). *In a world of COVID-19, what factors drive false information in Nigeria?* Report by Dubawa: The Fact-Checker, Issue 19.

Richtel, M. (2020). *WHO fights a pandemic besides Coronavirus: An "Infodemic"*. https://www.nytimes.com/2020/02/06/health/coronavirus-misinformation-social-media.html. Accessed 7 Feb 2020.

Roberts, A. (2017). Humour is a funny thing. *British Journal of Aesthetics, 56*, 355–366.

Roberts, A. (2019). *A philosophy of humour*. Palgrave Macmillan.

Ross, A. (1998). *The language of humour*. Routledge.

Shelley, C. (2003). Plato on the psychology of humour. *Humour, 16*(4), 351–367.

Shifman, L. (2014). *Memes in digital culture*. The MIT Press.

Siapera, E. (2018). *Understanding new media*. Sage.

Solon, O. (2013). Richard Dawkins on the internet's hijacking of the word 'meme'. http://www.wired.co.uk/article/richard-dawkins-memes

Ukomadu, A. (2020, May 11). Nigerian comics fight COVID-19 with gags and slapstick slaps. *Reuters*. https://mobile.reuters.com/article/amp/idUSKBN22K1LI

Wardle, C., & Derakhshan, H. (2018). Thinking about "information disorder": Formats of misinformation, disinformation and mal-information. In C. Ireton & J. Posetti (Eds.), *Journalism, fake news and disinformation* (pp. 44–56). UNESCO.

Williams, A. (2020, April 22). Laughter, however hollow, is one of the main coping mechanisms during periods of sickness, death and anxiety. So, don't feel guilty. *The New York Times*. https://www.nytimes.com/2020/04/22/style/coronavirus-humor.html. Accessed 10 Feb 2021.

CHAPTER 7

Social Media Audience's Interpretation of Selected Humor Memes on Coronavirus Pandemic in Nigeria

Gloria Chimeziem Ernest-Samuel

Introduction

In February, 2020, Nigerian Minister for Health reported that the country had had its first case of COVID-19 infection. The announcement brought Nigeria on the same pedestal with other nations in Asia, Europe and America battling with the pandemic which claimed millions of lives. The Centres for Disease Control and Prevention in its weekly report in April, 2020, placed the incidence of coronavirus cases at above 890,000, with about 45,000 deaths annually. The statistics includes 239,279 cases and 5443 deaths in the United States at that period. Although COVID-19 was alleged to have originated from Wuhan, China, in late 2019, many conspiracy theories and debates have generated controversies which raise doubts and suspicion. However, one clear fact is that the coronavirus is not new. Fielding (2020) reports that there have been earlier cases of coronavirus in 2003 and 2012, respectively. The 2003 virus was known as

G. C. Ernest-Samuel (✉)
Department of Theatre Arts, IMO State University, Owerri, Nigeria

S. Mpofu (ed.), *Digital Humour in the Covid-19 Pandemic*,
https://doi.org/10.1007/978-3-030-79279-4_7

the severe acute respiratory syndrome coronavirus (SARS-CoV) outbreak which occurred in mainland China and Hong Kong. The 2012 outbreak was in Saudi Arabia and in the United Arab Emirates and was known as the Middle East respiratory syndrome coronavirus (MERS-CoV). While the coronavirus of 2003 and 2012 took place in specific locations and were easily contained by scientists and researchers, the 2019 coronavirus was global, which informs why the World Health Organization labeled it a pandemic. According to Sarah Bosely et al. (2020), COVID-19 is caused by a member of the coronavirus family that has never been encountered before and transferred to human from animals. Some of the symptoms include fever, tiredness and cough. At other times, some patients may have runny nose, sore throat, nasal congestion, aches and pains or diarrhea. Report from the American Centers for Disease Control and Prevention (CDC) says that some strains of the coronavirus are asymptomatic. However, it does not prevent the patients from infecting others. The CDC COVID-19 Response Team suggests that 'Social distancing and everyday preventive behaviour remain important for all age groups as patients with less serious illness and those without symptoms likely play an important role in disease transmission' (2020, 1).

Recognized by world Poverty Clock, as the world capital of poverty, with over 40% of its population living below the poverty line, Nigeria needed a serious intervention to curb the spread of the coronavirus in the country. Kalu (2020) reports that in response to the increasing cases of coronavirus infection in Nigeria, on 18 March, 2020, the federal government enforced an initial two-week lockdown on 30 March 2020, for three of its 36 states (Lagos, Ogun and Abuja) and, on April 13, extended the lockdown. The government approved the closure of all schools, both private and public, and other institutions. By the directive, citizens were urged to 'stay-at-home,' maintain social distancing, wash hands on a regular basis, avoid touching their faces or others and so on. Movements within and outside the states were restricted. The citizens relied on the National Centre on Disease Control (NCDC) to access information and tips of surviving the coronavirus pandemic. Established in 2011 with a bill signed into law in 2018, the NCDC, according to information on the institution's website, is Nigeria's public health institute, 'with the mandate to lead the preparedness, detection and response to infectious disease outbreaks and public health emergencies' (NCDC 2020). Under the lockdown, although many receive text messages on a five-hourly basis from NCDC, the confined citizens learned to share their experiences, thoughts, anxieties and fears on the social media, which proved to be a veritable voice and platform for expressing their frustrations and information sharing, transmission and dissemination.

It was not surprising that there were noticeable increase in the presence of memes on the social media, particularly, Facebook. Varis and Blommaert (2015) credited the term, *memes* to Richard Dawkins, author of *The Selfish Gene* (1976) who analyzed a meme as a gene because it serves 'as small cultural units of transmission…which are spread by copying or imitation.' Memes are composed of images and texts on issues. The quality of copying and imitation is a feature common to memes on social media which inform why they are liked and shared by social media users. Varis and Blommaert rightly observe that 'social media interaction patterns show an amazing density of phatic interactions, in which signs are shared and circulated without an a priori determination of the meaning' (2015, 31). In another development, Wang et al. (2015, 2378) observe that by 'sharing photos, users could also express opinions or sentiments, social media images provide a potentially rich source for understanding public opinions/sentiments.' Memes voice the opinion of the generator and are shared by people who identify with the opinions. Thus, logically, the memes for this study voice people's feelings on the coronavirus, social distancing, the sit-at-home, quarantine, watching of hands and so on and were selected based on the number of *likes* and *shares* they generated among social media users affiliated to this researcher. This study is interested in analyzing selected popular user-generated memes on Facebook considered as humorous, to ascertain how the messages or information on COVID-19 were interpreted by the social media users. The study will attempt to substantiate if this class of communication actually serve the functions attributed to humor. Finally, it attempts to theorize on its use by social media users in Nigeria. The memes selected for this study are mainly African. This implies that they contain images, icons and languages which Africans can identify with, because as John Meyer (2000, 316) observes, there is need for the symbols to be familiar to the user in assessing humor, 'if the concepts that create the humor are so familiar as to be already known, or not familiar at all, the audience cannot "get" a joke.'

Due to the newness of coronavirus, very few studies have been conducted on coronavirus in the humanities. In fact, most of the available studies are in the field of medicine and microbiology. For instance, a study by Bergmann et al. (2006) examines the effect of the coronavirus on the central nervous system and attributes the disease to having devastating consequences on T-cells and adversely affects non-lytic humoral immunity which suppresses the disease. In another study by the CDC Response Team on coronavirus infection in United States, the team found out that children are less vulnerable than middle-aged adults and old people and with respiratory problem. The study recommends that people with children exposed to patients with coronavirus should maintain social distancing irrespective of signs or symptoms. Kalu (2020) argues that government's intervention in coronavirus infection is connected to poverty and hunger; thus measures put in place to fight coronavirus must take cognizance of providing palliatives for the citizens. Some studies have attempted to examine online memes. Varis and Blommaert have analyzed phatic forms of interactions on social media and focus on viral memes. Simmons et al. (2011) in their study of online memes observe that the credibility of the originator of an online meme may alter the content. In another study on social media images, Wang et al. (2015) conduct a sentiment analysis of social media memes and discovered that language and improper annotation play challenging roles in the appreciation of such images. A couple of studies have been done on humor. Meyer (2000) studies humor as a double-edged sword and attempts reading the functions. In a study related to this current study, Taecherungroj and Nueangjamnong (2015) examine humor in some viral memes from the Global South. In another study, McCreadie and Wiggins (2007) investigate the use of humor in health practice between physician and patients. Although there were positive effects, they observe that there is dearth of studies on humor in health practice and education. So far, there is currently no study on interpretations of social media-generated memes on coronavirus, particularly within the African context. This makes this study very significant and a contribution to knowledge.

Objectives of the Study

The coronavirus pandemic had generated lots of conversations and discourses which affect humanity. The objectives of this study include the following:

(a) To identify some popular African memes on aspects of coronavirus pandemic circulating on the social media, particularly Facebook.
(b) To understand how social media audience interpret selected memes on coronavirus pandemic.

(c) To examine the classifications of memes on coronavirus with the view of understanding heuristic representations and interpretations of such memes in Africa.

Research Questions

Considering the interest of this study, some questions are very important in this research investigation. The research questions include the following:

(a) How do social media audiences view selected COVID-19 memes and what aspect of the pandemic does the memes reflect?
(b) What satirical or humorous undertones are embedded in the memes?
(c) Are there other communicable messages attributable to the memes as forms of communication?

Research Methodology

This study is a socio-cultural investigation which examines the symbolic construction of memes on aspects of coronavirus pandemic. Twelve social media users who viewed and shared ideas on ten independent memes on Facebook were drafted into a WhatsApp group, in order to extract their opinions on the memes without the distraction of comments from the free public. The themes of the memes fall under the following: education, humor, satire and health concerns on the pandemic. The memes address issues on corona virus such as social distancing, self-quarantine, coughing in public, lockdown effects and so on. The memes were shared in the platform for the participants to interpret.

Because the study focuses on mediated communication on the internet, particularly on Facebook which is a social media, digital ethnography was adopted. The adaptive nature of ethnography called for the use of digital ethnography, also called ethnography of the internet (Hine, 2008). Murthy (2008) recommends social media such as Facebook as a field for ethnographic investigations for many reasons among the fact that it acts as a platform for social connections among people and allows for interaction and many social activities. Especially, it provides opportunities for millions of other social engagements which an ethnographic researcher can understudy with its multi-million users globally. Digital ethnography is considered suitable because it is a new mode of engagement which will allow us 'develop an in-depth understanding of the textures of social experience that arise as people engage with various technologies that comprise the contemporary internet' as Hine (2008, 29) observes. Other methods like observation, archiving documents and interviewing were also applied as forms of data collection in order to enrich the research outcome. The advantage of these methods is that it offered balanced result, instead of myopic views or opinions based on one-sided information. The data collected was analyzed through two methods: (a) thematic analysis and (b) discourse analysis. Thematic analysis is a method of identifying, analyzing and reporting patterns (themes) within data (Braun & Clarke, 2006) and involves using a theme to capture research issues in relation to the research question. Thematic analysis is deemed appropriate for analyzing the data acquired from the WhatsApp chats on the memes. The memes were selected because of their popularity on Facebook, and the data was organized according to themes to aid its analysis. The researcher communicated with the participants on Messenger and WhatApp and sought their permission to discuss the memes for the research. Of the 15 persons communicated initially, only 12 were finally chosen for the interview because of their interest in the discourse. Moreover, all 12 participants are educated and knowledgeable to a good extent on COVID-19 as well as humor. In the course of the documentation, the data was interpreted according to the positioning of the memes. Concrete issues emanating from the interviews were re-addressed to understand their relationship with issues on the research subject. The chats were copied and the responses were grouped according to themes in order to make meaning out of the data. The thematic data analysis was predominant in this analysis.

Discourse analysis is the second method used in analyzing the data. It involves 'the organization of texts and talk in practices, and with the discursive resources that those practices draw on' (Potter, 1996, 38); thus it unveils the hidden meaning of a text, which may be written documents, transcribed interviews, field notes and so on. It provides a means of analyzing and interpreting the intent of language. The critical discourse analysis was adopted in reading meaning to some of the texts generated in conversation with the research participants who are the respondents in this study. The adoption of discourse analysis thus enables the analyst-researcher to focus on the role of language as a communicative agent.

Theoretical and Conceptual Framework

As a major interest in the study, the concept of humor was used in analyzing the subject, while the study is based on relief theory which involves release or relaxation (also known as psychoanalytic theory) and has Sigmund Freud as one of its most outstanding representatives (Krikmann, 2006). The theory focuses significantly on humor recipient and its psychological effects on them. Arvo Krikmann observes that Freud considers humor as one of the so-called substitution mechanisms which enable the conversion of one's socially tabooed aggressive impulses to acceptable ones and thus avoid wasting additional mental energy to suppress them (see link). In examining the memes, this chapter argues that the memes result from the originators' desire to suppress the pains, disappoints and predicaments of living through COVID-19 experience. Thus, the memes were shared in order to provide alternative forms of appreciating and living with the coronavirus without fear.

The Memes and Respondents' Interpretations

The memes used in this study are varieties of public commentaries related to COVID-19 issues which were considered humorous because they generated laughing emojis and likeability from the public and were shared by many social media users on Facebook. The participants were requested to interpret the memes with the view of investigating if the memes were indeed considered by the participants to be humorous and to aid the public assessment and understanding of the memes given its engagement on COVID-19. The first of the ten memes selected for this study is a cartoon illustration of a discussion between two emojis: One of the emojis was assigned a text 'Hmm, the politicians are testing COVID-19 positive, while their wives are testing negative. How come?' The second emoji replies: 'I think they are testing the wrong 'spouses', they should check the side chics!' Humorously, the meme focuses on politicians and women. According to one of the respondents, the meme suggests that 'politicians are usually "away" from their wives but available for their side chicks.' Ultimately, as one of the respondents observes, 'politicians are highly exposed targets in this matter.' The meme suggests that 'the manner of tracking potential COVID-positive contacts could be more challenging than we already think.' This is because 'side chicks are rarely listed as contacts by their politician friends and sugar-daddies.' Moreover, as one of the respondents rhetorically asked, 'How many side chicks will they (politicians) acknowledge? Are they keeping records?' The meme highlights the growing importance of side chicks (mistresses) over wives among African political leaders. As another respondent observes, the meme suggests that 'most of our politicians are not close to their spouses the same way they are not close to the people... they are keeping mistresses whom they are more intimate with than their spouses. It also tells how they marginalize certain sections, groups – ethnic or geopolitical in the distribution of developmental projects.' The meme made health and social comments which suggests that 'efforts should be made to trace concubines of politicians, and have them tested, isolated and managed to curb the spread of the virus.' The humor lies in the fact that spouses of politicians are distant to them, while the side chicks (who are supposedly distant and outside their homes) are closer to them than their spouses. This meme is a discourse on the challenge of tracking of infected or potentially exposed contacts for isolation.

To further elaborate on the hidden communication, a respondent reveals that 'the two emojis are used here as derisive symbolic expressions of abnormalities in the life of the political class.' Another respondent observes that:

> The questions posed by the two symbols refer to the dominant issues of gross infidelity associated with the political class. The possibility of contracting COVID-19 through a relationship of infidelity might lead to a situation where a politician might test positive and his or her partner tests negative. The virus like HIV and Ebola, as a potent instrument of social disruption, is likely to heighten the trend of mutual suspicion among couples.

Thus, the meme highlights part of the social revelation of the pandemic. As another respondent observes, 'Paradoxically, the legitimate spouses of politicians do not share their infections; their mistresses instead do, suggesting that the side chics are in reality closer to the erring and wealthy politicians than their spouses and so share their afflictions.' It's remarkable to note that the meme 'foregrounds the fact that initially, Coronavirus afflicted the affluent in the Nigerian context, as the disease came from overseas and so struck politicians and other categories of the Rich who travelled abroad or came into contact with foreigners or travelers.'

The second meme is the humorous picture of a child with folded hands and gloomy face overtly expressing an abnormal situation. Accompanying the picture is the statement, 'One cannot cough in peace again…everybody will be looking at you coronically!' The visual posture of the young boy is humorous, and more so, with the accompanying text. Meyer observes that humor involving children often serves enforcement function (2000, 320). In other words, it helps to enforce social norms in a society. As a respondent observes about the meme:

> The fact is that the coronavirus pandemic or COVID-19 has created an abnormal situation in every aspect of our social life. The subtle ways in which the virus spreads through human contacts makes every person a suspect. As a result of this, normal human acts of yawning, coughing and sneezing are no longer taken as simple conditioned reflex actions, but are now regarded as the symptoms of infection from the virus. This has rendered some of these involuntary acts of the human being quite problematic. People are now afraid of yawning, coughing or sneezing in public; and this will certainly affect the normal modes of social relation for years to come.

When one is symptomatic of COVID-19, coughing is one of the symptoms. Due to the panic concerning the pandemic, when one coughs, people get suspicious. The unanimously acclaimed humorous meme passes on the message of cough as a major symptom of COVID-19. In the community, coughing effectively puts everyone on alert of a possible or potential COVID-19 patient. As a respondent notes, it suggests that it's 'Better to keep away from anyone with an "innocent" cough than to ignore and be put at risk by someone with COVID-19 induced cough.' Thus the meme frowns at people's inability to separate the two, so people can live their normal lives.

As another respondent observes,

> The meme makes an obvious reference to the belief that droplets set free through coughing and sneezing can cause Coronavirus infections. This portentous fact thus transforms coughing into a grave act deserving public attention, if not condemnation. Humour is derived basically from the neologism "coronically" that deliberately puns on "Corona".

Thus, 'graphically, the complainant's grave countenance—as though the whole world was against him—equally elicits laughter.' To another respondent, the message suggests that the outbreak of Corona virus has 'created a level of hygiene consciousness. The social message is that personal hygiene and decency is encouraged.' In a way, it addresses stigmatization of people with cough and reminds the public that not every cough is as a result of coronavirus.

The third meme is picture of a child carried at the back of an adult with a pouting tongue that is traditionally interpreted as an expression of joyful acknowledgment of another person's inclusion or sharing in one's difficult situation or misfortune. Accompanying the picture meme is the message: 'GOD DON CATCH ALL DADDIES AND MUMMIES. All of you will now understand how we children feel when you tell us to sit in one place… You too, sit in one place….' This meme expresses children's perception of their caging or restriction by adults, especially, by their parents. Thus, the meme is one of the classic images of the COVID-19 period in the minds of children. As a respondent in a chat observes:

> Actually we know that the child was not the author of the sarcasm attributed to the meme, but the parents who found themselves in the situation of their children, were forced to reflect and imagine what their kids have been going through. Therefore, this might be seen as one of the positive effects of the COVID 19 – it has helped so many people to reflect deeply over certain issues of life, and mostly, it has helped parents to understand the consequences of certain unnecessary rules and regulations they impose on their children.

In other words, the respondents admit that 'the lockdown has meant that both parents and their children are confined at home.' While this places a greater burden on parents, most of who have to take a break from their usual responsibilities but are still expected to provide food for the family; for the children, the meme affirms that 'it is indeed an opportunity for parents to share the pain of the children's routine confinement.' It addresses children's concerns with how they are treated. Arguably, one may claim that the meme is not related to the virus; however, it ridicules the new position of adults who are confined in various homes with children due to COVID-19. Graphically, the meme in fact passes wrong message with the infraction of social distancing. The child's mischievous grin is used as a social corrective, devised to 'discipline parents,' as Duncan (1962, 187) opines. According to one of the respondents, 'the meme suggests that children have been in "bondage" and are now happy that their parents who kept them in bondage are in bondage with them.' It is therefore a play on isolation. Children are instructed to sit in a place forgetting how active they are and should be. Ironically, COVID-19 has forced adults to take the 'medicine' they had forcefully made children to take. It ideally endorses the sit-at-home message. It's ironical that the meme uses a child who has not obeyed social distancing to ridicule adults confined to staying at home due to COVID-19. Significantly, it applies humor in interpreting children's appreciation of the stay-at-home period, simply because it restricts parents and adults.

The meme highlights some health and social lessons: It is not good to confine children and restrict their plays because, if they don't engage in such activities, it will be difficult to tell when they are sick, especially with those health issues without feverish symptoms. It may adversely affects their social life in later years, especially, in expressing themselves. The grin on the boy's face may be suggestive of two things: that 'what is good for the goose is also good for the gander,' and 'the confinement serves you all well.'

The fourth meme is a picture of a man who built his house at the peak of a very tall tree with a lengthy ladder to serve as a bridge to navigate the distance. At the base of the picture is the inscription 'self-quarantine!' Critically examining the meme, a respondent observes that 'the COVID-19 preventive injunction to observe social distancing in order to avoid Coronavirus infection is taken to a rather ridiculous extreme!' Another respondent aptly observes that 'Humans are social creatures and can hardly take full leave of the earth to avoid infection. It is interesting that the man seeking to take leave of the world has the wisdom to keep a ladder handy!'

The meme illustrates and may be compared to Diala (2019) narrative of the posture of Stylites who sought to avoid the contamination of sin by leaving the world (Fig. 7.1). The picture of a man isolating himself in a house hanging on top of a tree is an 'expression of abnormality,' according to a respondent because the picture is an expression of something highly strange within the African context, because Africans do not build houses on top of trees. It is a graphical discourse of extreme case of quarantine and presents quarantine or self-isolation as the best option at the COVID-19 era. The meme depicts that 'the fear of coronavirus can drive some Africans to the height of insanity, thus people are taking exaggerated steps in observing the simple rules of social distancing.' The imaginable question raised by this is 'how far can I go in order to escape this deadly disease?' As a respondent notes, this is the type of question that will be bordering so many minds until this virus is comprehensively contained. Undoubtedly, people are truly afraid of coronavirus and would do

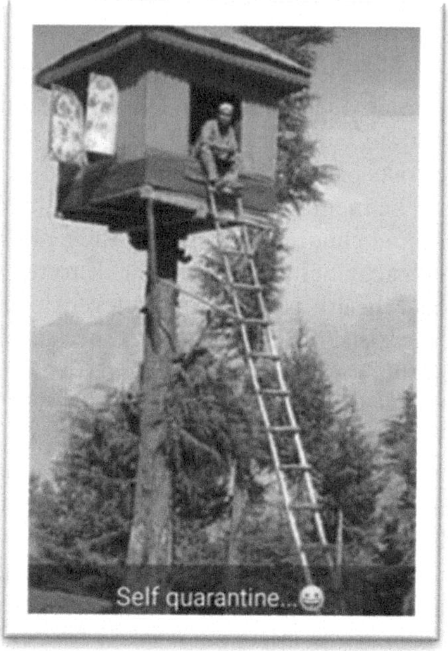

Fig. 7.1 A man distances himself from the society for self-quarantine

anything to survive the pandemic; thus the social message is 'the fear of Corona virus is real,' hence the effectively illustrated social distancing. The picture breaks the 'big' phrase to a level nearly everyone can understand. Equally, it best illustrates the self-isolation or quarantine scope of the government, which leaves everyone simply on one's own. The humor embedded in the picture shows the risk and strange measures taken by the man in order to safeguard his life from the virus.

The next meme presented for this study is a picture of members of a corporate organization standing far apart for a 'staff meeting' taking place outside the office complex with the observance of social distancing. The meme is a very captivating portrait of the present situation of abnormality. The outbreak of COVID-19 has changed dramatically the dynamics of the landscape of social humanity. The lesson of this is quite simple; the basic patterns of our social life have been essentially disrupted and will never be the same again for years to come. A respondent observes that 'the unorthodox staff meeting highlights the impact of social distancing, although what such a meeting can accomplish is doubtful.' It acknowledges that social relationship and interaction is important but requires to be revisited if people must survive the pandemic. The meme highlights the rising challenge of meeting up with the need to contain the challenge of COVID-19 disease. In the opinion of another respondent, it is a 'humorous way of expressing social distancing, and social distancing tremendously reduces the spread rate of the virus when it's applied'; thus, the meme is considered by all to be 'Humorous, apt and appropriate, and passes the message well.' However, another respondent observes that although there is humor in how people implement safety standards, the meme may be 'misleading because there is no indication of how staff will behave after the meeting.' One of the memes was a clear case of social distancing, the meme is a picture of a natural maize stalk with few undeveloped corns spaced out between one another with the inscription, "Even maize is observing social distancing. Please stay safe!" The meme is a classical use of a strange phenomenon in nature to indicate the strangeness of the situation humanity finds itself. All the respondents admit that 'The image is quite apt as a natural expression of what is now expected at the social level of human existence.' In fact, the scourge of the coronavirus pandemic has forced human beings to look at the malformation of things in nature—as a perfect depiction of what humanity is going through with the outbreak of coronavirus.

The rather malformed maize cob provides a graphic illustration of what social distancing should mean for humans. Admittedly, the respondents perceive humor as a consequence of a deliberate misapplication of a term relevant for an infectious disease to an agricultural product. For maize as for humans, the ideal is existence in communities rather than in isolation. John Meyer observes that 'humor in communication is a subject that seems difficult to analyze. After all, if one has to explain a joke, it is probably no longer funny' (Meyer, 2000, 310). The explanation applies to the meme. A respondent observes that 'the corn co-distancing shows aptly how media forms keep expanding; and illustrates that the abstract communication of social distancing is relatable for messages to rural audiences' and exhibits humor by exploring the natural phenomenon. In another meme, a man and a woman (apparently, his wife) were sternly staring at each other with an expression of mutual suspicion and distrust. Below them was an inscription: 'Kizito, who is NCDC and why is she texting you everyday asking you to wash your hands? Answer me now. Who is she? Who is NCDC?' The meme is a classic expression of what many families are going through within the COVID era. COVID-19 brought couples close to monitoring the doings and undoings of their spouses. Even among the happily married couple enjoying a harmonious living, there is always a possibility of mutual suspicion. Ironically, such 'suspicion that lies below the surface in the lives of happily married couples has been raised to its highest level with the erroneous interpretations of the bombardments of text messages brought about by the coronavirus pandemic.' In this meme, Kizito's wife who did not know the meaning of NCDC was suspicious of NCDC's frequent text messages to her husband. She concludes without prompting that NCDC is a 'she,' thus demanding to know why she instructs Kizito to wash his hands daily. 'This is a classic example of the heightening of the case of mutual suspicion among couple.' The meme introduces jealousy, which is such 'a goldmine for the humourist, because it invariably beclouds one's perception and consequently one's interpretation of reality' (Goldstein 1976: 108). Coupled with this fact is also the woman's basic illiteracy, ignorance and naivety. Consequently, 'the ritual hygienic washing of hands to stave off infection assumes a grave sexual connotation. The woman's countenance is truly hilarious!' Goldstein opines that humor is applied to encapsulate communicators' view into memorable phrases and short anecdotes, which results in clarification of meaning. In the meme, 'the Nigerian agency in charge of prevention and control of COVID-19 – (NCDC) is on top of the Corona virus matter, with respect to its bombardment of text messages to Nigerians.' While giving NCDC an important mention for obviously communicating issues of coronavirus to citizens, and creating humor out of Kizito's wife's ignorance, as all the respondents observe, the meme is wasted because the message is empty because it assumes everyone knows who NCDC is. One wonders why the messages kept were not addressed, for instance, disclosing that the messages actually came as a preventative measures by NCDC to protect the people from contacting and spreading the virus. A respondent observes that 'the meme addresses the issue of wrong conclusions and also infidelity in many homes/marriages today.' Cases as the accusation of Kizito's wife may not be ignored as the respondents observe because some rural population may be ignorant as Kizito's wife.

The next meme is a picture of a child in a thoughtful mood expressing concern of being forced to share in something that was brought about by the Chinese. Above the picture of the boy is the inscription, 'Only China chop lizard, frog, snake, and rat. I come dey wash hands for wetin I no follow chop. I tire.' The meme points expressively to the origin of the coronavirus pandemic. In the maze of the pandemic, many people are

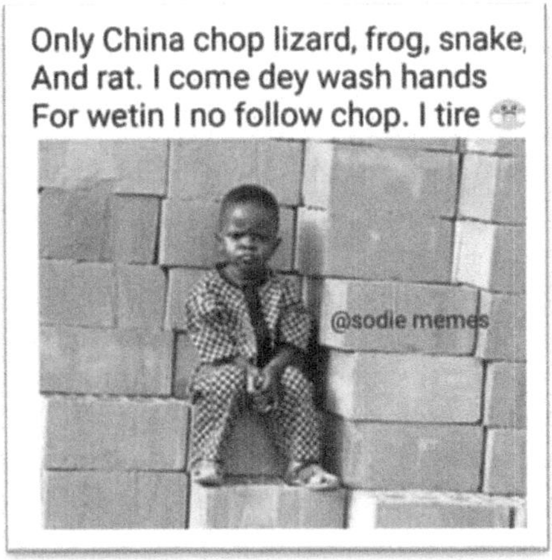

Fig. 7.2 The Child and China Wahala meme

concentrating on the reality of the virus and its effects without thinking about the source of its emergence (Fig.7.2). As one of the respondents observes, 'the meme beckons people to have moments of sober reflections over the entire reality of COVID-19 and learn very good lessons from it, especially, how some of our evil actions affect others in the social landscape of humanity.'

A respondent notes that the meme is 'Quite illustrative of the fact that the world is a village now, and someone's action nearly 5000kms away becomes suffered by a person who has no passport and has never travelled outside the locality.' The weird assortment of assumed Chinese delicacies of lizards, frog, snake and rat eaten as food by Chinese refers to an alleged origin of the coronavirus through a Chinese bat meal in Wuhan. By the indulgence, the world became infected although not partakers in the delicacies. The meme however underscores the fact that 'the global village has a greater proclivity to share liabilities rather than assets.' Another respondent observes that 'China has actually done unthinkable and unimaginable experiments; whether with animals or biological weapons which has put the global community in a "hand washing" paranoia-thus the world is washing hands for the unwholesome deeds of China.' The meme regrets that 'everyone should not be punished for the sins of others, and China should suffer the nemesis of their own actions and habits.' It generates humor by attributing the cause of the corona virus to the uncommon food eaten by the China people. While humor communication with children informs norms delicately by leveling criticisms as Graham et al. (1992) aver, this meme at the same time identifies with the audience.

The ninth meme is on the caricature images of an obese couple who are worried about how to get out of the room after the lockdown. 'The meme thematically focuses on the dire consequences of the coronavirus lockdown.' The respondents admit that the bloated images of the couple results from the lockdown and makes normal life impossible. This is a potent signal of the social difficulties that will emerge as the aftermaths of COVID-19. Indeed the socio-psychological problems created by the coronavirus pandemic will continue to affect the dynamics of social humanity for many years to come. The social message of the meme, according to one respondent, is that 'people should control their appetite and food intake during this period.' And as another respondent observes, 'exercise is necessary.' The humor is derived from the fact that the couple has survived the coronavirus, but is battling with obesity, another health challenge. Undoubtedly, the lockdown order has health implications because it restricts people from going to gyms or workplaces which would automatically serve as an exercise. As a respondent observes, the meme is 'a reminder that if people are not careful with the appetite or eating habits, gaining weight or being obese is imminent.' The meme is explicit and easy to understand. A respondent admits that the meme offers two lessons: 'One is the anticipated self-quarantine as a recipe for staying safe; and weight gain from excessive feeding and little or no physical activities as measure for avoiding COVID-19 infection.' All respondents admit that the meme passes the messages graphically and appropriately.

In the last meme, a quote was written referring to the existence of quarantine in the Bible, with an extract from Isaiah 26 verse 20. It reads, 'Go home, my people, and lock your doors! Hide yourselves for a little while until the Lord's anger has passed.' The quote ends with a smiling emoji. The meme provides a 'religious interpretation of the pandemic as a consequence of God's anger.' According to a respondent, the meme suggests that 'God is aware of the virus.' In another reading, a respondent affirms that 'The social message is that Divinity approves the lockdown.' While a respondent queries, 'Please, who says this is funny? I can't see why this is considered humorous!' and another observes that 'the message is heavy on exclusion,' yet another respondent opines that 'The humor is in the fact that there is a biblical back up to everything that happens on this planet, even Corona virus.' COVID-19 symptoms of diseases, ailments and so on are inadvertently signs of the *Lord's anger*. This is linked to

Africans' deep connection to religious beliefs. The respondent links the coincidence of the duration of the federal lockdown for 40 days and the biblical 40 days and 40 night connotations. Another respondent observes that 'there are two sides to the meme – serious matter and a joke. For the over religious, it makes quarantine biblical but I think in the most part it is a joke playing on a Bible verse.' The meme thus portrays Africans' penchant for attaching spiritual meaning to almost all human predicaments.

Discussion and Conclusion

In investigating humor in the memes, one needs to seek for what Reyes et al. (2012) term, 'the presence of amusing effects, such as laughter or well-being sensation.' However, many scholars believe that these effects can only be traced to the humor types. Martins et al. (2003) identified four styles which may be used to identify humor. These include self-enhancing, affiliative, self-defeating and aggressive humor. Affiliative humor involves the use of funny things, jokes and witty banter to devise humor. The meme on malformed maize is a good example of affiliative humor including the one on politicians and their mistresses because they involve the use of natural seed in making fun while addressing an important COVID-19 issue. Self-enhancing humor, according to Taecharungroj and Nueanjamnong (2015), involves amusing people through incongruities and maintaining a humorous perspective even in adversity. Consequently, memes like those with children expressing their opinion on COVID-19 predicaments aptly share self-enhancing humor, whereas the memes on the obese couple and the politicians and their mistresses may be classified as self-defeating humor. Catanescu and Tom (2001) however listed seven types of humor often used in the broadcast and print media, which aptly suits the social media. These include comparison, personification, exaggeration, pun, sarcasm, silliness and surprise. Taecharungroj and Nueanjamnong observe that 'silliness memes usually have funny faces or behaivours on the subjects in the memes.' Practically, most of the memes used in this study fall within these types. For instance, the children's memes fit into the silliness type of humor with the ridiculously funny expressions on the faces of the young boys used in the memes. The memes on self-quarantine on a house on top of a tree, staff meeting and malformed maize are various forms of exaggeration designed to generate laughter and fun while subtly opening conversation on COVID-19. The Biblical quotation on social distance is surprising likewise the meme on politicians and their mistresses. The use of 'coronically' in the meme about coughing uses pun to share humor. By sharing various forms of humorous attributes, one may argue that the memes are indeed humorous, although still critical about the coronavirus pandemic and its effect within Africa.

However, by using humor in the discourse of coronavirus, the originators of the memes adopt relief theory in their communication by allowing 'laughter operate like a safety valve in a steam pipe, (which) releases built up nervous energy' (Morreall, 2009). Consequently, what each participant reads from the memes are ideas designed to subtly control the fears, pains and anxieties generated by the coronavirus pandemic. Those communications thus provide opportunity for new meaning making out of the memes.

The emergent memes circulating among African social media users reflect socio-cultural and environmental issues and ideologies facing Africans. They are new and contemporary means of expression and communication; thus they are used to share feelings which overwhelm the originators. These memes share varieties of public emotions influenced by the COVID-19 pandemic. As social concepts and development, humor and pains are related. People may feel pain without suffering (Lorena Antonovici, 2015). The memes are mainly humorous because people need to laugh in order to reduce physiological tension from time to time (Berlyne, 1972). The humour memes are therefore new forms of communication for controlling the pains and apprehensive feelings derived from the coronavirus pandemic. Whereas coronavirus in Africa remains a scary healthy challenge; the coronavirus-induced humor memes confront public fears, apprehensions and difficult conditions induced by the disease and provide the public with a window of relief. The disadvantage is in its escapist role. The memes encourage Africans to see the health challenge from another perspective and to adjust to fate, while accepting difficult life situations as 'fun' and joke which come with lessons.

References

Antonovici, L. (2015). A theory of humor. In *Discourse as a form of multiculturalism in literature and communication* (pp. 417–430). Arhipelag XXI Press.

Bergmann, C., Thomas, L. E., & Stohlman, S. A. (2006). Coronavirus infection of the central nervous system: Host-virus stand-off. *Nature Reviews and Microbiology, 4*, 121–132.

Berlyne, D. E. (1972). Humor and its kin. In J. H. Goldstein & P. E. McGhee (Eds.), *The psychology of humor* (pp. 43–60). Academic.

Bosely, S. (2020). Lockdown can't end until COVID-19 vaccine is found, study say. *The Guardian*. London, 8 April 2020.

Braun, V., & Clarke, V. (2006). Using thematic analysis in psychology. *Qualitative Research in Psychology, 3*(2), 77–101.

Catanescu, C., & Tom, G. (2001). Types of humor in television and magazine advertising. *Review of Business-Saint John's University, 22*(1), 92–95.

CDC COVID-19 Response Team. (2020, February12–April 2). Coronavirus disease 2019 in children-United States. *Morbidity and Mortality Weekly Report (MMWR) Early Release, 69*. April. 1–6.

Diala, I. (2019). Dionysius, Christ, Agwu and the African Writer. In *23rd Inaugural Lecture*. Imo State University.

Duncan, H. D. (1962). *Communication and social order*. Bedminster Press.

Fielding, B. (2020). Africa: A brief history of the coronavirus family – Including one pandemic we might have missed. https://allafrica.com/stories/202003250027.html. Accessed 16 Apr 2020.

Goldstein, J. H. (1976). Theoretical notes on humor. *The Journal of Communication, 26*(3), 104–112.

Graham, E. E., Papa, M. J., & Brooks, G. P. (1992). Functions of humor in conversation: Conceptulization and measurement. *Western Journal of Communication, 56*, 161–183.

Hine, C. (2008). *Ethnography for the Internet: Embedded, embodied and everyday*. Bloombury Academic.

Kalu, B. (2020). The COVID-19 in Nigeria: A disease of hunger. *Lancet Spotlight., 8*(6), 556–557.

Krikmann, A. (2006). *Contemporary linguistic theories of humour*. http://www.folklore.ee/folklore/vol33/kriku.pdf. https://doi.org/10.7592/FEJF2006.33.krikum

Martin, R. A., Publik-Doris, P., Larsen, G. J., & Weir, K. (2003). Individual differences is uses of humor and their relation to psychological well-being: Development of the humor styles questionnaire. *Journal of Research in Personality, 37*(1), 48–75.

Meyer, J. C. (2000). Humor as a double-edged sword: Four functions of humor in communication. *Communication Theory, 10*(3), 310–331.

McCreadie, M., & Wiggins, S. (2007). The purpose and function of humour in health, healthcare and nursing: A narrative review. *Journal of Advanced Nursing, 61*(6), 548–595.

Morreall, J. (2009). Humor as a cognitive play. *Journal of Literary Theory., 3*(2), 241–260.

Murthy, D. (2008). Digital ethnography: An examination of the use of new technologies in social research. *Sociology, 42*(5), 837–855.

NCDC. (2020). *About NCDC*. https://ncdc.gov.ng/ncdc. Accessed 14 Apr 2020.

Potter, J. (1996). Discourse analysis and constructionist approaches: Theoretical background. In John T. E. Richardson (Ed.). *Handbook of qualitative research methods for psychology and social sciences.* BPS Books.

Reyes, A., Rosso, P., & Buscaldi, D. (2012). From humor recognition to irony detention: The figurative language of social media. *Data & Knowledge Engineering, 74*, 1–12.

Simmons, M. P., Adamic, L. A., & Adar, E. (2011). Memes online: Extracted, subtracted, injected, recollected. *AAAI Weblogs.* https://www.aaai.org

Taecherungroj, V., & Nueangjamnong, P. (2015). Humor 2.0: Styles and types of humour and virality of memes on Favebook. *Journal of Creative Communication.* https://doi.org/10.1177/0973258615614420

Varis, P., & Blommaert, J. (2015). Conviviality and collectives on social media: Virality, memes and social structures. *Multilingual Margin, 2*(1), 31–45.

Wang, Y., Wang, S., Tang, J., Liu, H., & Li, B. (2015). Unsupervised sentiment analysis for social media images. In *Proceedings of the twenty-fourth international joint conference on artificial intelligence (IJCAI, 2015)* (pp. 2378–2379).

PART II

Gender, Race and Family: Identity Politics in the Pandemic

CHAPTER 8

Coronavirus Satire: A Dissection of Feminist Politics and Humour

Millie Phiri

Introduction

What can we make of the humour that Felistas Chido Murata showcases on her Facebook page, Mai Ts Diaries, under the coronavirus pandemic in Zimbabwe? This chapter examines the period from March 2020 when the hard lockdown measures to manage the COVID-19 were imposed in Zimbabwe to December 2020, a time when African countries began to worry about the second wave and variants of the disease. Feminist humour is a recent phenomenon in this economically ravaged country of 14 million people where the masculinisation of the coronavirus disease has resulted in the feminisation of poverty. Felistas' humour replaces the notion that places women as only target of jokes and as receivers of male-framed comedy. It is a counter to hegemonic masculinity media spaces that fail to consider the needs of women in society. Her humour is also a disruption to masculine ways of appropriating knowledge that we have been accustomed to.

Murata, who is known as Mai Tt, is an award-winning comedian born in Mufakose, a black township in Zimbabwe's Harare capital. It is

M. Phiri (✉)
University of Johannesburg, Johannesburg, South Africa

S. Mpofu (ed.), *Digital Humour in the Covid-19 Pandemic*,
https://doi.org/10.1007/978-3-030-79279-4_8

common to use Mai as an epithet for a woman with children and to accompany it by the name of the first-born child, which is why she is known as Mai Tt, short for Mai Titi. This is commonly a sign of respect for women in Zimbabwe cultures. Mai Tt also represents black township women who are an alienated group because they undergo various levels of suffering that include water and food shortages, lack of health access and unemployment (Kubatana, 2020); yet, their voices are often not heard in the media or in the political space. She is also an epitome of women born and bred in townships, many of whom have grown up without the hope of ever making it given that Zimbabwe has been experiencing hardships since 2000 after its controversial land invasions that resulted in economic damage. Some of these women have since emigrated where they mainly work in agriculture, construction, domestic work and service industry (Forced Migration Studies Programme, 2009). In her Facebook posts, Murata often calls herself an "advocate", 'born-again Christian", "preacher" and "single mother", although at the time of writing she had remarried, further giving hope to single women that marriage is possible after divorce. Social media journalists commenting on her page describe her as inspiring, motivational, powerful, talented, fun, heavenly, teacher, multi-talented and Zimbabwe's Brenda Fassie, among other attributes. The late Brenda Fassie was a South African musical icon.

Secondly, her humour shows us that the lines between the public and the private realms, the social and the domestic, the personal and the political and the visible and invisible are blurred. Mai Tt's humour reveals how intimacy is political and also raises taboo subjects such as division of household chores among married couples and the controversial subject of violence against women and religion. She touches on how Zimbabwean men weaponise coronavirus to retain hold of patriarchal power in the household and perpetuates the concept of small houses, a Zimbabwean term describing men who have secret or unofficial wives or girlfriends (Muchabaiwa, 2018). The chapter further argues that humour and social media in Zimbabwe are helping women to chart a new identity trajectory that is shifting the representation of women and their issues in the media. Mai Tt's humour is not just comic but a discourse that helps women to connect with other "real women with real problems" who use social media as a place to air their views and get moral support, solidarity, help, counselling and advise on a wide array of issues that women would not ordinarily speak in public. This is central to the articulation of black feminism. Black feminism adds the black female voice into the dominant discourses. It helps capture—in a nuanced way—the realities and cultures specific to black women (Phiri, 2019).

Feminist humour portrays women as an empowered group. It promotes the idea of black *sisterhood* which is important in healing fractures and division. It is divide-and-rule tactics, after all, that exacerbate the abuse of African/black women. Black feminism is by no means homogenous, neither are black women's experiences of oppression monolithic. There is constant rewriting of feminism itself because it is never static or fixed. It is contextual and culturally specific. I chose it as a lens to frame feminist humour in this chapter so that I have a theoretical starting point and coherence without which the field of feminism becomes a conceptual jungle. The theory also serves to accommodate as much of the black female experience as possible.

Findings reveal that if humour is a form of communication and a statement about our surroundings, Mai Tt risks losing identity with her audience in the long run. She understands how women feel, and she is viewed as a champion for women and children. She is an inspiration and symbol for women who suffer adversity. Her ability to joke her pain away kindles hope in many women who feel like giving up. It is cathartic for her as much as to her dominant female audience who go through what she has experienced, but in doing so she lets out her dark side that leads to misogyny and hate speech. Hate speech is one of the main reasons why some women do not participate on social media.

The chapter will show that, sadly, this humour is also at times coloured with misinformation that comes with infodemic common during pandemics. The danger about falsehoods is that they are 70 percent more likely to be shared than accurate news (Kincaid & Pattison, 2020). They outperform the truth on every subject and travel "further, faster, and deeper". This is a conundrum considering Mai Tt's page has over 600,000 online subscribers scattered globally, and as evidence shows, her posts are shared more than other popular female comedians in the country who are also using Facebook as a tool to disseminate humour.

Theoretical and Conceptual Framework

The terms humour, laughter and comedy are used interchangeably in this chapter, although there is recognition that laughter is the physical action that often, but not necessarily, arises in response to humour. According to Lockyer and Pickering (2009) humour is one of the most pervasive elements of public culture and a central aspect of everyday life that is "obligatory", "ideological" and a "persistent desire" (Billig, 2009, 13).

Humour is under-investigated in Africa according to Källstig (2020) who wrote about Zimbabwe stand-up comedy. This is a paradox considering that humour is a resistance tactic to elite and dominant power (Obadare, 2016). The role of feminism is to help saturate society with constructive feminist frames such as what this chapter attempts to do. Her jokes are a social critique. For example, by being laughed at, institutions lose their perceived power. Segal and Demos (2019) talk of agency-affirming places which women use to "talk back" or express anger over injustices they experience, and Mai Tt's Facebook page can be classified as such. Social media is one of those places where women have become free to express their views about hard-to-discuss topics such as the ones which Murata addresses in her humorous skits pertaining to coronavirus on her Facebook Fan page. Segal and Demos (2019) also refer to overtly hostile or agency-denying places that deny women free speech. Social media can also be that place because of its misogynistic nature. Generally, it has been extraordinarily difficult for women to construct their identities in the mainstream media, for example, despite that it plays a critical role in information dissemination and is influential in shaping individual knowledge, attitudes and behaviours. Despite its misogyny nature, social media, unlike traditional media, helps to disrupt and reframe women's issues as we shall see with Mai Tt's feminist humour during the COVID-19 pandemic.

Since 2016, female comedians in Zimbabwe have been gaining popularity due to social media (Minjenjema & Mazvarirwofa, 2017). Whereas statistics on social media usage in Africa are not readily available, Facebook reports indicate that Facebook interactions increased up to 70 percent more in the USA since the coronavirus pandemic started. Globally before the crisis, billions spent most of their time on social media, with Facebook alone getting 1.6 billion daily log ins, 134 million were spending time on Twitter and a billion hours of video a day were being watched on YouTube (Schultz & Parikh, 2020). Murata's Facebook fan page was opened in 2016 and had over 600,000 subscribers at the time of writing.

Female comedians worth mentioning in Zimbabwe are Samantha Kureya, popularly known as "Gonyeti", and Tyra Chikocho, who is called "Madam Boss" by her fans. Kureya is popular for stand-up comedy and is acclaimed for focusing on topical political issues, while Chikocho specialises on online skits on trending issues in Zimbabwe on her Facebook page. Källstig (2020) describes the female comedians in Zimbabwe as rebellious artists taking up the comedy space to express themselves. This is despite Zimbabwe's perilous political space that wants to silence them. The framing of humour by female comedians now competes with the patriarchal dominant frames that control the narratives in the Zimbabwean society. Some of these frames are harmful to women. Ndlovu and Ngwenya (2010), while reviewing public transport stickers for humour, discovered that they depicted negative stereotypes about women and were more derogatory towards them than towards men, which made women vulnerable to violence against them. Female comedians in Zimbabwe have found themselves in trouble for mocking the proviledge. In August 2019, Kureya was beaten up and abducted for her critical skits of the police and the government (BBC, 2019). Social media is thus a meeting point of power, agency and oppression (Davies & Ilott, 2018).

Historically, humour in Zimbabwe has been used to test the openness, accessibility and riskiness of sensitive issues, as described by Lang and Lee (2010). The study of humour and particularly of how women are reflected is underexplored generally. This is where black feminism becomes meaningful because it considers how black women see the world. This is important because it is not enough to imagine empowerment for black women in isolation from deepseated changes in the overall social structure (Hill Collins, 2004). In this chapter we explore how humour represents black women's experiences and issues that affected them during the coronavirus pandemic. Subjecting humour to a feminist analysis helps to view humour from a unique and different perspective from that of the traditional male gaze.

We know through the theory of Superiority founded by Thomas Hubbes that humour is generated when there is a sudden realisation of supremacy with respect to another person or situation. Humour is a site of ridicule that serves to reaffirm existing structures of power and ways of being (Holm, 2017). Humour styles associated with the Superiority Theory are, among others, ridicule, teasing and sarcasm. Representation in comedy thus matters because that is where power relations are confirmed, negotiated or undermined (Szutenberg, 2012). How characters are represented structures the audiences' responses—to laugh with or laugh at them (Davies & Ilott, 2018). This theory taps on our emotional side. Mai Tt's humour touches on the masculinisation and weaponisation of coronavirus that resulted in feminised poverty and worsened the small house problem in Zimbabwe. It also portrays sexual feminist humour as an important part of feminist politics that is essential and that can no longer remain a taboo topic which cannot be discussed.

Historically, humour in Zimbabwe objectifies women as sex tools, evil, liars, gold diggers, own worst enemies, talkative, cheats, troublesome, stupid, jealous, gossipers, among other negative stereotypes (Ncube, 2020). According to Chambers (2005), feminist discourse is a system of representation that challenges these sexual objectifications and subordination of women which is what this chapter is about.

For its part, the incongruity theory views humour as a substitute of an unexpected event or remark because it is something that they are not accustomed to in their world, and so it fails to match their expectations (Davies & Ilott, 2018). The incongruity touches on the cognition side because you need to have the capacity to understand the differences and what part makes the joke. This includes the fact that rumour is also cultural and contextual. For example, knowing the language and culture is critical to understanding a joke (Davies & Ilott, 2018). Humour is a way of thinking which impinges upon representation. The coronavirus came at a time when Zimbabwe was experiencing harsh sociopolitical and economic problems. Humour as politics is concerned with understanding of contemporary society. It often exposes "foolishness" or "hypocrisy" of politicians and powerful public figures or highlights serious social issues such as religion and crime, and we see this on Mai Tt's Facebook fan page. It offers an effective way to critique entrenched values about identity politics and social power inequalities as we shall see when we analyse Mai Tt's sexual humour.

Then there is the relief or release theory which is laughter released as a form of nervous energy.

According to Freud (1960, 103), laughter at taboo subjects matter because it reveals a lot about a particular society's "constructs, its boundaries, rules and taboos". Davies and Ilott (2018) also let us know that when it comes to comedy and humour, "the political becomes personal". For example, the many issues that Mai Tt raises in her comedy such as husbands who use coronavirus as a tool for infidelity; sexual complications that couples face and which are exacerbated by the fact that under the lockdown, couples were forced to stay under one roof; and the issue of poverty. These are real issues that women in Zimbabwe faced as a result of the political decisions taken under the COVID-19 regulations. Lockdown regulations did not take into consideration that not all homes are safe for women; challenges such as access to reproductive health services; lack of water services; the informal sector in which many Zimbabwean women draw their livelihood from; and shortages of basic commodities (Kubatana, 2020).

Although humour in comedy reflects a society's norms and values, it has the potential to reconstruct social identities as Mai Tt's humour does. That is why women's comedy plays a crucial role in paying attention to the ideologies being perpetuated by the humour we laugh at. Humour is also contagious because it has the capacity to spread, especially via social media.

Methodology

I used a Facebook tool called CrowdTangle to gather data and analysed Mai Tt's humour on coronavirus. I searched for the words coronavirus, corona, COVID19, COVID, quarantine, lockdown, pandemic and "mbutu". According to the Shona dictionary, mbutu is a pet name for a cat, also an endearing name for a girl, but in this case this word refers to "pussy" or the female sex organ (vagina). It is included in the search as part of Mai Tt's coronavirus humour because what starts as humour by Mai Tt on whether or not people should have sex during the COVID-19 pandemic results in women opening up about marriage and sex relationship problems.

I decided on reviewing a 12-month period, although the actual period analysed is from March when Zimbabwe recorded its first COVID-19 case to December 2020. The 12–month period is chosen because CrowdTangle search options are 60 minutes, 3 hours, 12 hours, 24 hours, three days, one month, last 12 months and custom. I opted for the longest period so I may have more information. I searched photos, links, statuses, Facebook videos, Facebook live sessions, other videos including those shared on YouTube and a host of mixed bag messages that included talks on coronavirus.

CrowdTangle is a Facebook public insights tool that helps to show activities happening across social media. It makes content from public pages "more discoverable" and engagement data on that content—shares, views, comments and reactions—easy to sort through (Fraser, 2020). It is used to track all public Facebook pages, verified profiles and groups with more than 100 k likes. Mai Ts Diaries is a verified public page which had 344,753 likes by December 05, 2020. The CrowdTangle tool helps one to see how much a post has been commented on, the shares and clicks on Facebook's reaction buttons such as love, wow, haha, said, angry, care.

However, the limitation of CrowdTangle is that it does not show the content from followers due to privacy reasons. To deal with this shortcoming, I used posts generated by CrowdTangle to go on the actual Mai Ts Diaries to conduct a qualitative netnography exercise, manually scrolling for public comments about the posts in question. The other limitation is the fact that certain classes of women often miss out on conversations on Facebook platforms such as Mai Tt's because of lack of access to the Internet and high cost of data packs and smart devices in a country where unemployment is almost 90 percent, with food shortages and lack of medicines (Kubatana, 2020).

Reconstructing Feminist Politics Humour in Zimbabwe

Total interactions about coronavirus-related humour on Mai Tt's Facebook fan page on topics mentioned in the methodology were 394,464 in 87 posts over a 12-month period, although coronavirus pandemic started to peak in mid-March 2020. This is when Zimbabwe recorded its first COVID-19 case and announced its first hard lockdown measures to manage the pandemic. There was again a peak in April after which the lockdown measures were extended, followed by another peak in June when Zimbabwe tightened the coronavirus lockdown regulations as the number of cases increased. We saw the peak again in July after which another curfew was imposed (Moyo, 2020) (Figs. 8.1 and 8.2).

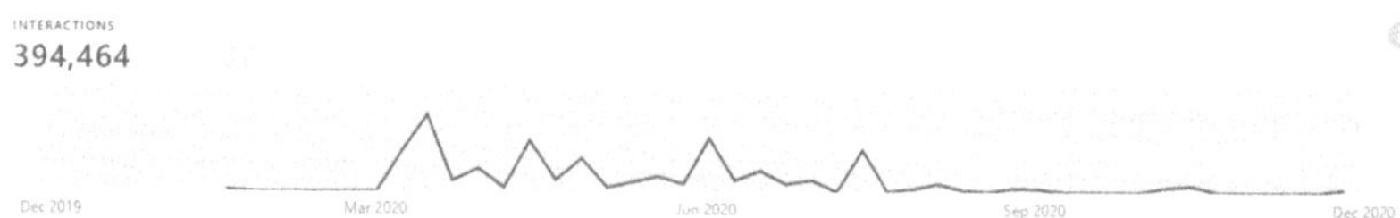

Fig. 8.1 Showing total interactions regarding the coronavirus pandemic on Mai Tt's Facebook Fan page. (Source: CrowdTangle)

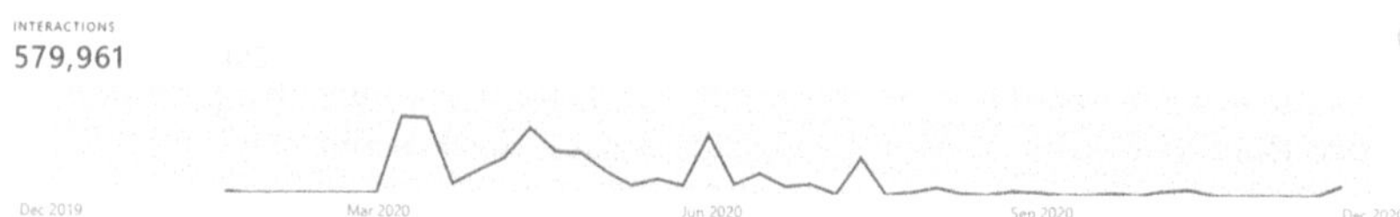

Fig. 8.2 Showing total interactions regarding coronavirus pandemic conversations on Mai Tt's, Madam Boss's and Gonyeti aka Samantha Kureya's Facebook pages. (Source: CrowdTangle)

I also conducted a combined search that included Mai Tt's Facebook page and female comedians, Chikocho and Kureya, using the same search words mentioned earlier, but taking out the word "mbutu" which is unique only to Mai Tt. The results reveal there were 579,961 interactions for 113 coronavirus-related posts in the same period. This indicates that Mai Tt commands by far more following and interactions. It was Mai Tt who seemed to directly address women's issues, particularly about sex, female singlehood and small houses. Not many results appeared for Kureya who is a stand-up comedian; Mai Tt and Madam Boss concentrate on online comedy. Mai Tt's humour is laced with dance, fashion, song, live talk shows, prayer and acting. Dancing and laughing at struggles is considered a feminised way of coping with adversity. Her acting makes her appealing to people who do not understand the Shona language she frequently uses in her jokes. For example, one commenter says, "I love this lady", referring to Mai Tt, then she puts the love emoji. The commenter further praises Mai Tt, highlighting that although she does not understand Shona, "the messages is there for everyone". Another one remarks that without Mai Tt, Facebook is "boring". Mai Tt's use of the Shona language and sometimes broken Ndebele, spoken north of the country, seem to help convey meanings to a wider audience and promote more dialogue.

In addition, I also conducted an intelligence research looking at all Facebook posts for the three female comedians including Mai Tt's over a 12-month period. The statistic confirms that Mai Tt by far out-performs other female comedians as she accounts for over 11 million interactions out of a combined total of 17.13 million.

Generally, Mai Tt draws a lot of content from her own experience, which makes her humour relatable, believable and a mirror of reality. She uses humour to either convey hard truth to the authorities or make fun of them. She uses the imaginary phone call talk, perhaps a suggestion that authorities should establish a way to communicate with ordinary women about issues that affect them before making decisions that impact them. Her Facebook page is a place where her audience discuss sensitive taboo subjects and where they find their own solutions, adding to indigenous feminist knowledge. Mai Tt's audience is mostly women, at least judging from the responses she gets, and most of her butts are cheating husbands and occasionally political figures. A butt is the focus of the joke, that is, the person who is made fun of (Davies & Ilott, 2018). Mai Tt's jokes fall into various forms such as narrative, satire and comic monologues. She focuses more on sexual humour and single women. Humour regarding coronavirus on Mai Ts Diaries can thus be thematised into the political and socio-economic issue groups; these include failings of political leaders; social issues and taboos such as sex, single women and small houses; the economic impact of the disease; and the health messaging and misinformation theme in which the jokes contain misinformation about the disease.

What Is Personal Is Political

By far the post that got the most comments (4670) and shares (10387) focused on Mai Tt joking on how coronavirus creates family time, which was previously almost nonexistent in most homes, resulting in couples having to share household chores. Household chores are femininised in Zimbabwe, and Mai Tt challenges this status quo by portraying household chores as gender-neutral. The home is part of the private realm. Feminist politics argues that the public realm is characterised by activities such as paid work and travel. In a broader framework, it includes enjoying rights of full citizenship and exercising political and democratic rights (Phiri, 2019). On the other hand, the private realm consists of anything that man demarcates as woman's natural space. This includes child-bearing, satisfying male conjugal needs, motherhood and domestic labour. Here the feminine is perceived as private and removed from politics (Pateman, 1989). Sharing of household chores is a controversial subject in Zimbabwe's culture where masculinity places emphasis on the public realm where men are viewed as breadwinners and heads of the homes. Mai Tt laughs at this patriarchal system that is blamed for the "small houses" syndrome in Zimbabwe. The following humorous prayer is politically loaded. It depicts Zimbabwe's failed political patriarchal system responsible for the shortages the country experiences and how this permeates into homes. She laments:

> We know that quarantine is not good but we know that it is to our advantage the main houses. We know our husbands are not happy, they are very angry…but father you did it for a reason so that we can spend time together. Even if we are not talking, we want to thank you…no more small houses, no more excuses, lies, no more fuel queues.

Even though the husband is just sitting on the sofa like a "bulldog", Mai Tt says, "we are at least happy our husbands are home". Phiri (2019) notes that the bull is the manifestation of masculinity par excellence. As a symbol, it expresses the display of blind male machismo and masculine virility. Bulls do not see or care when they hurt females, and at the same time, they justify it as being part of their nature. In the skit, Mai Tt demystifies the notion that the home is not personal or private, but is political and public. She ends the skit by instructing the husband to help with the laundry and the ironing. Mai Tt is deconstructing gender roles and making culturally taboo subjects that are deemed private, public. Her humour confirms (Davies & Ilott, 2018) assertions that humour brings out what is personal into the public realm.

Sexual Humour and Singlehood

Mai Tt reshapes the lives of single women through comedy by addressing taboo topics such as sex, dating and single parenthood. Issues of independence and sexuality of single women are hardly talked about in Zimbabwe except in dirty jokes. Chambers (2005), who addresses comedies of sexual morality and female singlehood, notes that single women are generally targeted in comedies as a "source of profound pleasure for audiences" (p.162). Being single and having sexual independence is synonymous to being a "slut" (Chambers, 2005, p. 171). Mai Tt is changing the narrative of single women to "carve out an identity that transcends the conventional married, domestic role", as Chambers put it. As Mai Tt rightly points out in her humour, traditionally, single divorced women in Zimbabwe are stigmatised and often blamed for marriage breakdowns and for a variety of reasons such as miscarriages, failure to bear children, failure to satisfy her partner in bed, lack of cooking skills, not able to perform household chores to the satisfaction of men and failure to treat the husband's relatives well because when a woman is married, she marries her husband's whole community. While there is a lot of focus on single women, the single status of men is largely uncontested unless it is in the context of post-divorce or mid-life crisis.

Singleness is frowned in the Zimbabwe culture where marriage is associated with stableness. Mai Tt helps to remove the anxieties and uneasiness associated with the state of being unmarried. Her jokes are a challenge to patriarchal discourses that portray single women as deviances who break social rules and transgress cultural boundaries according to Chambers

(2005). Single women are often portrayed by society as sad, lonely and socially subordinated. Mai Tt, who lived a single life for a long time before her December 2020 marriage, has been criticised before for being in a relationship with a younger man and mocked for her HIV status she publicly speaks about.

To address the matter of singlehood and sex, she started a live show which she calls "mbutu station" that in a funny way tackles topics which are often not talked about publicly in the Zimbabwe culture, such as small houses, sex problems, sex styles, oral sex, premature ejaculation, threesome, how women can seduce their own husbands/partners so that they do not go to small houses and how to coexist with small houses. The station also discussed whether one can contract the coronavirus if they have sex. Naming it "mbutu" instead of "vagina" as that is what the show is about would be culturally incorrect and offend her audience. When she started the show, she announced on her Facebook page status:

> So, I noticed a lot of couples are in a lot of disagreements in their relationships. Especially sex wise. These issues are very hard for a lot to discuss even in churches, sexual guidance is not given properly There is absolutely nothing wrong in discussing such topics because a lot of people are breaking up. So, I decided to do a program called Mbutu FM where couples come through and we all participate.

Although mbutu itself sounds stereotypical because it means "pussy", "cat" and "girl", Mai Tt uses it to address sexual taboos in a way that is not explicitly offending. Comedians strive to use humour that is culturally acceptable and appropriate.

Not only is Mai Tt's humour a form of resistance to male oppression but it helps in the construction of new feminist identities in both empowering and weakening ways. It is empowering because sexual humour is part of feminist politics that promotes free will for women which helps them make informed choices about their sexual and reproductive health and saves lives. Mai Tt uses the stereotyped notion that women are sex tools to their favour. For example, Mai Tt shares tips on how to sexually satisfy men, for example, what to wear and trending sex positions. This is important because the inability to negotiate safe sex results in women traditionally contracting sexually transmitted diseases such as HIV at higher rates than men. This humour is didactic because it imparts what may be considered by many women as life lessons. Mai Tt pursues a narrative that sex must be a terrain for negotiation, not a site for struggle. To illustrate the popularity of Mbutu station, she boasted on her Facebook status:

> I must say since we started this live stream it has received overwhelming reviews, sometimes we reach up to 3 k viewers on live meaning it's a very interesting topic.

Her Facebook page serves as a townhall where women lay their fears and anxieties, to be empowered not only through Mai Tt but through others on the forum. For example, a married woman shares that her husband is demanding a threesome, which is when a man has sex with two women, or vice versa. Although the advice from the audience on the platform is an overwhelmingly a "no, no", it is also made clear to the woman in question that after weighing the advice she receives, the final say on whether or not to keep the marriage lies with her. This just goes to prove how black feminism is evolving and cutting through cultural barriers to empower black women. Social media is helping women by showing them that feminism can break what is considered culturally sensitive and taboo and that they have choices and rights. Her humour delves into real-life issues of women, and by doing so Mai Tt's Facebook page takes the place of the social places that were traditionally used to crack jokes in Zimbabwe such as the time when women planted or harvested crops in the fields, at the well when fetching water or gathering firewood for cooking and at traditional ceremonies or other places where women gathered. But with modernisation and migration into cities, these traditional spaces are dwindling for black women, only to be revived by social media. Even with social media there is the problem of access to data and affordability of smart devices, so a majority of black women are still left out of online conversations.

However, Mai Tt's narrative is weakened through the trepidation of culture she often advances in her live humour shows that expects women to be the ones to put more work to prove their sex skills to their partners and keep their marriages working. The sex skills are viewed as a strategy to stop the so-called small houses, but do they? Writing from a sociological point of view, Muchabaiwa (2018) discovers that small house households are part of deeply entrenched patriarchal hegemony and are mired in problems that include GBV and financial constraints, among others. While Mai Tt teaches women self-respect and to exercise open-mindedness towards some unconventional methods of sex such as oral sex, these are not a panacea until hegemonic masculinity is eradicated. The skit in which Mai Tt uses a ruler to measure social distance in bed with her husband is an illustration of the patriarch/masculinity power relations that still exist between men and women. Controlling women's sexuality and reproduction is actually the heart of the patriarchy (Jaenes & Marques, 2019, 0:38:16–0:38:22) in the Netflix documentary about feminism called *What the f*is going on?*. Men have never accepted women setting limits for them. Their mentality is: "You don't want to sleep with me? I will find a whore" (Jaenes & Marques, 2019, 0:38:37). Mai Tt's skit is also mirroring the marital realities of couples who are distanced in real life and hardly have intimacy.

As Davies and Ilott (2018) say, it is not only the personal which is political when it comes to humour but the private runs the risk of becoming public as well. We see Mai Tt opening her personal life to her fans and vice versa. She uses confession humour where she discloses on some of her mistakes, highs and lows in her love life in a hilarious way. According to Chambers (2005), places such as Mai Ts Diaries do not only become spaces of women's hystericalisation but they are also spaces of feminist politics because they expose taboos, confer solidarity between women and debunk traditional narratives of sex and intimacy narratives such as the ones Mai Tt raises.

On the other hand, her jokes may be viewed as problematic by those who consider prostitution as their right, in that she castigates women who have sex with married men and advocates abstinence which is easier said than done. Singlehood has no easy answers but is an ever-changing terrain that women would need to constantly negotiate with. After all, feminism is not homogenous. While Mai Tt's humour is liberating for women, it also poses complications for sexual independence. It, however, disrupts traditional patriarchal discourses on femininity and singleness. This humour would be impossible were it not for social media that allows people to listen or watch it in their own privacy using their smart phones or other devices. The number of shares and comments attests to the attention the humour attracts (see Fig. 8.3).

Ridiculing Political Power

On the political front, Mai Tt uses skits to mock the privilege or those in the position of power. She utilises euphemistic humour where she exposes the truth that would not otherwise be discussed out there. For example,

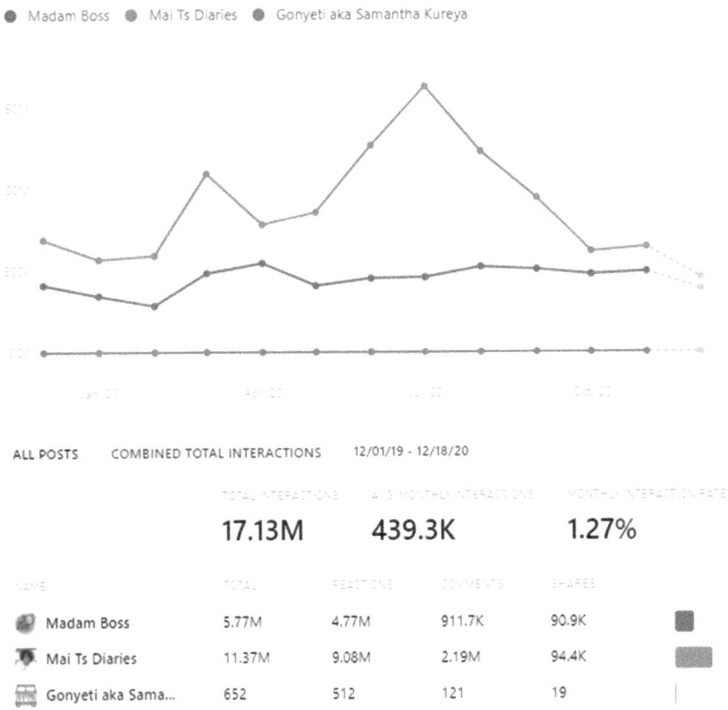

Fig. 8.3 CrowdTangle Intelligence report that compares account performance of activities of the three female comedians on all posts on their Facebook fan pages over a 12-month period from January 2020. (Source: CrowdTangle)

she mocks or laughs at politicians, and in one skit she addresses them as "stupid people" where she questions why the disease is named after a "crown", which means corona in the Shona language. Names of disasters such as cyclones are usually femininised. Mai Tt laughs off at world political figures for feminising disasters. She rejects this representation of women and makes fun of the coronavirus describing it as "evil corona". In a phone call to a politician, she demands to know why the disease is known by that name and orders that person to advise the president to change it.

> How can you crown an evil thing. You cannot just wake up to crown something so terrible, tell the president I'm not happy. You will look into it. Look into it if you don't we will do it ourselves.

She also calls the president regarding the serious gender-based violence. "You are a man of wisdom and integrity but I just saw that you banned alcohol. You want us to be sober?", she asks. She continues:

> We cannot be sober, we are stressed. We are staying with people whom we don't want to see every day. If we drink alcohol we just look at them and we see nothing. It's a wrong decision. Enemies are quarantined in one room. Make me your advisor. You will consider, thank you.

Although alcohol is ironically considered an instigator of GBV, Mai Tt hints at the problematic position of women who have to stay in the same home with their abusers. Perhaps out of desperation, they would rather drink their problems away. She mocks the lack of consideration of women's views, and by calling the authorities, she is demonstrating the dire need to provide a platform for women to be heard. Statistics say one in three women aged 15 to 49 have experienced physical violence in Zimbabwe and about one in four women have experienced sexual violence since the age of 15 years (UNFPA, 2020).

In yet another call, she asks president of Zimbabwe, Emmerson Mnangagwa, to consider sending a plane to pick her up from UK where she was stuck during the first lockdown regulations in March and bring her back home to Zimbabwe. This was in reference to other nations who were evacuating their nationals from countries around the world during COVID-19. She pokes fun at the president for being insensitive to the needs of ordinary people, especially women, in a nation that is rife with corruption.

COVID-19 Humour: Economic Impact on Women

She also uses humour to show how coronavirus affects women and men differently. This humour serves a psychological function whereby Mai Tt provides laughter amid the closing of businesses and people losing their sources of livelihood. In this kind of humour, she portrays women as caregivers and as burden lifters to those who are in state of panic and anxiety caused by the many unknowns of the disease, although this is considered unpaid work. Some women view her as a “sanitiser”. A commenter likens her jokes to how a sanitiser kills COVID-19. She metaphorises Mai Tt’s audience as the “covids” who need to be sanitised by her jokes. She raises issues that have an economic impact on women, such as homelessness in the pandemic, child-headed homes, failure to pay rentals and challenges of working from home. She therefore ridicules government policies that are insensitive to women. In one of the skits Mai Tt accuses her landlady of breaching the COVID-19 regulations by coming to her house to ask for rent and by not observing social distance. This was after the government directive at the height of the lockdown in April imploring landlords to stop collecting rentals until the COVID-19 lockdown has been lifted.

Her humour, however, gave birth to a number of online philanthropic activities where her audience would participate in helping to donate cash and goods to orphans, single female-headed homes and women in prisons and providing water to women in black townships. She uses her page to offer free promotions to boost female-headed businesses.

She also pokes fun at pastors who take advantage of the coronavirus situation. By pretending to be a prophetess, her humour is directed towards fellow women who normally fill church pews and who are viewed as gullible when it comes to giving money to church and who often want to be prayed for. In the skit, she advises givers not to put the money in the church account, but in her personal account. In a similar skit, she says, “don’t forget that if you don’t want this coronavirus to come to you, pay your tithe and offering”.

Misogyny

Mai Tt feels she is often misjudged and misunderstood, but unfortunately at times she fights the misogyny with more hate speech. Confession about her lived experiences exposes Mai Tt to humiliation and misogyny, although her strategy to deal with misogyny is often to block offensive comments as they come and to answer back. “Showbiz is like politics it’s a dirty game. I don’t offend people, all I do is fight for my rights”, she says. “Been abused for long and misunderstood because people start me then I end up retaliating”, she once pointed out on one of her Facebook page statuses. At one point her page was hacked. She has been attacked for her relationship with a younger man and for her HIV positive status. In turn, she has used her platform to attack those who cross her path. “I am a single mum who works for her children effortlessly”, she remarks in one of her videos as defence to an attack by a male pastor. She calls the pastor "junk" and says she is ready for a "fist" fight with him. She has on several occasions called other women "whores", "nobodies", "rats". Yet she claims to fight for women and that she is not a person of violence. In October 2020 she was slapped with a half a million US dollar defamation lawsuit after labelling a Harare businesswoman a "prostitute" (Machakaire, 2020).

There is also risk that her fame may alienate her from the very same women who look up to her. Although she continues to say she is not rich and not a politician, she does exhibit flamboyancy and opulence that creates a gap between her and the women she purports to be a voice for. For example, she recently underwent a liposuction and skin-enhancing procedures worth thousands of US dollars in neighbouring South Africa. At times, she wines and dines with the very politicians who are part of the system she mocks in her humour.

Comedy and Misinformation

Sadly, Mai Tt's humour is also littered with falsehoods and conspiracy theories, which is dangerous especially when it applies to a health pandemic such as the coronavirus. Misinformation is common with health pandemics or epidemics. It involves unknowingly spreading false information, while conspiracy theories are false stories repeated over time (Senft, 2020). During a cholera outbreak in Zimbabwe in 2018, people made humour out of the situation as a means to cope with the disease at a time when there was a shortage of water and other basic commodities (WHO, 2020). Research shows that there were rumours in 1918 during the Spanish flu, but now with social media, rumours spread faster, according to Barry (2020) during a presentation at the 2020 WHO Infodemic Management Training course. Barry is the author of the *Great Influenza,* that chronicles the history of the Spanish flu. New diseases are scary when there are still many unknowns, which is why people need humour to laugh it off. In 1796 when polio vaccine was invented, rumours started that cow heads would erupt from the bodies of people who received the vaccine (Wilson & Wysonge, 2020). Wasserman and Frost (2020)) postulate that people are drawn to conspiracy theories when there is a lot of uncertainty and lack of trust, and as a result they turn to humour, gossip and pavement radio. Mare (2019) alerts us to the fact that the Zimbabwe context, where public communication is generally constrained, popular art such as comedy is performing journalistic functions.

Jokingly Mai Tt tells her female audience during a live-in phone show to spray or apply disinfectants such as Dettol, anti-bacterial soap and other bleaches to the vagina to protect themselves from contracting the coronavirus during sex. When others asked if they should dilute the disinfectants, she repeatedly tells them to use the disinfectants undiluted. It is only at the end of the Facebook live comedy show that she informs her audience that it is just a joke. Although some of her audience point out that it is wrong information, from the onset, it is not clear how many could have been fooled by such jokes and how many listened to the show till the end to understand that she was joking. The particular video had been shared 31 times at the time of writing and had 60 k views and 3200 likes.

Mai Tt also posted anti-vaccination clips, one of which had been shared 307 times by the time of writing. "Amen he is telling the truth, say no to vaccine", one commenter says. "Amen, I stand with you…no unless they test it on them first (meaning the West). The pastor in that particular video vows to "die than being vaccinated". This was coming at a time when World Health Organization and nations globally were and are still fighting misinformation that is preventing people to protect themselves against the disease and promoting vaccination hesitancy. In her skit in which she laments how COVID-19 is preventing women's gossip, she remarks: "When they put you that chip you can't gossip anymore". She was referring to the misinformation that the proposed COVID-19 vaccinations come with chips that allow governments to remote-control individuals (Goodman & Carmichael, 2020).

In Zimbabwe, conspiracy theories around COVID-19 include that the disease was created in a lab in Wuhan and being spread by 5G networks and vaccination myths. What is more dangerous is that Mai Tt is viewed as an influencer and role model to women in Zimbabwe. Senft (2020) speaks of the ideological spiral model which explains how information reception, circulation and trust work. Basically, people join Facebook because of personal identity which basically says: here's how I determine right and wrong; or these are issues/values that are important to me. They are influenced by social identities that say: I feel included in what I understand as my group; I know how to distinguish my group from others, or social media preferences such as in my group nobody follows/supports/believes this; this topic is something I should know about or this platform/channel is what everyone uses. So, there is a great deal of danger for Facebook platforms such as Mai Tt to convey humour that carries misinformation. It is the same danger that arises when patriarchal discourses carry humour that is false about women. So as an influencer, what Mai Tt says has the potential to be believed, and if it is misinformation, it is likely to lead to confusion, risk-taking and harmful attitudes and behaviours (Purnat & Wilhelm, 2020). It can also increase stigma, hate speech and violence.

Conclusion

Mai Tt plays a role in shaping the women's worldview and by so doing creates a new feminist politics that is helping to change the narrative of women. Her humour mocks patriarchal myths and provides an emancipatory strategy to women. It mirrors everyday lives of women in Zimbabwe. Mai Tt is turning this male-dominated arts culture into a site of meaning, politics and life itself for women. Women are no longer just recipients of jokes but are also creating humorous texts embedded with feminist ideology, enabling women to participate in the construction of socially shared systems of interpretation. Women are able to articulate, negotiate and challenge matters that concern them. Mai Tt addresses marital conundrums such as "small houses" and taboo subjects such as sex, single women as well as controversial subjects such as sharing of household chores, gender-based-violence and false prophets and pastors. She demonises and rebukes the disease but more so the government for causing untold hardships to women. She laughs at politicians for failing to be sensitive to women's needs and to provide basic necessities such as clean water, food and sanitary products which would help to relieve stress and demonstrate government's commitment to cushion the poor and needy. Her humour is misogynistic sometimes, and her association with the political system that she mocks is contradictory and smacks of double standards.

References

Barry, J. (2020). *Learning from 1918 Spanish flu for better infodemic response in COVID-19*. Paper presented at the WHO Infodemic Management Training, Zoom.

BBC. (2019, August 22). Zimbabwean comedian Gonyeti 'abducted and beaten' in Harare. https://www.bbc.com/news/world-africa-49433387

Billig, M. (2009). Comic racism and violence. In S. Lockyer & M. Pickering (Eds.), *Beyond a Joke: The limits of humour* (pp. 25–44). Palgrave Macmillan.

Chambers, D. (2005). Comedies of sexual morality and female singlehood. In S. Lockyer & M. Pickering (Eds.), *Beyond a Joke: The limits of humour* (pp. 1–24). Palgrave Macmillan.

Davies, H., & Ilott, S. (2018). Mocking the weak: Contexts, theories, politics. In H. Davies & S. Ilott (Eds.), *Comedy and the politics of representation: Mocking the weak* (pp. 1–24). Palgrave Macmillan.

Forced Migration Studies Programme Wits University. (2009, November). *Zimbabwean migration into Southern Africa; new trends and responses.* http://www.migration.org.za/wp-content/uploads/2017/08/Zimbabwean-migration-into-Southern-Africa-new-trends-and-responses.pdf

Fraser, L. (2020). *What data is CrowdTangle tracking.* https://help.crowdtangle.com/en/articles/1140930-what-data-is-crowdtangle-tracking

Freud, S. (1960). *Jokes and their relation to the unconscious* (James Strachey, Trans. and ed.). Routledge and Kegan Paul.

Frost, M. (2020). *Risk communication and community engagement.* Paper presented at the WHO Infodemic Management Training, Zoom.

Goodman, J., & Carmichael, F. (2020, June 26). *Coronavirus: 5G and microchip conspiracies around the world.* https://www.bbc.com/news/53191523

Hill Collins, P. (2004). *Black sexual politics. African Americans, gender, and the new racism.* Routledge.

Holm, N. (2017). Introduction: Living in comic times. In *Humour as politics. Palgrave studies in comedy.* Palgrave Macmillan.

Jaenes, M., & Marques, R. (2019). *What the F*is going on?* [Film] Pokeepsie Documentary AIE, Pokeepsie Films SL, The other side films SL.

Källstig, A. (2020). Laughing in the face of danger: Performativity and resistance in Zimbabwean stand-up comedy. *Global Society.* https://doi.org/10.1080/13600826.2020.1828295

Kincaid, J., & Pattison, A. (2020, November). *Working with media, journalists and tech industry in message dissemination.* Paper presented at the WHO Infodemic Management Training, Zoom.

Kubatana. (2020, April 10). *COVID-19 lockdown: Gendered impacts, implications and effects on women and girls as primary caregivers.* http://kubatana.net/2020/04/10/COVID-19-zim-lockdown-gendered-impacts-implications-and-effects-on-women-and-girls-as-primary-caregivers/

Lang, J. C., & Lee, C. H. (2010). Workplace humour and organizational creativity. *The International Journal of Human Resource Management, 21*(1), 46–60.

Lockyer, S., & Pickering, M. (2009). Introduction: The ethics and aesthetics of humour and comedy. In S. Lockyer & M. Pickering (Eds.), *Beyond a Joke: The limits of humour* (pp. 1–24). Palgrave Macmillan.

Machakaire, T. (2020, October 06). *Mai Titi to pay 500k for defamation*. https://dailynews.co.zw/mai-titi-to-pay-500k-for-defamation/

Minjenjema, S., & Mazvarirwofa, K. (2017, September 18). *In Zimbabwe, female comics are succeeding in a male-dominated field*. https://deeply.thenewhumanitarian.org/womensadvancement/articles/2017/09/18/in-zimbabwe-female-comics-are-succeeding-in-a-male-dominated-field

Moyo, J. (2020, July 22). *Zimbabwe president declares curfew amid spiralling virus*. https://www.aa.com.tr/en/africa/zimbabwe-president-declares-curfew-amid-spiraling-virus/1918073

Muchabaiwa, W. M. (2018). *Gender dynamics of the small house phenomenon in the Harare Metropolitan province, Zimbabwe*. University of South Africa. http://uir.unisa.ac.za/bitstream/handle/10500/25554/thesis_Muchabaiwa_W.pdf?isAllowed=y&sequence=1

Ncube, G. (2020, May 20). *Eternal mothers, whores or witches: The oddities of being a woman in politics in Zimbabwe*. https://www.tandfonline.com/doi/full/10.1080/10130950.2020.1749523

Ndlovu, L., & Ngwenya, T. (2010). Public transport stickers: Degrading Zimbabwe womanhood. In I. Muwati, Z. Mguni, T. Gwekwerere, & R. Magosvongwe (Eds.), *Rediscoursing African womanhood in search for a sustainable renaissance* (pp. 17–23). College Press.

Obadare, E. (2016). *Humour, silence and civil society in Nigeria*. University of Rochester Press.

Pateman, C. (1989). *The disorder of women*. Polity.

Phiri, M. (2019). *Social media "talk" & gender violence: Discourses of gender violence on Facebook by audiences of E-tv's Scandal*. University of Johannesburg.

Purnat, T., & Wilhelm, E. (2020). *Misinformation and infodemic management: A framework approach to infodemic management*. Paper presented at the WHO Infodemic Management Training, Zoom.

Schultz, A., & Parikh, J. (2020, March 24). *Keeping our services stable and reliable during the COVID-19 outbreak*. https://about.fb.com/news/2020/03/keeping-our-apps-stable-during-COVID-19/

Segal, M. T., & Demos, V. (2019). *Gender and the media: Women's places*. Emerald Publishing Limited.

Senft, T. (2020, November). *Ethics in planning interventions and researching for infodemic management*. Paper presented at the WHO Infodemic Management Training, Zoom.

Szutenberg, Z. (2012). *Humour and feminism- A research into the whereabout of British Comediennes*. https://www.grin.com/document/202023

UNFPA Zimbabwe. (2020). *Gender-based violence*. https://zimbabwe.unfpa.org/en/topics/gender-based-violence-0

Wasserman, H. (2020, June 30). *Cultures of misinformation: Media, motivations responses.* Keynote talk, opening plenary 1st WHO global infodemiology conference.

Wilson, S. L., & Wysonge, C. S. (2020, December 3). *Misinformation on social media fuels vaccine hesitancy: A global study shows the link.* https://theconversation.com/misinformation-on-social-media-fuels-vaccine-hesitancy-a-global-study-shows-the-link-150652

World Health Organisation. (2020, October 05). *Cholera-Zimbabwe.* https://www.who.int/csr/don/05-october-2018-cholera-zimbabwe/en/

CHAPTER 9

'A Nation that Laughs Together, Stays Together': Deconstructing Humour on Twitter During the National Lockdown in South Africa

Nonhlanhla Ndlovu

Introduction

No need for Big Brother Naija this year, we're all housemates already #lockdownextension (Tweet, 23 April 2020).

This humorous tweet was posted in response to the announcement of an extension to the first lockdown period in South Africa in order to capture the exasperation that people felt at that time. The president had just announced a phased-in approach to easing the regulations characterized by 5 levels of lockdown after a much-anticipated end to the initial hard lockdown (see next section). The allegorical representation of the popular *Big Brother* reality show pronounced by the equally humorous responses to this tweet depicts how different elements of the show were being played

N. Ndlovu (✉)
Rhodes University, Grahamstown, South Africa

S. Mpofu (ed.), *Digital Humour in the Covid-19 Pandemic*,
https://doi.org/10.1007/978-3-030-79279-4_9

out in reality under lockdown. Users discuss how, just like the housemates on the show, people had lost track of the order of days. The "big brother voice behind the scenes" is attributed to the coronavirus and so "anyone that goes out will be eliminated", whilst the "isolation centre" is said to be signified by the actual eviction from the house. Interestingly, the person who would claim the grand prize in the end, as suggested somewhat sardonically, is none other than the president himself, never mind the fact that the meme accompanying the tweet paradoxically captures his dejected expression. I have chosen this particular tweet as an entry point into my discussion because it reminds me of Jeremy Bentham's panopticon in its metaphorical representation of disciplinary power (Foucault, 1977a, 1977b), a conception I find useful in framing my approach to critically deconstructing humour on Twitter during lockdown. The aim of disciplinary power is to produce bodies that are useful and docile, productive and subjected (Rabinow, 1984; Sarup, 1993). Therefore, construing themselves as housemates in the *Big Brother* Nigeria house, I argue, South Africans are constituted as 'willing' subjects of the rules pertaining to the house rules (lockdown regulations) and as the 'winner', Ramaphosa, representing the state, wields power over the housemates who, in essence, participate willingly in their own subjection. This instance demonstrates the fact that we are often constituted by the very power relations against which we struggle.

Taking a critical humour studies approach, this chapter provides a cartography of humour on Twitter between March and June 2020 in South Africa. A critical approach to humour means establishing a concern with how power relations are produced and reproduced in and through humour. I therefore employ critical discourse analysis perspectives to explore some of the humorous moments through selected tweets and hashtags that were trending during this period. The high level of engagement with humorous tweets and memes as demonstrated by an equally high level of retweets, likes and comments arguably demonstrates a sense of unity and camaraderie which, in turn, fosters an unrivalled sense of community. Their humorous take on social and political institutions as well as political leaders, not least among them the president himself, is telling of how South Africans understood themselves at this critical juncture. I therefore attempt an intersectional analysis that acknowledges that Twitter was used as a tool for negotiating identity across the social categories of gender, race and class during the national lockdown, and my discussion is limited to these discursive parameters. The chapter concludes by making inferences about how analyses of humour in this context destabilize the notion of the 'rainbow nation' and implications for social belonging and knowledge production within these discursive parameters.

Context

As the global spread of the COVID-19 pandemic became apparent in sub-Saharan Africa, South Africa emerged as the hotspot with the country reporting more than 2.6 million cases (South African Government, 2021) at the time of writing. South Africa recorded its first case of COVID-19 on 5 March 2020, and within two weeks, as local transmission started being recorded, government announced measures to combat the pandemic and subsequently declared a national state of disaster in terms of the Disaster Management Act (Ramaphosa, 2020a). This Act is provided for in Section 37.1 of the current constitution and partly provides for the suspension of the normative order when there is a threat to state security; COVID-19 represented the first real enemy since apartheid against which a national campaign could be launched (Kotzé, 2020). Accordingly, President Cyril Ramaphosa initially announced a raft of regulations including social distancing, closure of schools, limited social gatherings and suspension of travel to and from identified high-risk countries as well as quarantine procedures, among other measures. These regulations were amended on 25 March which saw an introduction of a strict national lockdown phase beginning on 27 March for a period of 21 days (Ramaphosa, 2020b). During this phase, all businesses were closed except for those identified as producing and providing essential goods and services. There was to be no movement between provinces, metropolitan areas and districts; hence, people were to be confined to their residential areas except when seeking essential goods and services.

The national lockdown was extended again on 16 April for a further period of 14 days, but the revised regulations allowed the operation of refineries and mining at reduced capacity in preparation for the gradual reopening of the economy. On 23 April, the president announced a phased-in approach of easing lockdown consisting of 5 levels in which "the National Coronavirus Command Council (NCCC) will determine the alert level based on an assessment of the infection rate and the capacity of our health system to provide care to those who need it" (Ramaphosa, 2020c). The country consequently moved on to level 4 on 1 May, level 3 on 1 June, level 2 on 18 August and level 1 on 21 September, with the president announcing amended regulations applicable in each phase. However, with the onset of a second wave, South Africa moved back to alert level 3 on 29 December 2020. South Africa's response has been lauded as swift and extensive as compared to other countries on the continent (Carlitz & Makhura, 2020). However, critical evaluations have also noted how the state has assumed its power over the citizenry by taking away their freedoms, then giving the citizens back their freedom piecemeal in a manner that depicts the functioning of disciplinary power (see Kotzé, 2020). In this scenario, the state effectively absolves itself of responsibility by shifting the responsibility of dealing with the threat of the pandemic on individuals. Individuals are forced to self-discipline (by adhering to all regulations) in order to redeem their freedoms or bear with the consequences of refusal. As such,

> In its disciplining, the state organizes and classifies; it establishes standards to which both ruler and ruled must be obliged. Both sides of the power relation have a determined behaviour to demonstrate. This correct behaviour is always known to the other and visible in space and time. Herein power is accountable in both directions. (Kotzé, 2020, 401–402)

Twitter constitutes this space mentioned above in which citizens discuss various issues related to lockdown. This argument is consistent with the emphasis of 'conduct of conduct' in Foucault's governmentality approach which is useful in unpacking the operation of disciplinary power on Twitter during the first three months of lockdown in South Africa, as users deployed humour which ultimately served to police each other's behaviour.

Humour and Identity in South Africa

Studies on humour in South Africa have tended to focus on stand-up comedy and the role it plays in critiquing dominant norms and discourses (Kallstig & Death, 2020; Musila, 2014; Parker, 2002). Recently, researchers have shown an interest in the role of humour in cinematic representations (Crigler, 2018). Crigler also attempts a historical overview of humour studies in South Africa, noting that the deployment of humour as social commentary dates back to precolonial indigenous cultures through apartheid to the present. Attempts to link humour explicitly to the nation-building project were common just after the end of apartheid when the ruling party, African National Congress (ANC), had the pressure of developing a sense of a 'national culture' (see Roome, 2002; Parker, 2002). Whilst acknowledging that there is scant literature that contextualizes laughter and community in South Africa, Crigler argues that humour has often been employed as a "means of representing and performing 'South African-ness'" (2018, 156).

Of course, the very meaning of 'nation' is highly contested (Anderson, 2006; Billig, 1995), and the ambiguities associated with its derivative terms—nationhood, national identity and national culture—are well documented in literature (see Ahluwalia, 2008; Hall, 1992; Schirato & Webb, 2003). I therefore employ these terms loosely, recognizing that South African identities are various and multifaceted and cannot be reduced to essences assumed in the constitution of national culture. For instance, in her discussion of race relations as represented in stand-up comedy, Musila (2014, 148) notes that "the rainbow project remains fractured along racial fault lines by contestations over the social, cultural, economic and political landscape of the country". The concern here is with how meaning and identity are negotiated discursively; I therefore consider humour as a disciplinary practice through which assumptions about gender, race and class are not only discursively produced and reproduced but also negotiated and contested with a view to change these hegemonic power relations. Understanding that the world is shaped by interlinked power relations, an intersectional critique of identity at this critical juncture is pertinent for a formulation of how these facets of South Africans' identity intersect to construct their social positionings.

Taking a cue from Obadare's (2009) view that ordinary people have harnessed the power of humour to construct and deconstruct meaning out of a reality that is decidedly surreal, I argue that lockdown and the associated restrictions present such a reality. The analysis of the deployment of humour during lockdown allows us to think critically about the contours of that moment when the future was uncertain. As such this chapter presents a momentous intervention as it grapples with the dominant discourses on Twitter emerging within the precarious context of COVID-19. Allowing that discourses 'speak us' (Foucault, 1978; Hall, 1997), I argue that discourses on Twitter during the lockdown in all their complexity, not least through humour, signify the point when South Africans became self-reflexive. They started questioning not only their social and political institutions, but also their identity. Crucially, at this moment of acute vulnerability, Twitter presented an agonistic sphere where not only a sense of community was cultivated through jest, but where identities were performed, contested and negotiated.

Resistance, Power and Discourse

This chapter builds upon critical approaches to the study of humour that conceptualize humour as resistance (Mbembe, 2001; Obadare, 2009; Musila, 2014; Odysseos et al., 2016), to argue that jabs thrown at political figures and institutions functioned as subversive ways of engaging with the state. Notably, Twitter users did not only take aim at politicians during the lockdown, they also critiqued dominant social discourses relating to gender, race and class and even mocked themselves in the process. Understanding that discourses not only shape but also enable social reality (Jäger & Maier, 2009), my approach also takes into account Foucauldian insights on power and resistance. Foucault contends that any society has its own set of discourses that it makes function as true, and hence "there can be no possible exercise of power without a certain economy of discourses of truth which operates through and on the basis of this association" (1980, 93). Individuals therefore are in constant struggle to conform to or resist the 'truth' of their society in the form of counter-discourses. By seeking to resist dominant discourses, members of a society engage in acts of counter-conduct in the form of "laughing at or about 'serious' issues such as race, disease and poverty" (Kallstig & Death, 2020, 5).

Counter-conduct is an important element of governmentality in which individuals constantly struggle against being governed, against the very processes that constitute them as subjects of certain discourses. I therefore harness the possibilities offered by these concepts to probe how the use of humour within the precarious context of lockdown serves a disciplinary function given that critical discourse analysis is "not only about the retrospective analysis of meaning, but also about the analysis of the ongoing production of reality through discourse, as conveyed by active subjects" (Jäger & Maier, 2009, 37). This critical perspective enables an examination of the experiences of South Africans as shaped by taken-for-granted social assumptions and expressed through the discursive parameters of humour. I show how they are constituted by the very discourses and structures which they struggle against. I argue that while humour brought much needed relief, a discursive interrogation of this humour unveils underlying social tensions and contradictions in South Africa's young democracy. Humour has the potential to illuminate not only the persistent conditions of inequality but also the emergent relations of power and precarity exacerbated by a global pandemic.

Consequently, the question to ask pertains to how engaging in everyday cultural practices such as tweeting has the power to contest and/or reinforce certain relations of power. As Foucault puts it:

> Let us not, therefore, ask why certain people want to dominate, what they seek, what is their overall strategy. Let us ask, instead, how things work at the level of subjugation, at the level of those continuous and uninterrupted processes which subject our bodies, govern our gestures, dictate our behaviours etc. (Foucault, 1980, 97)

Accordingly, in this chapter I pay attention to those utterances and memes generated on Twitter during lockdown to probe the resistances and the subjectivities that they enable. In order to illuminate the discursive aspects of social inequalities, this study employs critical discourse analysis perspectives (Wodak & Meyer, 2009; Fairclough, 1995; Van Dijk, 2001). The eclectic approach that I adopt combines methods of textual analysis that complements both critical linguistics and media studies (Janks, 1997; Dewa & Prinsloo, 2012). I therefore pay attention to transitivity choices and narrative analysis, including rhetorical analysis. In the sections that follow I discuss the analytical process in detail in an analysis-cum-discussion of these tweets that have been categorized and presented under identified themes. Given the sheer volume of tweets on a single day, I purposively selected those tweets that attracted conflicting views in order to capture the different positionings related to different social and political issues, particularly when new lockdown levels were announced.

There are ethical considerations to be taken into account when conducting Internet research, which are related to privacy and obtaining consent from research subjects. As a public platform, there was no obligation to obtain consent to conduct this research on Twitter as users of the platform agree to the terms and service agreement when signing up. These terms state that users consent to their information being collected and used by third parties (Williams et al., 2017). Twitter's terms of service and privacy policy also allow for the reuse of data. However, in the spirit of 'doing no harm' I sought to depersonalize data by not using actual names and Twitter handles (Fiesler and Proferes, 2017; Markham & Buchanan, 2012).

Cyril Ramaphosa: Friend or Foe

As the president of the country and inevitably the face of lockdown, Cyril Ramaphosa frequently bore the brunt of citizens' frustrations regarding the various stringent measures associated with the implementation of lockdown. This is demonstrated by him being the butt of jokes, most often coupled with nicknaming, which in turn arguably demonstrates the uneasy relationship between the president and the citizens of South Africa. Of course, these jokes were not all negative, as there are some people who constantly showed him their unwavering support. Perhaps the relationship between the president and the citizens during this time can best be described as turbulent, as it fluctuated with every new announcement made. People took to Twitter to debate new measures and to try to make sense of the president himself by using humorous memes and engaging in light banter to give perceptions on his governance.

Understandably, at different phases of the lockdown Ramaphosa had different epithets attached to him as responses to particular events. At the beginning of lockdown, he was endeared by the nation as he was perceived to have responded positively to calls to #LockdownSA. He was therefore referred to as "Uncle Cyril" as a sign of respect, and "Rammy" and "cupcake" as a sign of affection. However, as he came to be known for being late for national addresses—at what has come to be metaphorically known as the "family meetings" and Ramaphosa signifying the "breadwinner"—the monikers came to be laced with biting sarcasm to signify growing resentment. He therefore earned himself the nickname "Ramapunctual", while some comments suggested "if there was an award for late coming, this man deserves it". To express displeasure at being kept waiting, some suggested that being president was actually his "side hustle". Notably, there is an implicit reference to Ramaphosa's personal wealth which suggests that he did not prioritize the general well-being of South Africans at a time when they were agitated against the background of massive job losses. This stands in stark contrast with the construction of a metaphorical father figure and breadwinner mentioned above who unites South Africa as a family and commands respect.

In the same week that the president announced a R500 billion relief package, he also announced a phased-in approach to easing lockdown, two incidents which naturally ignited sustained interest. In the first instance, he was nicknamed "RamaBillion" after he announced the breakdown of how the relief package would be allocated. Notably, this was a light-hearted appreciative name at first, which a few months later assimilated negative connotations when there was massive corruption reported around its allocation. However, in response to the phased-in approach there was a lot of praise and admiration:

Thank you very much Mr President for your leadership. Your announcement shows that you're taking care of South Africans

What a move by our president...that was absolutely fantastic. Not many of us expected that! All I knew was that a coin only has two sides, but he proved me wrong...there is another side. Many believed it is either end or extend, but he precisely balanced them all...thank you CMR

We are well and truly led!

He's a leader among leaders and put his country first.

And of course, there was no shortage of humour:

Am I the only one seeing that level 4 lockdown is just a continuation of lockdown and our President is using levels to make us think that nothing has changed #lockdownextension #CyrilRambillion.

A lexical analysis of this tweet and responses to it shows the importance of linking texts to the wider social practices in meaning-making. The suggestion that "we're still in lockdown but this one is educated" not only plays on the infamous joke about different levels of education and the opportunities enabled and/or disabled by such, but also makes implicit reference to the president's educated background. Ramaphosa is often 'teased' for his good command of English which is usually construed as a sign of superiority, particularly in a country in which the apartheid system disadvantaged the majority of black people in terms of access to education. In this instance, the comments suggest that they have seen through him and therefore remark "he's tricking us", he is using a "strategic approach" and "dealing with us levelically". Note the intentional conversion of levels into an adverb by deliberately breaking the English grammatical rules. The effect of these rhetorical devices is to add emphasis and elicit humour but also within this context, it is a silent play of power. As Fairclough (1995) argues, it is important to consider the opaque relationship between language, power and discourse because these linkages often go unnoticed.

Coincidentally, it was the very same day that Ramaphosa also struggled to put on his mask at the end of his address, initially covering his eyes instead of his nose and mouth. By the end of the day, viral memes and videos circulated under the #MaskChallenge, and he had several nicknames attached to him. Of note was "RamaMzekezeke" deriving from a popular South African artist who had managed to hide his identity from the public for a long time by always wearing a mask and "RamaBirdbox" in intertextual reference to the Netflix film BirdBox. Some comments captured the funny episode thus: "*kahle kahle* (in actual fact) you're not supposed to see the virus, once you see it you catch it", and employing hyperbole: "President trying to warn us about level 7 of Corona". So humorous was the incident that Ramaphosa responded equally jokingly the next day, saying those who were laughing at him should sign up for his new TV channel where he would be teaching people how to wear a mask.

What is striking about this incident, besides the humour, is that it served as an apparent uniting force considering the difficult circumstances people were under. Ramaphosa was lauded for laughing at himself, and interestingly, this was immediately equated to "good leadership":

> *Shows he's human like the rest of us #RamaphosaMyPresident.*
>
> *I like the fact that he doesn't take things personal. His humour is what we need as a nation.*

What should be noted here is how humour is deployed to construct a particular image of the president. It functioned ideologically as a symbolization of unity. Ramaphosa is lauded by his supporters for responding casually to ridicule, a characteristic that rubber-stamps his leadership in their eyes. Furthermore, as suggested by the aforementioned comments, he is seen as unifying the nation by his mere act of being able to laugh at himself and acknowledge his vulnerability. However, considering the delicate situation that existed, I argue that in responding to this incident, Ramaphosa was performing goodwill in order to reinforce the relations of power. His response functioned as a reminder that he is still in charge, and in these particular responses people enacted deference to his rule. He is therefore deified as demonstrated by the quoted tweets.

If at the beginning of lockdown the relationship between the president and the citizens was flirtatious, the relationship turned sour when, eventually, deep in the throes of a seemingly never-ending lockdown, reality began to set in with most citizens as they dealt with massive job losses. The relationship became confrontational such that hashtags moved from #CyrilFridays (to celebrate the president) to #*Voetsek*Cyril and more broadly #*Voetsek*ANC to poke holes at the leadership. It gave people a chance to criticize his presidency, the policies of the ANC and corrupt ministers and therefore narrate alternative 'truths'. Humour in this instance became an avenue to resist and critique state power (Obadare, 2009).

Clearly, the seeds of resentment were slowly taking root. However, what I want to draw attention to is that even when people were demanding accountability from ANC, Ramaphosa seemed to be absolved from accountability by his supporters. This tweet sums up this argument succinctly:

> *I'm no ANC fan. In fact, I despise it. BUT when Pres Zuma was wreaking havoc, YOU said #ZumaMustFall, not #ANCMustFall. This Pres is wreaking havoc with the economy. YOU spout #VoetsekANC? No. If you're honest, you'll use the same sword that fell on his predecessor. #VoetsekCyril.*

His supporters emphasized his good characteristics and juxtaposed them with the former president Jacob Zuma who was linked to numerous corruption scandals. The argument was that it was the system that was corrupt and not Cyril Ramaphosa, which arguably served to reinforce his sainthood. For example, they argued: "Ramaphosa is sabotaged by the same cadres he is advocating…The man is working hard, but the so-called cadres are milking him down, instead of being used as a pawn in the game of factions. I think we should have empathy towards the President".

Whilst one cannot draw clear conclusions on whether Cyril Ramaphosa was perceived as a friend or foe during this period, what I have attempted to capture in this section are the different constructions of Ramaphosa and the growing resentment towards the ANC. My argument is that the lockdown has illuminated the wrongdoings of the ANC and the citizens are beginning to see Ramaphosa in a different light and to critique his policies. Whereas at the beginning of lockdown there was a certain docility and acceptance of government-imposed restrictions, it later changed when citizens demanded individual agency. Two divergent and often conflicting discourses emerged regarding community which entailed obligation to government on the one hand and recourse to neoliberal principles on the other hand which emphasizes individual rights. Navigating between these two discourses is what, in many cases, caused the discursive contestations.

A Female President?

When the nation was becoming highly agitated against Ramaphosa and calls for #CyrilMustGo were gaining momentum on Twitter, a few individuals toyed with the idea of having a female president. Naturally, a few female leaders were suggested but dismissed on (largely) sexist grounds. This is demonstrated most clearly through Nkosazana Dlamini-Zuma, the Minister of Corporate Governance and Traditional Affairs, who bore the brunt of criticism.

In his national address announcing the phased-in approach to lockdown, the president had announced that tobacco products would be sold at level 4. Having been banned at level 5 along with alcohol sales, this was a welcome news to most people. Yet a few days later, Minister Dlamini-Zuma announced that after consultations, the government had decided to continue with both the alcohol and cigarette ban under level 4. Understandably, this sparked a lot of criticism from the general public and the minister suffered scathing attacks. She was accused of making unilateral decisions and undermining the president. So controversial was the issue that the president was forced to make a statement clarifying that it had been a cabinet decision and not an independent decision. This did little to salvage the hatred spewed towards the minister as observed in the constant flippant references to her being the actual president behind the scenes, such that in the national addresses that followed, it was argued that the president was simply reading the speeches that she had prepared.

Several expletives were thrown her way and she was variously characterized as "witch", "devil" "wicked", "devious" and "swine". These predicational strategies employed here bear the imprint of value judgements by linguistically assigning qualities to their referent (Richardson, 2007). Such labels are often deployed as symbolic sanctions against women who perform non-mainstream femininities (Abedinifard, 2016). Disguised as light banter, gender humour functions to police the patriarchal gender norms currently operating within the South African gender order. In this case Minister Dlamini-Zuma is assigned all the negative characteristics of a witch and a devil in order to undermine and vilify her so as to 'erase' her from the public sphere reserved for men in a patriarchal society. Consider these comments:

So tired of #NDZ 'jokes' that are mostly racist and misogynistic. She may be dull and hate smoking but she's stepped up and is trying to address this pandemic unlike @DDMabuza

The same vicious #NDZ whose ally & ex-husband deliberately sow hate in SA through Bell Pottinger? An #NDZ who is causing untold harm through illicit cigarette sales? Collecting a salary from the black market & tax payers. You have a heart of Jesus

A problem when you're led by a woman who thinks that she controls everyone because she controls her husband at home

Maybe she should lose weight because she's a health risk @DlaminiZuma

What a devious disgusting useless woman - this while thousands go hungry?

The tenor of the language in these tweets is hostile and suggests an unforgiving attitude towards Dlamini-Zuma. While the first comment is laudable for calling out racist and misogynistic attitudes using a logical argument, it fails to achieve its purpose by labelling her "dull", thereby endorsing Dlamini-Zuma's criticism. She is elevated only so that she can be simultaneously brought down. The next two responses draw upon a patriarchal discourse by making a connection to her ex-husband as if to suggest that she is only relevant in reference to him. This reference serves to strip her of agency and is further emphasized by the sexist stereotype that a woman who is in a position of power is often accused of being in 'control' of her husband. Typically, most gender humour draws on hegemonic gender norms in order to be effective. As if this is not enough, Minister Dlamini-Zuma is also trolled for her weight and the way she dresses, of which she earns the nickname "*Kopdoek*". To emphasize this point, several memes of the president wearing her doek also made the rounds much to the amusement of many. In this instance, the president is effectively emasculated while the ridiculousness of the images serves to underline the fact that Dlamini-Zuma should not be in public office.

As argued by Shifman and Lemish (2010), sexist humour tends to ridicule women for the purpose of emphasizing their inferiority to men. It also employs traditional stereotypes in which women are constructed as stupid and illogical, and also described according to their physical characteristics so as to emphasize a hierarchical difference between men and women. Language, as a site for the cultural production of gender identity, therefore becomes a central site of struggle (Talbot, 2010; Weedon, 1997). The supporters of Dlamini-Zuma therefore crucially defended her, pointing out that "we can disagree with people but body shaming and all the insults are lame" and exclaiming "it's almost like people want to believe that CR does not lead NCCC or cabinet". Clearly invoking a feminist discourse, some argue that Dlamini-Zuma is a powerful woman who has achieved a lot by herself and should be recognized in her own right. Feminist discourses continue to struggle for visibility, and platforms such as this are critical for illuminating discourses that challenge and denaturalize social realities. To conclude this brief section, it is notable that what is made discursively salient here is the constant disavowal of women in power based on their sex, which is why the criticism levelled against Dlamini-Zuma is much harsher than that levelled against the president discussed in the previous section. Laughter is often deployed as a tool of punishment for women who embody pariah femininities in order to vociferously 'guard' hegemonic gender norms (Abedinifard, 2016).

Humour as Disciplinary Practice

On 1 May when South Africa moved to level 4, several restrictions were eased and part of these included restrictions on exercise. Exercise was permitted for 3 hours between 6–9 am. It is quite striking that this 'simple' allowance became a trigger of much robust debate and served to illuminate the division of South Africa along class and racial lines.

A variety of perspectives were expressed in terms of the inequalities that were wrought by the lockdown. Briefly, to provide context, the South African National Defence Forces (SANDF) was deployed at the beginning of lockdown to ensure compliance with the stay-at-home rules. The fact that there was heavy presence of the SANDF in the townships was identified as a pointer to the class stratifications in South Africa captured in various news reports. Contained within this decidedly brutal deployment of the army and the forced adjustment to the stringent stay-at-home rules was a particular normalization of precarity by the state with little regard for the uncertainties that were brought by the pandemic, especially for those who could not just adjust considering that their survival was dependent on the informal sector. The army was accused of heavy-handedness in dealing with people who were found moving around, and various videos containing punishment of such people breaking lockdown rules made the rounds. What quickly became apparent was that the heavy-handedness of the army was attributed to a racial issue and a discursive contestation between blacks and whites ensued. For example, someone tweeted:

> *Since this #21daysLockdownSouthAfrica started, I have never seen whites being treated the way we as blacks have been treated. But I stand to be corrected if I am wrong.*

Others disputed the racial aspect, arguing that it elided the bullying instead which should be the focal point. Already, there were suggestions that those who were better off were managing the lockdown better, because they did not have to go out and look for food as they were privileged enough to have stocked enough supplies before lockdown began. Arguably, things came to a head when Sea Point residents in Cape Town were captured in droves going to exercise along the beach, an overwhelming majority of them being white people. Immediately a contrast was drawn between them and black people and the hashtags #whiteprivilege and #SeaPoint began to trend.

A tweet accompanied by an image contrasting white people and black people under lockdown captioned "Spot the difference" was posted by a user. Frame 1 captured Sea Point residents, while frame 2 showed black people queueing for social grants. In response to the major criticism that emerged for the image, although it was explained that the image was used to prove the point that neither black people nor white people were practising social distancing, many pointed out the inequalities that differentiated the two races. They pointed out that a line had been drawn between the haves and the have-nots. It was argued that white people had the luxury to exercise, whilst black people did not have that luxury as they had to queue for the R350 COVID-19 relief fund offered by the government which they needed for their survival. Exercising, the argument went, was not an essential part of living, and hence the two scenarios could not be juxtaposed fairly. The white people, despite trying to justify that exercise is important, were accused of being "ignorant" because "privilege is never more important than safety". Furthermore, because of their reckless behaviour and "their weak immune systems", they were going to go home and spread the virus to "innocent our mothers and grandmothers" whom they employ as domestic workers who in turn would take it to the townships. Clearly the arguments demonstrated the class differences that exist in South Africa which have the tendency of being pronounced in times of crises such as these. These concerns are captured in this tweet:

> *The sad thing about this whole Sea Point mass gathering of joggers is that these people will take the virus to the shops & infect everyone; incl. those who do not*

have access to better health care facilities. At the end of the day, the poor will suffer the most.

Note the lexical choices "mass gathering", "these people" and the modal truth claims signified by the repeated word "will". Taken together, these rhetorical devices function to create a pathotic argument that appeals to the decoder's emotions (Richardson, 2007) to make its full impact. In this case it is to persuade the black reader that the white people constitute the villain in this scenario and should be vilified for the sake of "everyone" (read poor black people). An interesting moment I want to emphasize pertains to when it had seemingly been established that indeed it was only white people who had been found exercising, someone posted a picture of a black man posing for a picture in the crowd, captioned "There's always that one person". In response to this tweet, a range of humorous responses were elicited:

We are disappointed in him
I am Lukhanyo but you can call me 'Luke'
Coconut
Ra mo tseba (We know him) *his kids only know English*
Afrikaans yona? (what about Afrikaans)
Such a disgrace
The black sheep
He is the #StrongerTogether brigade
Boet (bro)
With the Springbok shirt just so they know he's ok
I speak for abo darkie (blacks), *we disowned this guy. We don't know him…we never signed off on this*
This one is a mpimpi (sellout)
That one is a dangerous one. He does racism and suppresses the black man more than the white man so that he can be included in the white group. But they will never admit him in the white group. Use him yes. [sic]

Taken holistically this thread presents a discursive contestation against the dominant discourse of white superiority. There is a clear demarcation of us versus them (black vs white), with the aim of constructing a 'proudly black' counter-discourse. Construed thus, this young man is therefore a signifier of deviance from the 'normal', and therefore it is justifiable that he should be ridiculed. He is discursively expurgated as 'other' through the use of referential strategies that demonstrate that they do not identify him as black, and hence the metaphors "coconut" and "black sheep" to signify that he constitutes an 'epidermalized' subjectivity (Fanon, 2008) that construes white as superior. It is within this context that he is therefore constructed as a sell-out but will never be fully admitted in white circles. The implicit suggestion in these comments is that to identify as black, one's children should speak their native language as opposed to English and Afrikaans, one must not change their vernacular name to a similar sounding English name in order to fit in and one's favourite national team cannot be rugby because it has historically been a racial sport in South Africa. This stereotypical image constructed in this instance and in its justified confrontation of white superiority operates as a hegemonic discourse that proposes particular 'truths' relating to blackness, which serves to expurgate those who are not its subjects. This is problematic because, in speaking for *abo darkie*, there is a universalization of black experiences implied within that ultimately serves to police the behaviour of other blacks in a manner of 'conduct of conduct' (Foucault, 1982: 220–221). In confronting the power of the discourse of white privilege, there is the very real possibility that black people are constrained in the process by compartmentalizing what being black means in certain contexts and essentially disregarding cultural differences. To this end, I concur with Musila's (2014) argument that race relations remain the biggest threat to the rainbow nation which, she argues, remains 'mythically cohesive.' Indeed, barely a decade later, the illusion of a rainbow nation persists and is illuminated in instances such as these showing that racial (and gendered) identities are critical and nuanced and are contained in everyday utterances as they jostle for dominance.

Twitter as an Agonistic Public Sphere

One of the most significant findings that emerged pertains to how Twitter is perceived by its users. There has been growing interest in this area of research, and while I do not go into detail here, the results are consistent with studies concerned with the social use of technology. As depicted by the popular meme of a young man seemingly typing on a cellphone while his gaze is fixed elsewhere, Twitter is so central to South Africans' interpretations of Ramaphosa's televised speeches that they engage with both simultaneously, which equates to 'watching' the national address speeches on Twitter. Whilst some depend on Twitter for the breakdown of the speeches, others enjoy capturing the instant (humorous) reactions to the national addresses. These real-time contributions enhance meaning-making and the social use of television (D'heer & Verdegen, 2015). Twitter therefore offers a mediated social space where they can relax and have fun. This corroborates Duffy and Ling's (2000) argument that the sharing of news on social media helps to maintain social cohesion and users often share news for many reasons including entertainment, sharing information, helping and to elicit a strong emotional response. South Africans, in this context, found a space they conceive as a platform for critical social commentary that impacts on decisions made by the government. An example suffices:

> *Fikile Mbalula is actually responding to the comments he sees on Twitter [laughing emojis] the power of Twitter #Level4Regulations*
>
> *At least he is bringing concerns of normal South Africans to the fore, unlike being ignored by the government which some of you will cry about.*

Various responses in this thread concur "he *is* responding", and one comments, "funny you say that coz I picked up the same vibe from #angiemotshekga (Basic Education minister) yesterday, she was responding to Twitter comments…Lol Twitter is Power!" This confidence exuded of the perceived impact of Twitter serves to demonstrate the central role that the platform plays in not only shaping reality but also producing knowledge as well. If the two ministers in their speeches implicitly responded to comments on Twitter, this means that Twitter discourses shaped their policy responses in tremendous ways. Surveying the discourses on Twitter meant that ministers could read the pulse of society and respond appropriately. In the two instances mentioned, there was public outcry regarding how the transport sector was going to operate and how schools were going to reopen under COVID-19 regulations respectively. This is contrary to the argument that "Twitter users call for criticism *without consequence* as they feel the need to utter their discontents but do not expect or call for particular changes based upon their utterances" (D'heer & Verdegen, 2015, 232, emphasis in original). South African Twitter users see themselves as 'speaking truth to power', hence the conceptualization of Twitter as an agonistic public sphere.

The agonistic public sphere (Mouffe 1999) should be understood as a place of struggle which supports not only the reproduction of dominant social relations but also their contestations by subordinate groups. As such Twitter provides "a means for the formation of counter-publics, the articulation of identities and oppositional discourses, and the contestation of the discursive boundaries of the mainstream public sphere" (Dahlberg, 2007, 60). In this case, it also shapes the discursive terrain of the mainstream public sphere such that when the president addressed corruption claims relating to the R500 billion, Twitter users insisted he was directly responding to their concerns. Against this background, one can conclude that Twitter users harnessed the allowances afforded by the platform to set the agenda for public discourse during the lockdown, and these discourses function as forms of resistance.

Conclusion

Placing the jokes within a wider societal context, it is my conclusion that laughter is productive (in the Foucauldian sense); it is productive of relations of power as demonstrated by the discourses which we inhabit and the performances we enact thereof. In enacting these performances of power, we reinforce and challenge existing discourses in platforms such as Twitter which serve as agonistic spheres. In the same space that behaviours are policed, whether by those in power or by other users, dominant discourses pertaining to gender race and class are challenged and negotiated. The global pandemic has emphasized how identities are consistently contested in conversations that cut across race, gender and class and lockdown served to illuminate the complex intersection of these discourses. This study provides important insights into how South African-ness was performed amidst the discursive contestations that often resulted in chaos. However, amidst this chaos South Africans predominantly enunciated a discourse of togetherness. Lockdown presented a situation in which South Africans were trying to make emotional sense of drastic changes. What is made textually salient is that while Twitter constituted a place to relax and navigate this precarity through laughing together, in what I consider as 'performing togetherness'; this textually performed togetherness was compromised by deep inequalities which leave South Africa vulnerable as a nation. This vulnerability, in turn, has devastating effects for social belonging in the long term and should inform larger debates over identity and social change.

Considering the pandemic as a social and cultural phenomenon necessitates that we consider the material human effects the virus has left in its wake. This is an important issue for future research.

References

Abedinifard, M. (2016). Ridicule, gender hegemony and the disciplinary function of mainstream gender humour. *Social Semiotics, 26*(3), 234–249.

Ahluwalia, P. (2008). Empire and the "new" politics of existence. In R. Krishnaswamy & J. C. Hawley (Eds.), *The postcolonial and the global.* University of Minnesota Press.

Anderson, B. (2006). *Imagined communities: Reflections on the origin and spread of nationalism.* Verso.

Billig, M. (1995). *Banal nationalism.* Sage.

Carlitz, R., & Makhura, M. (2020). Life under lockdown: Illustrating tradeoffs in South Africa's response to COVID-19. *World Development, 137.*

Crigler, R. K. (2018). No laughing matter? Humour and the performance of South Africa. *South African Theatre Journal, 31*(2–3), 151–171.

D'heer, E., & Verdegen, P. (2015). What social media data mean for audience studies: A multidimensional investigation of Twitter use during a current affairs TV programme. *Information, Communication and Society, 18*(2), 221–234.

Dahlberg, L. (2007). The internet, deliberative democracy and power: Radicalising the public sphere. *International Journal of Media and Cultural Politics, 3*(1), 47–64.

Dewa, N., & Prinsloo, J. (2012). 'I am a man!' the *Daily Sun* campaign and gender violence. *Equid Novi: African Journalism Studies, 33*(2), 20–35.

Duffy, A., & Ling, R. (2000). The gift of news: Phatic news sharing on social media for social cohesion. *Journalism Studies, 21*(1), 72–87.

Fanon, F. (2008). *Black skin, white masks.* Groove Press.

Fairclough, N. (1995). *Critical discourse analysis: The critical study of language.* Longman.

Fiesler, C., & Proferes. (2017). "Participant" perceptions of Twitter research ethics. *Social Media and Society,* 1–10. https://doi.org/10.1177/2056305118763366

Foucault, M. (1977a). *Discipline and punish: The birth of the prison* (Trans. A. Sheridan). Penguin Books.

Foucault, M. (1977b). Truth and power. Interviewers: Fontana Alessandro and Pasquino Pasquale. In C. Gordon (Ed.), *Michel Foucault: Power/Knowledge. Selected Interviews and other writings 1972–1977 by Michel Foucault* (1980, pp. 109–133). Harvey Press.

Foucault, M. (1978). Governmentality. In J. D. Faubion (Ed.). *Power: The essential works of Michel Foucault 1954–1984* (Vol. 3, 1994, pp. 201–222). Penguin Books.

Foucault, M. (1982). Afterword: The subject and power. In L. Dreyfus Hubert & R. Paul (Eds.), *Michel Foucault: Beyond structuralism and hermeneutics* (pp. 208–226). Chicago University Press.

Foucault, M. (1980). Power and discourse. In *Selected interviews and other writings 1972–1977 by Michel Foucault.* Harvest Press.

Hall, S. (1992). The question of cultural identity. In S. Hall, D. Held, & A. McGrew (Eds.), *Modernity and its futures* (pp. 274–325). Polity Press.

Hall, S. (1997). *Representation. Cultural representations and signifying practices.* Sage.

Jäger, S., & Maier, F. (2009). Theoretical and methodological aspects of Foucauldian critical discourse analysis and dispositive analysis. In R. Wodak & M. Meyer (Eds.), *Methods of critical discourse analysis* (2nd ed., pp. 34–61). Sage.

Janks, H. (1997). Critical discourse analysis as a research tool. *Discourse: Studies in the Cultural Politics of Education, 18*(3), 329–342.

Kallstig, A., & Death, C. (2020). Laughter, resistance and ambivalence in Trevor Noah's stand-up comedy: Returning mimicry as mockery. *Critical African Studies*, 1–18. https://doi.org/10.1080/21681392.2020.1743191

Kotzé, K. (2020). Responding to COVID-19 Emergency Laws and the return to government in South Africa. *Javnost-The Public, 27*(4), 393–406.

Markham, A., & Buchanan, E. (2012). *Ethical decision-making and internet research: Recommendations from the AoIR Ethics Working Committee.* https://www.aoir.org/reports/ethics2.pdf. Accessed 02 Jan 2021.

Mbembe, A. (2001). *On the postcolony.* University of California Press.

Mouffe, C. (1999). Deliberative democracy or agonistic pluralism. *Social Research, 66*(3), 745–758.

Musila, G. (2014). Laughing at the rainbow's cracks? Blackness, whiteness and the ambivalences of South African stand-up comedy. In C. van Vyk (Ed.), *Civic agency in Africa: Arts of resistance in the 21st century* (pp. 147–166). James Currey.

Obadare, E. (2009). The uses of ridicule: Humour, 'infrapolitics' and civil society in Nigeria. *African Affairs, 108*(431), 241–261.

Odysseos, L., Death, C., & Malmvig, H. (2016). Interrogating Michel Foucualt's counter-conduct: Theorising the subjects and practices of resistance in global politics. *Global Society, 30*(2), 151–156.

Parker, Z. (2002). Standing up for the nation: An investigation of stand-up comedy in South Africa post 1994 with specific reference to women's power and the body. *South African Theatre Journal, 16*(1), 8–29.

Rabinow, P. (1984). Introduction. In P. Rabinow (Ed.), *The Foucault reader: An introduction to Foucault's thought* (pp. 3–29). Penguin Books.

Ramaphosa, C. (2020a, March 15). President Cyril Ramaphosa: Measures to combat coronavirus COVID-19 pandemic. *South African Government.* https://www.gov.za/speeches/statement-president-cyril-ramaphosa-measures-combat-COVID-19-epidemic-15-mar-2020-0000

Ramaphosa, C. (2020b, March 24). Statement by President Cyril Ramaphosa on escalation of measures to combat the COVID-19 epidemic, Union Buildings,

Tshwane. *The Presidency, Republic of South Africa*. http://www.thepresidency.gov.za/speeches/statement-president-cyril-ramaphosa-escalation-measures-combat-COVID-19-epidemic%2C-union

Ramaphosa, C. (2020c, April 23). President Cyril Ramaphosa: South Africa's response to coronavirus COVID-19 pandemic. *South African Government*. https://www.gov.za/speeches/president-cyril-ramaphosa-south-africas-response-coronavirus-COVID-19-pandemic-23-apr-2020

Richardson, J. E. (2007). *Analysing newspapers: An approach from critical discourse analysis*. Palgrave Macmillan.

Roome, D. (2002). The serious 'consequences' of comedy: Negotiating cultural change and difference through humour. *South African Theatre Journal, 16*(1), 44–62.

Sarup, M. (1993). *An introductory guide to post-structuralism and postmodernism* (2nd ed.). Harvester Wheatsheaf.

Schirato, T., & Webb, J. (2003). *Understanding globalisation*. Sage.

Shifman, L., & Lemish, D. (2010). Between feminism and fun(ny)mism. *Information, Communication and Society, 13*(6), 870–891.

South African Government. (2021). *COVID-19 statistics in South Africa*. https://www.gov.za/COVID-19/statistics

Talbot, M. (2010). *Language and gender* (2nd ed.). Polity Press.

Van Dijk, T. (2001). Discourse, ideology and context. *Folia Linguistica, XXXV*(1–2), 11–40.

Weedon, C. (1997). *Feminist practice and poststructuralist theory* (2nd ed.). Blackwell Publishing.

Williams, M. L., Burnap, P., & Sloan, L. (2017). Towards an ethical framework for publishing Twitter data in social research: Taking into account users' views, online context and algorithmic estimation. *Sociology.*, 1–20. https://doi.org/10.1177/0038038517708140

Wodak, R., & Meyer, M. (2009). Critical discourse analysis: History, agenda, theory and methodology. In R. Wodak & M. Meyer (Eds.), *Methods of critical discourse analysis* (2nd ed., pp. 1–33). Sage.

CHAPTER 10

Fear and Loathing and Laughter: COVID-19 as an Expression of Decolonial Love

Mvuzo Ponono

Decolonial love is political struggle against structures of dehumanisation and self-hate
—Glenda Daniels, *2021*

Introduction

After making a plea to the government for help, fellow South Africans were ultimately repatriated from Wuhan, China. However, prior to that successful mission, when the plan was first announced, a litany of jokes doing the rounds on social media made light of the situation. One user teased: "Stay there coz we've temporarily moved to Zim you won't find anyone". Another posted: "Stay there shuuuu, we can't build a hospital in 48 hours here". When considered deeply, those jokes revealed the anxiety and the fear South Africans had as the world braced for what was to come. Worse came to worse in March 2020, when the first case of the coronavirus was reported in South Africa. The mood shifted swiftly to anger as pictures of white people 'panic buying' at Makro did the rounds. "So

M. Ponono (✉)
University of the Free State, Bloemfontein, South Africa
e-mail: ponoNom@ufs.ac.za

S. Mpofu (ed.), *Digital Humour in the Covid-19 Pandemic*,
https://doi.org/10.1007/978-3-030-79279-4_10

grand gran abelungu (white people) abaphangeli (do not work) or what? How did they get time off to go clean the shops empty while we're forced to be at work and service them?" – a Twitter user observed. The proposed chapter will make the argument that, on the one hand, the coexistence of the laughter and outrage on social media shows a deep love for the country that is expressed through humour and appreciation for social media sites that provide such relief. And on the other hand, a deep hate or animosity that expresses a despair borne out of centuries of social divides. The point is that these extremes find a way to somehow coexist online, and this provides an avenue for an expression of deep trauma.

The best way to describe it is that people enjoy or love being South African and laugh at all sorts of peculiarities but also hate certain aspects of being South African. When making fun of the repatriation one user on Facebook wrote: "I love my country! Guys plzz I'm tired of laughing your comments makes me laugh". A month later a response to the spate of panic-buying noted: "Check who has the luxury of 'panic buying'. They will then get in their big ass cars and go self-quarantine in their comfy homes. My people are packed up at Noord taxi rank to get to their shacks, make plans to feed their families just for today". This is an intense love that lives next to intense hate. This is what can be termed a decolonial love. Sandoval (2000) argues that this is not a romantic love, but rather it is 'invented love, or love as a political technology'. It is, she explained, a body of knowledge, arts, practices and procedures for re-forming the self and the world (Sandoval, 2000, 4). Decolonial love is political struggle against structures of dehumanisation and self-hate (Daniels, 2021). What we often see on social media sites is that right next to the jokes that provide relaxation and a lessening of anxiety are proclamations of deep disappointment with the lack of transformation in the country. The lashing out by black people who are desperate to love a country and a partner that often does not love them back is interesting to note. The following chapter will investigate the coexistence of online humour and animosity and make the argument that social media provides a platforms for airing of views that speak to the heart of decoloniality.

Democratic Racism and Black Twitter

The relationship between races in South Africa is a fraught one. Any phenomenon, including laughter, takes place in social life that suffers from a long history of race-based oppression. Tomaselli (1997) provides a useful context, stating that even with the disappearance of overt racism from official discourse in South Africa post-1990, the racist structure of society remained the same. Critics argue that grand declarations such as South Africa's much lauded constitution belie the material reality of 'white' political and economic control (Tomaselli, 1997). This has been evident in the history of post-democratic South Africa, where the economy and wealth are concentrated in the hands of a few. To this point, Ramokhele (2018) asks: "Why is it that 24 years after democracy we (blacks) are still on the periphery? In six years time a child who was born in 1994 will be turning 30 – and if they have their first child on the anniversary of democracy, that child will be born into a country where they will still be a minority in the economic participation landscape, 30 years in".

Carr (2016, 65) contends that this state of being can be explained as a form of democratic racism, in which racist behaviour, actions and outcomes (including the poor remaining black) are codified in society. Carr (2016, 59) further explains that this is a reality where laws, courts, economic systems, institutions and legislative bodies, among others, "were developed by Whites from a distinctly White vantage-point". These partisan social institutions create a "normative, hegemonic underpinning of society, which is essentially White-based", and thus normalise unequal favour (Carr, 2016, 59). Furthermore, in such instances of institutionalised racism, where race is a central organising principle, its influence is felt in every aspect of a black person's life, including the economy and media representation (Hall, 1997). Media scholars qualify the critique by arguing that the problem is not the media system per se; it is more about the racial structure of the society, which continues to have white people or whiteness at the centre of attention and blackness relegated to the margins (Schutte, 2015; Duncan, 2013).

Larson (2006) argues that the moral guidelines followed by popular narratives may not be explicitly racist, but it can be argued that social discourse reinforces anti-black messaging. This is done through denying the extent to which racial inequality is prevalent and by offering discourses that maintain the inequality of the social structure (Larson, 2006). One good example of the aforementioned point and the complexity of the duality is the Marikana massacre that took place in 2012. Critics have pointed out that the mainstream representation of the conflict was clearly and unashamedly biased towards business, and pushed a narrative that delegitimised the legitimate, but legally unprotected, actions taken by the miners (Duncan, 2013). In the immediate aftermath of Marikana, the media were criticised for relying on police accounts to report on the incident, which were bent towards portraying the striking miners as the aggressors and instigators of the massacre (Hlongwane, 2016). South African media scholars and civil society activists have argued that the massacre showed that the colonial trope of the immoral or "primitive and savage black male" is not foreign to South African mainstream media representation and has been used in contemporary media reportage (Schutte, 2015, 8). What the reportage of the massacre demonstrated, in its distorted representation of the miners, is that the mainstream media automatically assumed fault with the marginalised.

Gray (1997, 92) adds that anti-black cultural, social, political and moral discourses continue to have "purchase in the collective common sense, because they continue to frame, reiterate, and make available a store house of meanings". These negative meanings, Gray (1997) continues, are still sharply focused on and animated in popular culture and media around race and sexuality. Copious academic research has revealed a consistent media bias against black people, both in the coverage of crime and more generally (Entman & Gross, 2008). Media representations are thus selected and constructed in ways that consistently promote the racial status quo of inequality and the subsequent injustices are construed as "common sense" (Larson 2006, 2). The result of this prejudicial gatekeeping is a systematic bias against young people, women, minority groups and subaltern groupings (Larson 2006). Furthermore, as Gray (1997) points out, this marginalisation also tends to favour the domination of most organs of media and television by the outlook of the upper-income whites and those who have been assimilated into this ideology.

The result is often distrust between races or black people distrusting white people in South Africa (in Ponono, 2019).

> Black people are frustrated in South Africa, and on top of that we are still carrying anger from the past. White people have not owned up to their mistakes. They have not so much as apologised. Black people still have a hangover from the past because some really horrible things happened. The psychological damage that has been done by white people on black people is immense. I have worked for white people at Just Property Group. White people will always remain the same, they will always see you as subhuman. So I don't have trust for a white person when it comes to developing a black person. I trust a black person to do that. A black person may have their mistakes, but they know what to do because they come from the same situ-

> ation. Helen Zille can dance for black people. The DA can install a black leader but we know that that is just a façade. We are not stupid; we can see what is happening. So while they think that they can play those mind games, that is what makes me distrust them even more. (*Bongani)

> The problem with South Africa starts with the fact that black people have long been discriminated against. Racism is something that affected me back then, but it doesn't any longer because it happens day in and day out. In the main we are poor and unemployed because we are black. Being unemployed has a big effect on our lives because you are implicated in many things in the community. It's not nice not to work because you find that if something goes missing or something bad happens, people say it is those dogs that aren't working. Sometimes, you cannot blame the poor for doing what is necessary to survive. People do things they never thought they would do only because they are poor. (*Wayne)

Due to the fact that South African mainstream media and political discourse is constructed through a lens of whiteness (Schutte, 2015), Black Twitter or collectivising online to push a positive narrative about black experience has gained popularity. Although defining Black Twitter is a difficult task, suffice to say the term refers to a particular collective of black identities and voices on Twitter taking part in collective, culturally specific jokes and dialogues that affect the community – "from discussing colorism to dishing out jokes about common 'black mom' phrases" (Wheeler, 2019). The term is used to describe a large network of black Twitter users and their loosely coordinated interactions, many of which accumulate into trending topics due to the network's size, interconnectedness and unique activity (Ramsey, 2015). Furthermore, Black Twitter can be seen as a temporally linked group of people, throughout the diaspora, who share culture, language and interest for specific issues, and who talk about specific topics with a black frame of reference (Clark, 2014).

The sensitivity those involved in online communities felt with media's representation of black life—which is negative or simplistic—lead to these collective engagements. Black Twitter and the humour we see are a reaction against the systems that encourage self-hate. Black Twitter communicators use the platform specifically to find redress or an avenue to field concerns about marginalisation amongst other things. This process, being part of this online community, starts with first identifying as a black person who is interested in the topic that is being discussed. This is followed by self-selection, which is deciding to participate in the conversation (Clark,

2014). Through that participation there's affirmation. The result is back and forth conversation between people about various topics. This constant engagement lets communicators know that they are not alone, and that there are others paying attention and engaged (Clark, 2014). This finally leads to "re-affirmation and vindication; the stage where participants are looking for some kind of change in the physical world". Clark (2014) argues this is where you often see online conversations reflected in offline spaces—when you see them being covered by certain news media personalities. This is when people lose jobs, people make public apologies for things that they have said that have been brought to light via Twitter (Clark, 2014).

Racism and Decolonial Love

This process of reaffirmation online can be understood as a way to love self in a world that encourages you to do otherwise—to self-hate. This is made necessary by the fact that colonialisation created a classificatory system that was used to classify subgroups of human types and to break up the diversity of society into distinct types according to essentialised characteristics (Hall, 1997). As much as classification is a fundamental aspect of human culture, as it allows the generation of meaning divisions according to race represent the negative aspect of classification because the systems can become a tool in the dispossession of power (Hall, 1997). The cultural function of colonial knowledge, in its drive to dominate for extraction, was to organise people based on their differences into hierarchical social groups (Hall, 1997). Racism is thus the use of classification as a system of power, where the markings of difference across populations become the reason for groups of people to be treated differently (Hall, 1997). The power of racism thus is to ascribe positive values to one group and negative values to another, and then to establish a system which becomes the basis of how to treat these various groups unequally (Hall, 1997).

Desai (2001) argues that racism was thus the legitimising force of colonial authority because the discourse of race and its subsequent power relations was such that whites gave orders and blacks obeyed (Desai, 2001). This was to rule by creating a dominant order, where the prevailing discourses relied on the representation of a savage 'other'. Mudimbe (1977) writes that the African was presented in European Enlightenment thought as an 'other'; with abnormal differences when compared to the white male, and, as such, race served to distinguish between savage and civilised. This secured a dominant position for the white race by assuring the control and exploitation of the subaltern population (Reddy, 2000). With the negative classification achieved, the dominant Western culture was free to pursue the project of colonialism which was billed an effort to save the dominated African culture from savagery (Desai, 2001).

Fanon (1952) observes that the black man (person) is black in relation to the white man (person). This point is similar to the one made by Mudimbe (1977) that Africa was formed as a series of oppositions in order to distinguish between the savage and the civilised. Fanon's (1952, 84) point is that the elements a black person uses to construct their being are provided for them by the other, the white man, who has "woven me out of a thousand details, anecdotes, stories". The crucial point highlighted by Fanon (1952) is that racism is effective because it operates on two levels: first on the "bodily and corporeal schema", which is physical domination, and second, below the surface, on the "schema composed of the stories and anecdotes and metaphors and images, which construct the relationship between the individual and the cultural space" (Fanon, 1952, 84).

The big takeaway from Fanon's (1952) conception of race is not just the negative understanding of stereotypes but also the perceived effects these have on the psyche of black people. Fanon (1952, 85) argues that the negative representations that the black person 'knows so well' enable a dislocation from his inherited sense of being. This dislocation then removes the self from the self, and imprisons the black individual in the world of whiteness, making them an object. Thus, when a black person is faced with the weight of representations that are placed on him, Fanon (1952) writes that it is possible that he ceases to be a person but becomes the subhuman and the construction the white world intends for him to be. This can be understood to mean that black people will suffer an inferiority complex caused by their skin colour, which might affect the way they engage in mainstream discourse. In addition, another possibility is of a deep-seated resistance to such depictions or oppression (see Bobo, 2004). The argument made is that, although the preceding might be true, it may also be true that, whether consciously or unconsciously, black South Africans who coalesce online are also engaged in a constant struggle to resist domination.

Contestation and Resistance

Even though colonial expansion was legitimated and largely accepted by both dominated and dominant people, there have always been undercurrents of ambivalence and anxiety (Desai, 2001). During the course of colonialisation, despite the evaporation of liberties and self-reliance, a critical awareness of colonial domination and the use of tropes for the purpose of legitimation was attained by the dominated (Prakash, 1991). It is in this respect that this chapter is intended to make the point that the process of domination and subordination is always a fracture and thus a point of friction between social formations. This is to say that dominated people have the possibility to accept, resist and reform the prevailing order. Magubane (1971) argues that because colonialism is economic, political and cultural domination, a process of acculturation—or of adopting the cultural traits or social patterns of another group—must be considered. In his regard, the process of domination is not solely about one culture being dominated by another. As such, any investigation into the behaviour of indigenous populations must take into account the 'total situation', which is to say domination and its inevitable counter point—resistance.

Such an analysis is to note that, although constructed in dominant discourses as essentialised objects of European history and exploitation, the subaltern refused the role of passive objects without a history (Reddy, 2000). Marginalised groups organised and articulated counter-discourses or an alternative tradition that constructed a history of resistance which reversed the narratives of the dominant group (Reddy, 2000). For example, nationalist organisations countered European domination by claiming a history of resistance that was traced back to the many wars fought between indigenous people and colonial forces (Reddy, 2000). This claim functioned as a way of positioning the counter-tradition of resistance, next to the dominant tradition of colonialism, as equal (Reddy, 2000). Like the dominant, the subordinate wished to secure a 'counter-identity' and appropriate as much control over social existence as possible (Reddy, 2000). These counter-discourses, therefore, produced an alternative 'tradition of struggle' and history, a tradition that also constituted a subaltern identity (Reddy, 2000).

Therefore, to acknowledge a history of resistance is to see colonialism as a mixture of two conflicting ideals rather than complete dominance. It is to see a tentative balance and to acknowledge that Africans have engaged with the discourses of the coloniser to produce their own inventions of

Africa (Magubane, 1971). Prakash (1991) argues that the subordinated can incorporate the principles and values of the social hierarchy, which continues to dominate them. They can do so while also, inadvertently, expanding its limits by resisting certain aspects of it. Therefore, Africa is not only invented in the negative or in the way suitable to the dominant. The concept of resistance allows us to see that people counter dominant discourses, and thus Africa, and any other situation of dominance, can be reinvented and turned into a positive conception (Desai, 2001, 7). This is to understand that colonial representations or stereotypes are a terrain of struggle and that the dominated have always sought and fought to represent themselves. The usefulness of this view to understanding black South Africans using social media to push back against negative representation is quite plain: through humour and anger people use available platforms to reimagine the bounds of social discourse.

Additionally, the theory of resistance is useful here because it points to the fact that it is unhealthy to assume or maintain easy binaries, such as domination and resistance. Reddy (2000) argues that the common assumption is that colonialism was about absolute dominance by the empire and the postcolonial period was about the triumph of revolutionary causes that fought on behalf of the subaltern. Such binaries allow themselves to easily fall into the tendency to think of resistance as the negation of domination, as something conceived and mounted in opposition and external to, if not autonomous (Haynes & Prakash, 1991). This is a tendency to delink the two moments as if there is first a period of domination, which is then followed by an independent time of resistance (Haynes & Prakash, 1991). The point of this account is to show that such a binary cannot be retained and to point out that there is often a conceptual divide between the colonial and postcolonial moments.

In this regard, Haynes and Prakash (1991) argue that the tendency to separate domination and resistance allows two assumptions to assert themselves. First, that relations of power enjoy an uncomplicated and unchallenged existence until moments of societal upheaval; and, second, that in 'normal' times, the cultural practices and identities of the dominated remain firmly grounded in a terrain mapped by the dominant. Such an understanding allows us to investigate power relations, whether colonial, postcolonial or post-authoritarian, not as singular or monolithic but rather as a practice fraught with contradictions and tensions (Reddy, 2000). Work done on the subject of resistance has argued that power must be seen as a tenuous exercise because it is constantly fractured by the everyday struggles of the subordinate because resistance is constantly present in the behaviours, traditions and consciousness of the subordinate (Haynes & Prakash, 1991). The online space, in the collectivisation of black people online to challenge ongoing subjugation through laughter and polemic, is an example of such struggles.

Multipositionality and Race

In light of the earlier discussion, Hall (1997) argues that the tendency for racial frameworks to allow appearance or an essence to stand in the place of what is, in fact, a deeply complex cultural system is the trap of racism. It is to seek the impossible: a guarantee of an essence from genetic features in a context of complex subaltern agency. Hall (1997) goes on to theorise that in the end racism cannot perform the function it is purposed, which is to fix a constructed 'truth' beyond any doubt. Therefore, a more adequate reading of race relations maintains that the challenges imposed on the subordinate by a racist gaze need equal consideration because, through responsive action, subaltern groups reform such boundaries (Guha, 1983). Social media has proven this to be the case with Black Twitter holding court on issues that affect black people—from the funny to the upsetting.

In the preceding sections, race has been discussed in reference to domination and resistance. The concept is again under discussion; however, this time it is in relation to its openness, which is due to the fact that domineering structures are often resisted. In this respect, Hall argues (Hall, 1997) that race can be likened to language because of the ideas it can signify. Similarly, Winter (2008, 18) writes that race is a "metalanguage because it serves as a global sign, since it speaks about and lends meaning to a host of terms and expressions". Therefore, since language is human in construction, race then is not a fixed concept but is socially and historically grounded (Hall, 1997). As an instance of trans-historic signification, race is only a sign that can be made to mean different things, in different cultures and at different times (Hall, 1997). Lewis (2008) emphasises that the meaning of all signs, including race, is relational because it is never fixed but subject to variation and thus multiple interpretations.

This discursive definition of race is important because it allowed the theoretical shift from an outdated understanding based on physical difference to an understanding of how ideas and knowledge of difference organise human practice (Hall, 1997). After initially subscribing to the science of race, Du Bois (1903) abandoned the scientific definitions that were prevalent at the time. He went on to favour more socio-historical approaches—writing that Africans and people of African descent share a common history, have suffered a common disaster and have one long memory of that misfortune (Du Bois, 1903). As such, Du Bois insisted that colour matters because its sense of meaning for black people is as a badge of social pain. It is important to arrive at this juncture because it adds to the earlier discussion that pointed to people of colour collecting around their historical tie to black pain and degradation. This is to say that by acknowledging openness of race, individuals have multiple realities and frameworks to draw from, including a shared black history. This shared black pain could then draw black people together and drive them to laugh at their countries' shortcomings or, equally, to express rage at the unequal systems that continue to benefit the white people the most.

Writing on the subject of domination and multipositionality, Biko (2004, 113) contends that in order to accommodate the problems they face, black people often develop a Janus face or an ontological split. This split is explained as, on one hand, being dominated or made to believe you are inferior, while on the other, resisting the domination by realising humanness.

One of the consequences of living life as both a person and a problem is a 'double consciousness'—"two souls in one dark body" (Du Bois, 1903). It is in light of this realisation that Du Bois (1903) postulates that black people are gifted at birth with a second sight, which is a way to see themselves using the lens of the dominant culture and their own: a life lived in a very complex manner (Du Bois, 1903). "It is a peculiar sensation, this double-consciousness, this sense of always looking at one's self through the eyes of others, of measuring one's soul by the tape of a world that looks on in amused contempt and pity. In other words, society makes difficulties for him because of his color, which thus means that the black man ever feels his two-ness, an American, a Negro; two souls, two thoughts, two unreconciled strivings; two warring ideals in one dark body, whose dogged strength alone keeps it from being torn asunder" (Du Bois, 1903, 8). With this sense of double consciousness, seeing the world from two states of mind, "the black man is always fighting to then understand his own self or attain a sense of self-consciousness. The life and history of the black man is the struggle to merge the two selves into one, into a "better and truer self" (Du Bois, 1903, 8).

Fanon (1952) furthers this analysis towards multipositionality in stating that the black person is a human being who knows himself to be complete because he inherits such understandings. However, he is convinced otherwise when dominated, and therefore he has to strive to reconcile these warring perceptions of self in order to find the "possibility of existence" (Fanon, 1952, 74). Fanon (1952, 84) goes on to call this the "triple person", which is to be in three places at once: subhuman, human and conflicted. The reason this insight is important is that it places emphasis on the fact that what takes place in the individual is not a simple merger of two cultures but different conceptions. The strength of such a view, to move beyond a double consciousness, is that it enables us to understand that black people occupy multiple positions. This could mean being totally dominated, being oppositional and negotiating through conflict, indifference or complete unawareness (Lewis 2008).

Multiple Realities of the Postcolony

Bhabha (1993) has remarked that the importance of multipositionality, or this idea of multiplicity of the colonial subject, is not about getting lost in plurality but rather about acknowledging a 'third space'. In his understanding of multipositionality, Bhabha (1993) follows Fanon's (1952) conception of the fluidity of blackness. The point is that the meaning of race is not singular but a constant and unending production of contested and contradictory meanings (Bhabha, 1993). Bhabha (1993) states that the in-between nature of blackness can be seen as a third space or a newness. What the framework articulates is a cultural difference that is defined as in-between space, a space in which areas of difference may overlap and thus create something unique (Bhabha, 1993).

The value of this discussion on multipositionality is not that a colonial subject draws from all available discourses simultaneously; it is that in having the option to do so, they create anew (Bhabha 1993). When applied here, the understanding is that the marginalised, those existing in the political society and those benefitting directly from the state through active negotiation outside the formal rules of citizenship might converse with power in many ways. They might, in one instance, engage in riots or rebellion, and in the next assume a language of deliberation rather than direct contestation. This is to move closer to what Chatterjee (2012) has called the need for a new conceptual framework in the analysis of postcolonial societies. Chatterjee (2012) argues that it is inappropriate to analyse political action in postcolonial settings as simply an uprising against the government or capital. Such has been the case in South Africa where many have falsely argued that the service delivery protests (or admonishment of the ruling party online) will result in a great loss of electoral power for the ANC (Friedman, 2015). This counter-view, which supports Chatterjee's (2012) position, argues that service delivery strikes in South Africa are launched by staunch supporters of the ANC, who have no intention of switching parties, but take to the streets in an effort to air their grievances (Friedman, 2015).

Chatterjee (2012) writes that since welfare and developmental functions are now widely recognised to be necessary tasks for the governments to provide for the poor, these functions are legitimately claimed by the poor. "This means that government officials and political representatives in rural areas are constantly besieged by demands for various forms of welfare and development benefits. It also means that poor citizens learn to operate the levers of the government system, to apply pressure at the right places or negotiate for better terms. This is where the everyday operations of democratic politics, organisation and leadership come into play" (Chatterjee, 2012, 132). This process of acquiescence and rebellion is more a play on the dominant power structure, and a way of manoeuvring, rather than attempts to revolutionise the system.

In this regard, Chatterjee (2012) argues that the power struggles that we see in postcolonial societies cannot simply be reduced to a dramatic confrontation between those in power and the 'contradictory consciousness' of subaltern classes who acquiesce to the power but also violently oppose it. It is when such a stance is taken that one can see that this process is more about the relation of people to power, in environments where inequality is prevalent and enduring. To comprehend such a context, Chatterjee (2012) maintains that critical scholars have to apply a new framework, one that is able to account for multipositionality of those that have to bear the brunt of an old history and a new history in the present world. In responding to Chatterjee's call, the framework that has been developed here is novel because it considers the varying types of online engagement (the laughter next to the rage) by black people not contradictory or passive but multifaceted and unique.

As a way towards a conclusion, the work done by Mbembe (2001) offers a further way forward. Mbembe (2001, 103) highlights the historical continuity, arguing that postcolonial African regimes did not invent government systems from scratch after independence. Rather, these states gained their social knowledge from several cultures, heritages and traditions, whose "features have become entangled over time" (Mbembe,

2001, 103). As such, Mbembe (2001) further argues that the postcolony is chaotically pluralistic. Although it has its own internal coherence, it has developed unique systems in re-forming the old systems. Building on the point of uniqueness caused by the mixture of several traditions, Mbembe (2001, 102) writes that the "postcolony is thus characterised by a distinctive style of political improvisation, a tendency to excess and a lack of proportion, as well as by distinctive ways identities are multiplied, transformed, and put into circulation".

Mbembe (2001) forwards the argument that has been drawn out in this chapter by writing that in order to understand and to account for postcolonial relations of power, "we need to go beyond the binary categories used in standard interpretations of domination, such as resistance vs passivity, autonomy vs subjection, state vs civil society, hegemony vs counter hegemony…" (Mbembe, 2001, 103). Doing so is to realise that what you have in postcolonial societies today is something "akin to a custom, which fronts as modernity but without being fully included in it" (Mbembe, 2001, 103). Therefore, although the colonial state model and its repressive tendencies have always lived side by side with a liberal civic order, the state has often practised the exact opposite of the liberal model of debate and discussion. Mbembe (2001) argues that this sense of uneasy split is more pronounced in the postcolony because its sense of divide between ruler and subjects is inflated to despotic levels.

It is in this regard that Mbembe (2001) argues that maintaining a framework of oppositions is unhelpful and instead clouds the nature of postcolonial relations. This is because, although postcolonial systems are characterised by extremes, these extremes still live side by side. It is thus better to recognise the postcolonial nationalist orders that were instituted after independence were operated within a mixture of systems and maintained hegemony in such a cacophonous environment by producing 'overblown' symbols (Mbembe, 2001, 103). Therefore, in the postcolony the 'overblown' and 'grotesque' are essential features of the society. Influenced by colonial structuring, the dominant power is obscene in using violence in its display of power. The subject population is also obscene and grotesque in voicing displeasure. Obscenity and grotesque are thus part and parcel of the space because they can be used for repression and as ways to undermine those in power and to show vulnerability of officialdom (through laughter and through protest). It is only through such a shift in perspective that we can understand that the postcolonial relationship is not primarily a relationship of resistance or collaboration but of newness and reformation (Mbembe, 2001).

This means that in order to understand online engagement by subaltern citizens and subjects in a postcolonial setting, we have to understand the multiplicity of their subject positions. This is "Because Africa is moving in several directions at once, this is a period that, at the same time, has been, is not yet, is, at once, in front and behind, inside and outside, above and below" (Mbembe, 2001, 241). With these insights in mind, Mbembe (2001) urges that we must realise that the postcolony and its subjects are far from being uniform and cannot be reduced to simpletons or contradiction. Therefore, what has to be understood is that although the marginalised making sense of the world might appear to be contradictory, the overlapping nature of systems in this society requires such a study to recognise that a person pulls from various frameworks in order to make unique sense of a changed and rapidly changing society. In order to understand this pendulum swing between fear, laughter and loathing, it is important we understand the multiposition of a black person. They are at once in love with the country of their birth, and in another instance loathe the very same country that is structured to oppress them.

Conclusion

The point that is drawn out is one comprehensively argued by Lewis (2008), who states that in the context of cultural conflict and social divisions, we have to understand that a black person is one person and many people, and this speaks to a 'multipositionality'. This means that we have to also realise that when we talk of a racialised subjectivity it means being aware of the textured nature of black subjectivity, and we thus have to reject simple constructions of black people as 'uni-dimensional' individuals capable of only a single and uniform consciousness (Lewis 2008). What the Mbembe (2001) and Chatterjee (2012) insights illuminate is that when examining black social life, it is important to keep in mind that it is rather a complex mixture of standpoints affected by history, oppression, culture, conquest and many other variables. It is an attempt to grant the oppressed agency, the ability to convert forms of oppression to ways of living. Everyday reality is an expression of deconial love—it is a daily attempt to love self in a world that encourages one to hate themselves.

Selected User Responses: Laughter

In an article titled, "I Just Want to Come Home", published by *TimesLive*, one of the people stuck in China said: "We are now completely stranded … I just want to come home, I just want to go back to my mom and give her a big hug".

1. One of the first responses to the article joked: Your mom gave me the message, she says you not worry about the hug, just stay there and be a big girl, she will send kisses with Instagram.
2. Your mother is also mothering all of us in your absence here, so we just can't risk her, we love u sis.
3. Nana listen we love you but don't come here, asseblief. We will send you whatever you need, OK? Biltong, magewu and inkomazi. Just let us know what it is you need. And don't write to us either because you've probably sneezed all over that paper and envelope. Please darling, we can't risk you coming here and making the vulnerable sick. Sending you love.
4. Stay there dear, we are busy fixing the problems that made you leave in the first place…So give us the opportunity to better ourselves like you did.
5. Just hang in there a bit longer, not easy at all Mzantsi is not ready for that Corona now,but always remember not just momy but the whole of South Africa loves you a lot, keep well.
6. South Africa is on holiday pls come when we back.
7. Just spoke to ur mom, well she said everything is fine so stay there until everything is cleared.
8. No need to stress about coming here my dear…we will transport your mother to you.
9. If only you knew that we are dealing with loadshedding you wouldn't come this side. You have a better chance of survival that side. Are you not excited about the new hospital? Go and take pictures. Don't forget to share please because sharing is caring. Enjoy.
10. Just buy a mask. You are safe with a mask.
11. Hai stay there, do you know how many tenders it takes to build a toilet here? Never shem.
12. Don't worry my darling. It was made in China,It won't last long.
13. They must stay there shuuuuu we cant build a hospital in 48 hrs here.
14. Stay there coz we've temporarily moved to Zim you won't find anyone here even mom has moved .

15. Plz Nana. We love you and don't come back. We have enough PROBLEMS and I don't think we can deal with Corona virus. We can't even manage Eskom; then what abt corona.

Selected User Responses: Rage

The supermarket Makro trended number one in South Africa in late March as when the first case of the coronavirus was reported in South Africa, it sparked panic buying.

1. The same people that brought the virus to our shores are now panic buying in bulk and emptying all the shelves in stores and leaving nothing for the rest of us. This is bullshit behavior.
2. When it whites it called 'Panic buying' when it black it called 'breaking the rules' by the way there is still queue at Makro even now.
3. Check who has the luxury of "panic buying". They will then get in their big ass cars and go self quarantine in their comfy homes. My people are packed up ko Noord taxi rank to get to their shacks, make plans to feed their families just for today #Makro #Coronavirussouthafrica
4. She is not talking sense when she lies this has nothing to do with black an whiteFace with tears of joyFace with tears of joyblack pple shop at makro I have a makro 4 km away from me an that's the shop I use a lot and they reported on makro lines during the panic buying what sense are u speaking off?
5. This is going to get increasingly annoying during this lockdown so let me say this. 1. Most low income people were not given time off to prep for #SouthAfricanLockdown. 2. Those same people cannot bulk buy so stores will see them more often.
6. While abo Piet was panic buying out the whole Makro at 11:15 on a random Tuesday, the people in this picture were working in CNA, as domestic workers, in a Fish and Chips shop not able to get more than 30 minutes for lunch.
7. Basically people with money are cleaning out shops- even big outlets like Makro- to fill their houses? What are you doing with 10 bags of 10 kg rice? I hope you're donating to different families in need cos this panic buying is too much
8. Corona is not gonna kill us... Starvation will....we will die of hunger because of panic buying #Makro

9. Who was shooting when white people crowded @Makro_SA Alberton panic buying few days before the announcement of the official shutdown
10. The difference in reporting now that some black people are paid and are panic buying vs when the whites clogged up Makro. Why are these reporters at townships telling us about people not abiding by the law? Suka
11. Why were you not at Makro when white people were panic buying like the world is coming to an end. Where was this fake concern? FYI we don't have cars, we live far from supermarkets. You are annoying.
12. By excusing criminals and criminality as part and parcel of "township life". Face with rolling eyes. Nothing has been more racist than the current governments low expectations about black folk. They don't take law enforcement and the rule-of-law seriously in poor, mostly black communities.

References

Bhabha, H. K. (1993). *The location of culture*. Routledge.

Biko, S. (2004). *I write what I like*. Pan Macmillan South Africa.

Bobo, J. (2004). The color purple: Black women as cultural readers. In J. Bobo, C. Hudley, & C. Michel (Eds.), *The black studies reader*. Routledge.

Carr, P. R. (2016). Whiteness and white privilege: Problematizing race and racism in a "color-blind" world. *International Journal of Critical Pedagogy, 7*(1).

Chatterjee, P. (2012). Gramsci in the twenty-first century. In N. Srivastava & B. Bhattacharya (Eds.), *The postcolonial Gramsci*. Routledge.

Clark, M. (2014). *To Tweet our own cause: A mixed method study of the online phenomenon Black Twitter*. PhD thesis, Chapel Hill.

Daniels, G. (2021, forthcoming). *The oppressive politics of place: How decolonial love could be a tonic for South African women journalists*. Unisa Press.

Desai, G. G. (2001). *Subject to colonialism: African self-fashioning and the colonial library*. Duke University Press.

Du Bois, W. E. B. (1903). *The souls of black folk: Essays and sketches*. A. Constable.

Duncan, J. (2013). South African journalism and the Marikana massacre: A case study of an editorial failure. *The Political Economy of Communication, 1*(2), 65–88.

Entman, R. M., & Gross, K. A. (2008). Race to judgement: Stereotyping media and criminal defendants. *Law and Contemporary Problems, 71*(93).

Fanon, F. (1952). *Black skin, white masks*. Pluto Press.

Friedman, S. (2015). The Janus face of the past: Preserving and resisting South African path dependence. In X. Mangcu (Ed.), *The colour of our future: Does race matter in post-apartheid South Africa?* Wits University Press.

Gray, H. (1997). What a story! Understanding the audience for scandal. In J. Lull & S. Hinerman (Eds.), *Media scandals: Morality and desire in the popular culture marketplace*. Polity Press.

Guha, R. (1983). On some aspects of the historiography of colonial India. In *Subaltern studies: Writings on Indian history and society*. Oxford University Press.

Hall, S. (1997). *Race, the floating signifier*. Media Education Foundation. Retrieved from http://www.mediaed.org/transcripts/Stuart-Hall-Race-the-Floating-Signifier-Transcript.pdf

Haynes, D., & Prakash, G. (1991). *Contesting power: Resistance and everyday social relations in South Asia*. Oxford University Press.

Hlongwane, S. (2016). Tatane, Macia, Marikana: South Africa's own #BlackLivesMatter moment is long overdue. *Mail and Guardian*. Published 14 July 2016. Retrieved from: https://mg.co.za/article/2016-07-14-00-tatane-macia-marikana-south-africas-own-blacklivesmatter-moment-is-long-overdue

Larson, S. G. (2006). *Media & minorities: The politics of race in news and entertainment*. New York: Rowman & Littlefield Publishers.

Lewis, E. (2008). Race, power, multipositionality. *Interventions, 10*(3), 340–358.

Magubane, B. (1971). A critical look at indices used in the study of social change in Colonial Africa. *Current Anthropology, 12*(4), 419–445.

Mbembe, A. (2001). *On the postcolony*. Wits University Press.

Mudimbe, V. Y. (1977). *The invention of Africa*. Indiana University Press.

Ponono, M. (2019). *Centralising a counter public: An ethnographic study of the interpretation of mainstream news media by young adults in Joza*. PhD thesis, Rhodes University. Retrieved from: https://vital.seals.ac.za/vital/access/manager/Repository/vital:28655?site_name=GlobalView

Prakash, G. (1991). Government and resistance in South Asia. In D. Haynes & G. Prakash (Eds.), *Contesting power: Resistance and everyday social relations in South Asia*. Oxford University Press.

Ramokhele, B. (2018). How we make Johann Rupert rich daily. *City Press*, December 11, 2018. Retrieved from: https://www.news24.com/citypress/voices/how-we-make-johann-rupert-rich-daily-20181211?fbclid=IwAR3spoAmxORe4LWK-OLeNYYgKdvZ7l4TftCFiAQ8kVtb9KowF_NeNA2K3XA

Ramsey, D. X. (2015, April 10). The truth about Black Twitter: Complex, influential, and far more meaningful than the sum of its social justice-driven hashtags. *The Atlantic*. Retrieved from: https://www.theatlantic.com/technology/archive/2015/04/the-truth-about-black-Twitter/390120

Reddy, T. (2000). *Hegemony and resistance: Contesting identities in South Africa*. Ashgate.

Sandoval, C. (2000). *Methodology of the oppressed*. University of Minneapolis Press.

Schutte, G. (2015). Colonial tropes and the media coverage of the Marikana massacre. *French Journal for Media Research*. Retrieved from: http://frenchjournalformediaresearch.com/index.php?id=610

Tomaselli, K. (1997). Ownership and control in the South African print media: Black empowerment after apartheid, 1990–1997. *Ecquid Novi: African Journalism Studies, 18*(1), 67–68.

Wheeler, A. (2019, December 23). Ten years of Black Twitter: A merciless watchdog for problematic behaviour. *The Guardian*. Retrieved from: https://www.theguardian.com/technology/2019/dec/23/ten-years-black-Twitter-watchdog

Winter, N. J. G. (2008). *Dangerous frames: How ideas about race and gender shape public opinion*. Chicago University Press.

PART III

Weapons of the Masses: Humour, Ridicule and Confronting Political Power

CHAPTER 11

#VoetsekANC and COVID Corruption: A Foucauldian Discourse Analysis of "A Song for the ANC"

Adelina Mbinjama

Introduction

In August 2020, many South Africans were alarmed by the extent to which the African National Congress (ANC) had deviated from the values of its veterans, as revealed by the number of corruption cases levied against its members. The party experienced a backlash in response to their misdealings when they were exposed for giving state tenders to deliver personal protective equipment (PPE), intended to assist those engaged in combatting the coronavirus (COVID-19) pandemic, to individuals within the ANC social circles. Columnist Bishop Sithembele Sipuka's (2020) *Corruption Has Become SA's Other 'Pandemic'* briefly explains how people expressed their discontent at a government and political party whose unscrupulous nature seemingly knew no bounds.

A. Mbinjama (✉)
Department of Media Studies, Cape Peninsula University of Technology, Cape Town, South Africa

S. Mpofu (ed.), *Digital Humour in the Covid-19 Pandemic*,
https://doi.org/10.1007/978-3-030-79279-4_11

Citizens reacted across various social media platforms, shunning and mocking with the hashtag #VoetsekANC, signifying that the ruling government had lost credibility. 'Voetsek', a South African slang term for 'go away', is a combination of Afrikaans and tsotsitaal (a township colloquial tongue) (see Bhana, 2016; Adjepong, 2020). The word is often used to shout at stray dogs and is considered a derogative term that is discouraged when interpolating a human being, especially in public. As mentioned earlier, at the apex of the COVID PPE corruption by ANC members, the #VoetsekANC hashtag started trending on social media, including on TikTok, among a population of Internet users (such as Generation Z and Generation Alpha) who typically do not comment on ANC actions.

Ridicule and humour, using memes, parodies, songs and videos, were increasingly being associated with the ANC during August–September 2020. Wasserman (2020) notes that, almost immediately after the national lockdown was announced in March 2020, South Africans took to social media, with memes featuring prominent politicians and negative puns, using TikTok (www.tiktok.com) video clips, Twitter (www.twitter.com), WhatsApp (www.whatsapp.com) and Facebook (www.facebook.com) statuses to make fun of the virus.

More recently, news of corruption by the ANC during COVID-19 resulted in social media users vetting #VoetsekANC online. To further mock and ridicule the ruling government in respect of its series of corruption cases that keep mounting, The Kiffness musician, Dave Scott, made a parody, called "A Song for the ANC", of English band Pink Floyd's "Another Brick in the Wall" (see The Kiffness, 2020). This chapter offers a Foucauldian discourse analysis (FDA) of the song as "an innovative qualitative methodology" (Sam, 2019). While Foucault himself never explored the relationship his work had with online movements, the chapter argues that the song and #VoetsekANC movement are manifestations of Foucault's 'governmentality' and of influencer culture. Theoretical debates on the usefulness of Foucault's notion of governmentality for online movements are in relatively short supply. Thus, governmentality as a theoretical tool in analysing the power relations that have manifested themselves on social media at micro- and macro-levels bridges the gap in literature on online movements.

Literature Review

Social Media and Politics in South Africa (2015–2020)

The convergence of social media and politics in South Africa is not new. Notably, it became prevalent during the 2015 and 2016 *#RhodesMustFall* and *#FeesMustFall* protests on university campuses (Baragwanath, 2016; Mpofu, 2017). Students had staged protests on campuses to lament the institutional racism they experienced and, later, the fee increases, both of which would continue to render universities a space that is only accessible to the privileged few (Baragwanath, 2016). Students used social media as a tool to mobilise themselves, which proved to be an effective form of political communication. Baragwanath (2016) further notes that although students used social media as a form of mobilisation, it did not replace physical participation. It merely supplemented it.

Another noteworthy intersection between social media and politics in South Africa has to be the Bell Pottinger disinformation campaign in 2017. This campaign was coordinated by the UK public relations firm, Bell Pottinger, at the behest of the then beleaguered South African President Jacob Zuma (Tannous et al., 2019). According to Tannous et al. (2019), the campaign was designed to exploit the racial divisions that exist in South Africa, on behalf of the Gupta family, who were associates of Jacob Zuma. The campaign made use of terms such as "white monopoly capital" and "radical economic transformation" as a way of drawing attention away from the Gupta family's nefarious business dealings with the state (Tannous et al., 2019).

Research conducted by Malila et al. (2013) reveals that young people in South Africa are distrustful of politicians and political institutions. Political cynicism and frustration with the performance of the current government provides an abundant space for elaboration of scandals and of conspiracy theories that provide more believable "explanations for people's current circumstances than political, economic, or scientific authorities" (Wasserman, 2020). Therefore, it is not surprising that (especially) young people take to social media to air their frustrations and to share their opinions about politics. Wasserman (2020) maintains that the increased ubiquity of the growing range of social media platforms exposes users to multiple editing tools which, in turn, enable media users to create and engage with news topics in more creative ways. Perhaps more cogent is the recognition on Wasserman's (2020) part of the various psychosocial, political and psychological reasons as to why South Africans choose to express themselves through humour—as opposed to despair—despite the many challenges that they face.

In Ellis's (1989) ground-breaking article "Tuning in to pavement radio", he defines an African phenomenon that has no official English term but can best be described in French as "radio trottoir", which directly translates to "pavement radio". Pavement radio, according to Ellis (1989, 321), "can be defined as the popular and unofficial discussion of current affairs in Africa". Unlike traditional media, such as press, television and radio, there is "no identifiable individual, institution or group of people" that controls it (Ellis, 1989, 321). Ellis (1989, 322) maintains that the "social role and pedigree of pavement radio" is qualitatively different to rumour and gossip and plays a different social and political function. It is also different to rumour in its choice of subject, as pavement radio usually discusses issues of public interest or importance (Ellis, 1989).

This latter point is pivotal to this study, as the root cause of the discontent towards the ANC is endemic corruption, which in and of itself is a matter of public interest and importance. Pavement radio, opines Ellis (1989, 329), should therefore "be seen in the same light as oral tradition and treated as a descendent of the more formal oral histories that are linked with ruling dynasties and national rituals". Wasserman (2020) argues that "these practises"— referring to the oral traditions of socio-political commentary—illustrate how the conviviality of African societies also influences their media use. At a political level, pavement radio often thrives when mainstream media are strictly controlled by authorities or where the distrust of official narratives is commonplace (Wasserman, 2020). In the South African context, media ownership and control are a contested matter and, while there is a significant number of South Africans who still trust mainstream media, there are factions, particularly amongst young people, who distrust it (Wasserman, 2020). Hence, social media has become an alternate means of communicating and receiving political information.

Foucault has been used in other academic texts to discuss digital media influencers, making his philosophical underpinnings suitable for this chapter (see Maples-Yap, 2020). Olivier (2010, 294) states that, by using Foucault, multiple subject positions can be constructed through media representation. Therefore, these contexts provide a basis for the discussions around online movements and their implications for what Michel Foucault calls 'governmentality' (which will be discussed later in the chapter).

Social Media and Influencer Culture in South Africa

Social media have provided accessible platforms to a new generation of political influencers, especially those individuals not coming from traditional political backgrounds or actors such as politicians, lobbyists or full-time journalists. The Kiffness song has made an impact on the way their audiences, and the broader social audience, think about politics. The Kiffness is a live electronic act from Cape Town, South Africa, founded by Dave Scott in 2011. Dave Scott, who is now a reputable producer, is important in the political sphere because of the influence he has on predominantly younger, more affluent users on social media. These individuals are, in their own right, particularly engaged and active online, with a moderate number of followers.

Wellman, Stoldt, Tully and Ekdale (2020, 68) describe social media influencers as individuals who seek to "leverage their social and cultural capital on social media to shape the opinions and purchasing decisions of others". Most of the literature relating to social media influencers and influencer marketing relates to the commercial aspects of this phenomenon. For example, consideration is given to the ways in which brands make use of social media influencers, as part of the marketing mix, to acquire more customers and to grow their market share. From a commercial perspective, scholars have come to question the value and impact of social media influencers on brand equity and positioning (van Staden & van Niekerk, 2018; Abratt, 2019).

However, literature on influencer marketing as it relates to politics in the Global South points to the existence of political parties who use social media influencers to garner votes during elections. Although there may be blurred lines in this regard—especially if one considers Singh's (2019) assertion that the modern science of politics sees voters as consumers who ostensibly have to "purchase" politicians and public servants in elections—they still serve as an apt point of departure from which to analyse influencer marketing. In 2016, South African celebrity influencers were implicated in an ANC-sponsored covert social media campaign that attempted to besmirch opposition parties and garner support for the governing party, the ANC, during the 2016 Local Government Elections (Comrie, 2017). Those who participated in the campaign were dubbed as members of "the war room", which was led by ANC member and activist, Shaka Sisulu, and public relations professional, Sihle Bolani (Comrie, 2017). The campaign, according to Comrie (2017), raised the ire of members of the ANC leadership and proved to be unsuccessful as the ANC lost the support in key metros during that election. This gives credence to questions raised by van Staden and van Niekerk (2018) and by Abratt (2019) relating to the efficacy of influencer marketing in achieving the desired objectives of its organisation.

The questionable results are attributed to the perceived lack of authenticity associated with influencer marketing; Wellman et al. (2020) hold that influencers have a tendency to operate outside of ethical frameworks and thus tend to skirt certain legal considerations. In contrast, political activists who have used social media to garner support for their movements have also garnered influencer status, but without their ethical frameworks being questioned. The social media activism demonstrated by TikTok users in South Africa as a means of expressing their discontent towards the ANC is an example of how ordinary South Africans have used social media influencer principles as a means of capturing the imagination of their audiences. Furthermore, because #VoetsekANC gained popularity through the organic sharing of content on TikTok and then, later, on other social media platforms, one can thus deduce that there was no alternative political force that was influencing this anti-ANC sentiment. This gives this movement a sense of authenticity that is not readily afforded to ordinary social media influencers who post content at the behest of a brand or political organisation.

TikTok Amongst Generation X and Generation Alpha

We can extrapolate from the #VoetsekANC movement that TikTok and other social media platforms in South Africa were used collectively for galvanising protests about political circumstances that citizens were displeased about. Experts say that TikTok is a place where individuals can share their thoughts, ideas, passions and humour online and where others can comment about it (Keeton, 2020). TikTok is a video-sharing platform that allows users to create fun, positive, humorous and joyful micro-videos, ranging from "several seconds to several minutes and then share it with the wider TikTok community" (Zhu et al., 2020, 2). The platform, now available in over 150 countries, was founded in 2017 and is believed to be the fastest growing social media application in the world, topping the list of "the most downloaded" applications in 2018 (Zhu et al., 2020, 2). According to We Are Social (2019), TikTok claims to have 500 million active users and over a billion downloads. A 2019 study suggests that

TikTok added 188 million new users in the first three months of 2019 (Yeh, 2019). This speaks to the growing popularity of the platform in South Africa, where the TikTok trend—in terms of popularity—is following a similar path.

World Wide Worx MD, Arthur Goldstuck, has stated, "TikTok has its own rules, and the first one is that all the rules of social media have changed" (Mzekandaba, 2020). He said this in light of the way TikTok gained traction faster than any other platform. The surge in TikTok usage was seen after the COVID-19-induced lockdown at the end of March 2020. The increased usage can also be attributed to people's need for home entertainment during this period (Keeton, 2020). This type of platform is something, according to McCoubrey (2020) (cited in Keeton, 2020), teenagers have always loved. Users as young as 13 have an opportunity to engage on the platform (Keeton, 2020).

A recent study conducted by World Wide Worx and Ornico states that TikTok in South Africa gained notoriety in 2019 and gained momentum amongst the youth in 2020 (Mzekandaba, 2020). In South Africa, TikTok was the biggest social media sensation of 2019, and in 2020 had the biggest youth market, with the majority of its subscribers being young people who were born post the apartheid regime and who make up what is known as Generations Z and Alpha. According to DeIuliis and Saylor (2021), Generation Z are those born after 2001 and Generation Alpha are those born after 2009. Both these population groups participated and were exposed to #VoetsekANC due to influencer culture.

One of the key associations that can be made is that TikTok users mobilised their social and cultural capital to shape the opinions of others about the political discourses in South Africa. Generation Z and Generation Alpha were politicising their views and those of their social networks—which include family, friends, influencers and politicians—by creating video content that included #VoetsekANC memes, parodies and songs such as "A Song for the ANC", all of which aimed to express their dissatisfaction with the ANC. The movement #VoetsekANC and song "A Song for the ANC" are manifestations of influencer culture and what Foucault calls 'governmentality'—a concept used by Wellman et al. (2020) when defining social media influencers. In the light of the evident distrust of political institution by young people in South Africa and their use of social media as a platform to express their discontent, the authors have elected to focus on the political reasons for "A Song for the ANC", providing a discourse analysis that aims to discuss the different types of language used in the song, and the purposes and effects of cultural rules and conventions used in the lyrics.

This chapter is significant because, historically, online movements in South Africa have been centred around gender-based violence, university fees and other social issues, but not against the governing political party—that is, until the recent #VoetsekANC. Whilst the chapter does not fully unearth all South Africa's sociopolitical discourses prevailing on social media, including in their humorous forms, it nonetheless provides analysis of reflection on the current government and its politics, as authored by The Kiffness musician and social media influencer, Dave Scott, and users of #VoetsekANC. This chapter contributes to the existing literature on online movements and argues that #VoetsekANC and the song by The Kiffness are manifestation of governmentality and of influencer culture, as what has transpired in the real world of politics has translated to the online environment. Thus, the focus of this chapter is the analysis of the #VoetsekANC movement that bridges social media and politics.

Theoretical Framework and Methodology

Foucauldian Philosophies and Humour in South Africa

What makes Foucault's ideas complimentary to this chapter is the fact that his major works [*A History of Madness* (1961), *The Birth of the Clinic: An Archaeology of Medical Perception* (1963), *The Order of Things: An Archaeology of the Human Sciences* (1966) and *Discipline and Punish: The Birth of the Prison* (1975)] represent an attempt to produce a historical account of the formation of ideas, including those that are philosophical. As a cultural theorist and philosopher, Foucault attempted to show how there have been shifts in our understandings from one epoch to another, separating our thinking in the modern age from that of earlier ages (Buckingham et al., 2011, 302). Thus, for example, the ideas of Generation X and Generation Alpha are very different from the ideas of those who are much older. Ideas are constitutive of the historical contexts. In modern societies, for example, salient aspects of context that influence idea formation are the greater division of labour, greater urbanisation, organic solidarity and greater growth of individualism (Buckingham et al., 2011, 303). Foucault's interest in psychoanalysis underpinned his concern for crime, the body, madness and sexuality. He analysed the emergence of modern institutions, such as prisons, hospitals and schools, that have played an increasing role in controlling and monitoring the social population. He wanted to show that there was another side to Enlightenment ideas about individual liberty—namely, the concern with discipline and surveillance. Foucault advanced important ideas about the relationship between power, ideology and discourse in relation to modern organisational systems. As a result, Foucault has been used in academic discourses to critique governments, systems of institutions and discursive practices (see Macleod & Durrheim, 2002).

Foucault's work has also been used to discuss the use of humour in various contexts (see Dolan, 1993). According to Wasserman (2020), the use of laughter to deal with the virus may also be a form of catharsis for African people. Humour is not a foreign concept to South Africans, particularly during times of crisis. Events such as the corruption characteristic of the Jacob Zuma era, later termed "state capture", and the ongoing power blackouts as a result of an inept national power utility, Eskom, are examples of crises where South Africans have chosen humour as opposed to despair (Wasserman, 2020).

Since discourses of humour and power may be approached by many avenues, this chapter focuses on Dave Scott's (The Kiffness) lyrics of "A Song for the ANC" and on #VoetsekANC to argue that they are manifestations of 'governmentality' and influencer culture. Poststructuralist thinkers like Foucault make it possible to critique some of the ideologies underlying these two social media phenomena. The "A Song for the ANC" contains meta discourses—it philosophically denotes discussion about a discussion.

'Governmentality' and Discourse in Social Media

Foucauldian discourse analysis allows for an interpretivist approach to how social media platforms provide a certain level of autonomy to individuals on these platforms. Olivier (2009, 2) states that Foucault's notion of discourse "seems to suggest that, because human subjects are discursively constituted, their actions can only be grasped in terms and on the basis of the (historical) discourses that comprise subjects' subjectivity exhaustively".

Olivier (2010, 294) states that "human identity is structured by language in the sense of discourse". He defines discourse as:

> *language insofar as meaning and power-relations come together in it. In other words, talking about discourse as that which makes humans distinctive, is an*

acknowledgement that the language we use is not innocent, but carries the imprint of power-relations, and the discourse that first structures our psyche configures it one way or another as far as these unavoidable (albeit revisable) interests or relations of power are concerned. (Olivier, 2010, 294–295)

According to Olivier (2010, 295) "Wherever discourse operates, a counter-discourse can be activated which means that dominant discourses can be discursively opposed from the position of the speaking subject, as opposed to that of the one that is 'spoken' or constructed" (Olivier, 2003, 2005).

Discourse, as defined by Foucault, refers to ways of creating knowledge, along with the communal practices, forms of bias and power relations which are inherent in such knowledges and relations between them (see Foucault, 1990; Foucault, 1995). Baumgarten and Ullrich (2016, 14) explain:

Discourses are more than ways of thinking about producing meaning. Discourses define the boundaries of what can be thought of and communicated at a given time in a given society. The suffragettes of the late 19th and early 20th centuries, for example, did not demand equal distribution of childcare between men and women, because at that time it was still generally unthinkable. They did, however, call for equal political rights, e.g. the right to vote. These claims fit well into the historical context of institutional reforms that extend the franchise.

As Lemke (2002, 12) asserts, "Discourses and other practices in power regulation, such as practices of government and the government of the self, shape the subjectivity of the people". According to Lemke (2002, 10), Foucault often defines governmentality as the "art of government". Lemke explains that

Foucault coins the concept of "governmentality" as a "guideline" for the analysis he offers by way of historical reconstructions embracing a period starting from Ancient Greece through to modern neo-liberalism (Foucault, 1997, *67). The semantic linking of governing ("gouverner") and modes of thought ("mentalité") indicates that it is not possible to study the technologies of power without an analysis of the political rationality underpinning them".* (Lemke, 2002, 2)

Baumgarten and Ullrich (2016, 15) explain that, in Foucauldian terms, discourses "shape the individual's relations to her/himself and thus affect the mobilization potential of social movements" (see also Rabinow, 1994;

Foucault & Ewald, 2003). Foucault's approach to subjectivity is correlative with a study of "techniques of the self" (Kelly, 2013, 517; Lemke, 2002, 4). The enquiry of technique was already prominent in Foucault's reflections of the 1970s on power—of all his works, he uses the term "technique" most recurrently in *Discipline and Punish* (1975) (Kelly, 2013, 511). In Foucault's trajectory of thinking, this idea is now applied to the self—that is, to what we do to ourselves rather than to others (Kelly, 2013). Examples would be obsession with oneself, and prioritsing oneself. This stance is openly evident on TikTok, where users make quick videos of themselves to convey personal, sociopolitical and cultural issues that they want their followers to grasp and be entertained by.

Neoliberal governments are a dominant form of government in which the understanding is that the market is the fairest mechanism in so far as it gives the most to those who achieve the most through self-promotion. Although there are dominant discourses that exist in such a system, people have a *choice* whether to question power. According to Foucault (1990, p. 84) this is so "whether it is the discourse of patriarchy, or that of capitalism". In effect, "we are not exclusively 'spoken' or 'constructed' by it [discourse], which is another way of saying that we are not slaves to it" (Olivier, 2010, 295).

Instead of being captives to and victims of the dominant ideologies, #VoetsekANC demonstrated that the mass population in South Africa were fed-up and against the ways in which the ANC government was governing. The government's ideas and behaviours shaped Dave Scott (The Kiffness) and the societies he represents. Attached to being a young, white male South African—as Dave Scott is—are a specific set of discourses. The commonplace negative discourses about his demographic convey that some of them are entitled, spoilt, racist and oblivious to the privileges they enjoy from being born 'white'. To make a valid assessment, one would have to unravel the individual's human identity to recognise and understand layers of discourses.

For centuries, whites (especially men) have controlled South Africa through slavery and colonial rule and then through the apartheid regime. After 1994, a black majority ruling party (ANC) took over the administration of the country and has since been in power. While subjectivation was used in the past to control and dominate people (including through technologies), many South Africans feel that the current government is taking advantage of the power bestowed on them (Malinga, 2021). Of note, Foucault (1978, 95) opines that "Where there is power, there is resistance". Through the hashtag, citizens publicly shared their political discourses against the ANC more widely online than via traditional media. This got the attention of leaders of the ANC, indicating that its supporters had made paradigm shifts and wanted more sovereignty and for government to be more responsible with the power the people had given them over the years through votes.

Foucault theorises the interwoven relationship of online movements and the ANC and helps comprehend "A Song for the ANC" as a form of resistance and as a manifestation of influencer culture and 'governmentality'. Foucault is concerned with the practices and tactics of power which are the foundation of social structures and organisations. Governmentality consequently permits us to observe the authenticated forms of knowledge and power complexes. In order to understand the #VoetsekANC and "A Song for the ANC" as manifestations of influencer culture and Foucault's 'governmentality', it is appropriate to turn to Foucault's ideas of discourse. This chapter focuses specifically on the value of Foucault's work for criticising sociopolitical ideologies prevalent in the digital sphere. The remaining section of the chapter provides discussion of the discourse of the song, "A Song for the ANC", in which the power relations in South Africa are expressed through language. Using Foucauldian tools, the sociopolitical and cultural contexts are briefly discussed through the analysis of the lyrics.

Findings and Discussion

Song as a Form of Resistance

Foucault uses the term 'power/knowledge' to signify that power is constituted through accepted forms of knowledge, scientific understanding and 'truth' (Olivier, 2009). 'Truth' is a thing of this world: it is produced only by virtue of multiple forms of constraint. Further, it induces regular effects of power. Olivier (2009: 3) states that "Foucault expressed the discursive link between actions and knowledge". Olivier (2009, 6) reports that "As Foucault puts it (1990, 84): 'There is no power without potential refusal or revolt'". South Africans have a history of using song as a form of resistance to those they deem oppressors. In particular, struggle songs, which emanate from the South African Apartheid past, are the point of reference here. Nkoala (2013, 51) states that struggle songs are an integral part of political past, present and future. While "A Song for the ANC" does not qualify as a struggle song per se, it echoes sentiments of a disgruntled population who have chosen to express their disdain through song. Pring-Mill (1987, as cited by Nkoala, 2013, 51) explains that "the sound of song is described as a blow at the invader, a rampart in defense, a weapon against injustice". The following are the complete lyrics of "A Song for the ANC":

> [LISTEN PROPERLY]
> *We don't need your administration.*
> *We don't need your drug control.*
> *You've left a chasm in the country.*
> *Leeches leave those funds alone.*
> *Hey! Voetsek.*
> *Leave those funds alone.*
> *All in all Mzansi, is just sick of it all.*
> *All in all Mzansi is just sick of it all.*
> *Tsek.*

While the song is not a struggle song, Foucault's discourse analysis explores it as a form of resistance, especially in light of the *#voetsekanc* movement.

"A Song for the ANC" Is Not a Struggle Song

Jokingly, fans of The Kiffness have remarked that the song should be the country's national anthem since it is a form of resistance against the ANC. Others have taken the song as a struggle song. However, Nkoala (2013, 52) notes that the efficacy of struggle songs is dependent on their ability to persuade. They achieve this by being "functional, inspirational, educational, instructional, ideological and political" (Nkoala, 2013, 52). According to Nkoala (2013, 52–54), when conducting an analysis on a liberation or struggle song, one must consider whether all three (orator, audience and text) of the modes of persuasion are present. Nkoala (2013, 53) cites Aristotle (1994) when defining the salient aspects of the modes of persuasion—an orator reflecting the personal character of the speaker, in this case The Kiffness; the audience which has to be in a certain frame of mind; and the text as the actual speech or song itself.

In the context of the "A Song for the ANC", the orator is the singer, Dave Scott (The Kiffness). Unlike struggle songs, which are usually sung within group settings so as to evoke certain emotions and thus be effective (Nkoala, 2013, 53), "A Song for the ANC" is sung by one person. This therefore makes it less likely to be persuasive. In addition to this, the personal character of the orator must be considered (Nkoala, 2013, 53). It must therefore be noted that The Kiffness was also embroiled in an online racism debacle in 2020 and is known to harbour views that favour "white privilege" (IOL, 2020). This makes the prospect of the song being persuasive more unlikely, unless it is possible to segment the audience with which Dave Scott is mostly communicating.

When it comes to struggle songs, the audience is most likely to be members of the sociopolitical group that would be singing the songs (Nkoala, 2013, 53). This creates an interesting dynamic because, according to Nkoala (2013), the orator(s) would be at once both the orator and the audience. And they would be charged with the responsibility of persuading both themselves and others, unless they were directing their songs against the authorities (Nkoala, 2013, 53). In the case of "A Song for the ANC", one can certainly deduce that the intended audience are the leaders of the ANC and the government. However, owing to the complex nature of race antagonism in South Africa, it would be worthwhile to consider that the audience that Dave Scott/The Kiffness was also targeting with his song included his majority white followers on social media.

While disdain for the ANC is shared across the racial divide, it is necessary in this analysis to consider the nuances in the context of The Kiffness's ideological inclination. The text of struggle songs was often unwritten and was modified to capture the emotions and conditions of the time (Nkoala, 2013, 54). As a result, the lyrics and structure of the songs changed so much that they would also alter the meaning of the song (Nkoala, 2013, 53). Because the text in this case is written and not performed, the possibility of being able to analyse it as a struggle song is limited. However, it is best analysed as one would a normal speech, as the persuasive intent is embedded within it (Nkoala, 2013, 53).

As opined by Nkoala (2013, 54) previously, in order for a text to be persuasive, it must be "functional, inspirational, educational, instructional, ideological and political". Of these criteria, "A Song for the ANC" satisfies the instructional, ideological and political requirements. The song is instructional in that it clearly rebukes the current administration and instructs the leaders to "*leave those funds alone*". It is ideological as it denounces the need for "*your administration*… and …*your drug control*". These are usually sentiments shared by libertarian conservatives who believe in a society that has less government control which, in this case, speaks to the orator's ideological inclination. The song is also political because it is directed at political actors who have the power to change the status quo and speak to sociopolitical issues that the country faces.

Political History of Corruption

In reference to the first two lines of the song, "*We don't need your administration… We don't need your drug control*", Foucault challenges the idea that power is wielded by people or groups by way of 'episodic' or 'sovereign' acts of domination or coercion, seeing it instead as dispersed and pervasive. 'Power is everywhere' and 'comes from everywhere', so, in this sense, it is neither an agency nor a structure (Foucault, 1998, 63). Instead, power is a kind of 'metapower' or 'regime of truth' that pervades society and is in constant flux and negotiation. A key point about Foucault's approach to power is that it transcends politics and sees power as an everyday, socialised and embodied phenomenon. For this reason, state-centric power struggles, including revolutions, do not always lead to change in the social order.

For some, Foucault's concept of power is so elusive and removed from agency or structure that there seems to be little scope for practical action (Foucault, 1998). Nonetheless, Foucault's work has been hugely influential in pointing to the ways that norms can be so embedded as to be beyond our perception, causing us to discipline ourselves without any wilful coercion from other actors. Prior to the lockdown, President Cyril Ramaphosa's 'new dawn' was being questioned by political pundits (Graham, 2020). Four million jobs were lost, and Eskom, the country's power utility, was experiencing power load-shedding due to equipment breakdowns. The country was downgraded by all three rating agencies. The derailment of the ANC, according to Graham (2020), continued to point to the party's links to corruption. In the course of the response to COVID-19, government corruption by ANC members and their allies was associated with resources that were meant to assist in the battle against COVID-19. The movement #VoetsekANC has been associated with the political ideology that the ANC is merely corrupt due to its failings to administer proper services to its citizens. "Foucault's work of governmentality extends this repertoire by augmenting the analysis of power at a micro-level to the myriad of ways in which power operates at a macro-level" (Macleod & Durrheim, 2002, 43). Foucault indicates that modern government is exercised through an "ensemble formed by institutions, procedures, analyses, reflections, calculations and tactics" (Macleod & Durrheim, 2002, 43). At local and national levels, these disciplinarian forms of power by the ANC have been openly rebuked and mocked through the online movement and "The Song for the ANC". The internal politics of the ANC infiltrated into various external structures within the state.

Election of Zuma as President and the Disbanding of The Scorpions

Derailment of the ANC became more obvious immediately before and after the Polokwane conference in 2007 (Malinga, 2021). At the conference the ANC elected Jacob Zuma as president of the ANC, following which he was appointed president of the country. Factions within the ANC used state intelligence services to spy on each other and create fake reports to discredit opposing factions, ultimately leading to the disbanding of the Scorpions (organised crime investigation unit) and the enforced resignation of Thabo Mbeki as president. In-fighting within the ANC had resulted in the misuse of budgets, resources and government agencies (Malinga, 2021). The Kiffness song implied a mocking of Zuma directly with the words, *[LISTEN PROPERLY]*. This is what Zuma had said while struggling to pronounce a large number written in his closing speech at an ANC party conference in 2015. Many South Africans found this equally embarrassing and amusing as Zuma was the president of the country and could not read out aloud the number of ANC party members. This incident magnified the notion of Zuma as incompetent. By using the words in the song, it subliminally extends the same message to the whole ANC. The song also suggests that #VoetsekANC is a manifestation of the many problems that citizens have been facing with the government since it elected Zuma as president. Online the song is accompanying hashtags *#ANCMustFall #CorruptionMustFall*. Foucault's governmentality is generally associated with the willing participation of the governed, but in this case the song and the movement represented citizens' unwillingness to be governed by the ANC.

In all the historical cases, such as the Kapembe Commission, State Capture and the Zondo Commission, a certain type of power is exercised, using certain methods mobilised by certain groups of people over others. Importantly, all of this was not the exercising of the juridical power. It was not simply the power of the law, but was what Foucault calls 'biopower'—that is, having power over people's bodies. For Foucault, biopower is a technology of power for governing over people in large groups, and the distinctive quality of this political technology is that it allows for the control of entire populations (Baumgarten & Ullrich, 2016).

The power to produce subjects that would operate in favour of the ANC is indicative of criticism that was implied during the #VoetsekANC movement. The lyrics to the song says *We don't need your drug control.* It can refer to the historical moment when the Scorpions (upon which South African citizens depended to arrest politicians and other superpowers for wrongdoing) were targeting mostly ANC members, as a result of which the party put pressure on President Mbeki to address the issue. In response, he appointed a Commission headed by Judge Sici Kapembe, who recommended that the Scorpions be under the administration of either the Minister of Justice or the police. As soon as Mbeki was forced to resign as president, the Scorpions was disbanded. Through the online movement and the lyrics to the song, it was obvious that people were not only resisting the ANC but also showing how the government's dealings had to be exposed on a more widespread, non-traditional platform. This was done by subjectifying individuals (i.e. through the lyrics: LISTEN PROPERLY) and posting humorous memes about ANC with #VoetsekANC, which then turned the once respected organisation into an object—through the use of technology.

According to Macleod and Durrheim (2002, 44) "governmentality is simultaneously individualising and totalising. On the one hand, governmentality is simultaneously subjectivising (i.e. it concerns itself with the constitution of individualised subjectivity) and objectivising (i.e. through the operation of bio-power the individual is transformed into an object or docile body). On the other hand, the individual is implicated in large-scale normalising structures and regulatory controls". The use of the song and the widespread use of #VoetsekANC are manifestations of 'governmentality' as there is an interlink between "the micro-effects of power (e.g. self-technologies) with the macro strategies of power without privileging one or the other" (Macleod and Durrheim, 2002, 44). The #VoetsekANC manifested the climate of the state and its resistance to the ANC through the power of technology. Adversely, one could also argue that the use of the various technological platforms and structures in themselves carry micro and macro forms of control and power. In accordance with Foucault, governmentality occurs on multiple, interwoven levels. On Twitter, the nature of the movement was more detailed and intertextualised with corresponding links to news articles about the ANCs mishaps, whereas on TikTok the corruption cases were merely mocked through humorous videos, which appeared on other social media platforms for a much older population to consume. This also indicates that young people's "disrespectful" views about the ANC are considered and shared across generations and their influence in political discourse might have to be taken in a more serious light. Technology has impacted the way that intuitions wield power upon other people and how power has an effect on those people.

COVID Corruption and "Tsek" Movement on TikTok

Dave Scott's "A Song for the ANC" was created from the #VoetsekANC movement that emerged from citizens gaining knowledge of the corruption centred around the funding and resources earmarked to control the global pandemic. About R500 billion for food parcels and social services was squandered by some ANC members and their counterparts (Sipuka, 2020). Scott's song becomes more humorous when he sings, *"Leeches leave those funds alone…"Hey! Voetsek"*. The lyrics suggest that the ANC is not worthy of being respected as a political party. This is significant in that many young and old social media users from various backgrounds (but most especially Caucasians) endorsed the song. While a few expressed their shock and disbelief that the ANC was openly being 'outed' and ridiculed for stealing money meant for the poor, others encouraged the young man for using his artistry to covey the distasteful way in which the party was conducting itself. Before this, citizens had to accept that South Africa has been under the management of the Guptas, a wealthy foreign family. In addition, evidence presented to the Zondo Commission revealed that underhand dealings infiltrated the judicial system—in so far as specially selected judges were adjudicating in favour of Zuma and the ANC (Martin and Solomon, 2016, 24). Therefore, the song was a form of resistance to the government's agendas and a call for the ANC to be responsible and serious about crime, corruption and fraud issues in the country.

The lyrics *"All in all Mzansi, is just sick of it all"* reflect citizens' feelings of being disappointed and frustrated with the ANC for its powerlessness to address many of the important socioeconomic issues affecting the country. The political party's inability to not misrepresent and misuse funds and resources needed to prevent COVID-19 is viewed as the most demoralising action of the ANC, leading to the breakdown of citizens' confidence in political institutions. The song's ending, "Tsek", an abbreviation of 'voetsek', links to #VoetsekANC as a symbolic portrayal of the low level of respect that citizens have towards the ANC and is also an indication of how the ANC leaders are interpellated and viewed as none caring corrupt individuals.

Foucault (1997, 73) explains that biopower does not have an effect on people physically, but on possible future actions—that is, their possibility and choices that are available. He says this power is an action upon action. It constrains and encourages. Judicial power is subtractive and, in a way, repressive, while biopower is productive. Institutions, such as the government, can also exert biopower by disciplining and training, which can result in rewards and can be achieved through cumulative measures. These actions have an effect on others (such as citizens) and their possible actions.

Prediction of behaviours, Foucault asserts, can only be done by analysing groups of people, where a set of norms and standards exist as a basis for analysis (Foucault, 1997). This can be done with reference to a population, where what people are doing and how they behave in certain contexts can be quantified. Subjects may be created through the exertion of power and knowledge on a specific population. In South Africa, citizens are forced to wear face masks and to adhere to lockdown regulations. However, citizens became tired of the discipline exercised on the bodies of individuals and security exercised over the population, so that when news broke out of the ways in which the ANC were misusing COVID-19 relief aids, citizens "rebelled" against the government through the hashtag. The political use of the hashtag #VoetsekANC demonstrated the resistance to and shifting of power against the ruling government. Although some content was represented in humorous ways across different social media platforms, points of resistance in the network of power relations were vocalised.

Conclusion

Foucault's theoretical ideas have been shown to be effective in analysis of "A song for the ANC" by referring to the brief political history of corruption by the ANC, which evoked the #VoetsekANC movement. By analysing the song lyrics, the chapter has shown how institutional power is affirmed not only by juridical means of the state but also through individual subjects. The chapter has shown that if these ambivalent forms of power are neglected, the specific power formations which have stabilised online movements and informed influencer culture may not be resolved.

Influencer culture impacts the way that political power is shared across social media platforms. Influencers have political power to drive others into being informed about sociocultural issues that affect human beings. TikTok, in particular, has taught South African users to view politics more humorously and creatively on social media. TikTok is now seen as a technology associated with power (Fung, 2020). The more followers one has, the more influence one has and the more one is considered credible or knowledgeable. Although individuals and their networks share similar thoughts about the government, such as in the case of the ANC, the #VoetsekANC movement went from a micro level of power to a macro level through the interconnectedness of technological systems that make it possible for various individuals and technologies to exchange knowledge.

According to Macleod and Durrheim (2002, 46), disciplinary technology has as its aim the regulation and normalisation of subjects. Although the individual ostensibly has more formal rights than before, taking into consideration South Africa's oppressive past, there is less room for deviance and disorder. Disciplinary technology operates through hierarchical observation and normalising judgement. What governmentality adds to this is the possibility of identifying and resisting concentrations of power. This is reflected in the actions of current Generations Z and Alpha, who have used TikTok as a form of expressing their discontent with the corruption related to COVID-19. The older generation, however, has used social media to sow divisions and further polarise societies (Fung, 2020) and further entrench Foucault's governmentality. This is true for both South Africa and the United States of America (USA) with regard to the Cambridge Analytica scandal. The USA is also at the epicentre of the current geopolitical battle with TikTok, as the former president of the USA Donald Trump's rhetoric continues to be anti-China.

Suffice it to say that a platform like TikTok gives leeway for political commentary by its creators, as seen during South Africa's national lockdown. The disdain for TikTok shown by former President Donald Trump led him to announce earlier in 2020 that he intended to ban the social media platform by September 2020 (Fung, 2020). Trump laments that US citizens' personal user data from the platform might end up in the hands of the Chinese government (Fung, 2020). This forms part of a wider trade war with the Chinese government, which is currently at its zenith. Fung (2020) also states that Trump's attempt at banning TikTok has been rejected by a federal judge and therefore has not come into effect. This is an example of the ramifications of the confluence between politics and social media. The issue of control is, however, contestable in the context of social media platforms as the control that platforms such as Facebook have has been widely reported following the Cambridge Analytica scandal of 2018 (Confessore, 2018).

It has recently become commonplace for social media platforms to use personal data as a form of control over audiences. These platforms have access to users' personal data and can infer psychological personas that can be used for both political and commercial purposes. This political insensitivity, as it pertains to platforms such as Facebook, can also be used to understand the current political quagmire within which TikTok finds itself. These examples illustrate that governmentality "links technologies of the self with technologies of domination" (Lemke, 2002, 3), an area that can be explored for future research with regards to online movements, especially in the wake of COVID-19.

References

Abratt, R. (2019). *The impact of influencer marketing on consumer based brand equity*. PhD dissertation, University of Witwatersrand.

Adjepong, A. (2020). Voetsek! Get [ting] lost: African sportswomen in 'the sporting black diaspora'. *International Review for the Sociology of Sport, 55*(7), 868–883.

Baragwanath, R. (2016). Social media and contentious politics in South Africa. *Communication and the Public, 1*(3), 362–366.

Baumgarten, B., & Ullrich, P. (2016). Discourse, power, and governmentality. Social movement research with and beyond Foucault. In J. Roose & H. Dietz (Eds.), *Social theory and social movements* (pp. 13–38). Springer VS.

Bhana, D. (2016). 'Voetsek!' Boys, violence, and the gendered negotiation of masculinity. In *Gender and childhood sexuality in primary school* (pp. 113–129). Springer.

Buckingham, W., Burnham, D., Hill, C., King, P. J., Marenbon, J., & Weeks, M. (2011). *The philosophy book*. DK Publishing.

Comrie, S. (2017, January 23). Top officials endorse ANC war room. *The Conversation*. https://theconversation.com/ramaphosas-famous-negotiating-skills-have-failed-him-heres-why-130393

Confessore, N. (2018, April 4). Cambridge analytica and Facebook: The scandal and the fallout so far. *New York Times*. https://www.nytimes.com/2018/04/04/us/politics/cambridge-analytica-scandal-fallout.html

DeIuliis, E. D., & Saylor, E. (2021). Bridging the gap: Three strategies to optimize professional relationships with Generation Y and Z. *The Open Journal of Occupational Therapy, 9*(1), 1–13.

Dolan, F. M. (1993). The philosophical laughter of Michel Foucault. *Qui Parle, 6*(2, Spring/Summer), 131–149.

Ellis, S. (1989). Tuning in to pavement radio. *African Affairs, 88*(352), 321–330.

Foucault, M. (1978). *The history of sexuality. Vol. 1. An introduction* (R. Hurley, Trans.). Random House.

Foucault, M. (1990). Politics and reason. In L. D. Kritzman (Ed.), *Michel Foucault: Politics, philosophy, culture. Interviews and other writings 1977–1984* (pp. 57–85). Routledge.

Foucault, M. (1995). *Discipline and punish. The birth of the prison* (Trans. A. Sheridan). Vintage Books.

Foucault, M. (1998). *The will to knowledge: The history of sexuality* (Vol. I). Penguin Books.

Foucault, M., & Ewald, F. (2003). Society must be defended. In *Lectures at the Collège de France, 1975–1976* (Vol. 1, D. Macey, Trans., M. Vertani & A. Fontana, Ed.). Macmillan.

Foucault, M. (1997). The birth of biopolitics. In P. Rabinow (Ed.), *Michel Foucault, ethics: Subjectivity and truth* (pp. 73–79). The New Press.

Fung, B. (2020, September 28). Judge rules TikTok can avoid a ban in the US, for now. *CNN Business.* https://edition.cnn.com/2020/09/27/tech/tiktok-ban-judge/index.html

Graham, M. (2020, January 23). Ramaphosa's famous negotiation skills have failed him. Here's why. *The Conversation.* https://theconversation.com/ramaphosas-famous-negotiating-skills-have-failed-him-heres-why-130393

IOL. (2020, September 8). The Kiffness faces backlash after referring to Clicks' racist advert as a 'mistake'. *Independent Online.* https://www.iol.co.za/entertainment/celebrity-news/local/the-kiffness-faces-backlash-after-referring-to-clicks-racist-advert-as-a-mistake-a2fa3768-627a-4b56-96bd-c18ce64e35c9

Keeton, C. (2020, June 23). TikTok taking off in SA under lockdown. *Times Live.* https://www.timeslive.co.za/news/sci-tech/2020-06-23-tiktok-taking-off-in-sa-under-lockdown/

Kelly, M. G. E. (2013). Foucault, subjectivity, and technologies of the self. In C. Falzon, T. O'Leary, & J. Sawicki (Eds.), *A companion to Foucault* (pp. 510–525). Wiley-Blackwell.

Lemke, T. (2002). Foucault, governmentality, and critique. *Rethinking Marxism, 14*(3), 49–64.

Macleod, C., & Durrheim, K. (2002). Foucauldian feminism: The implications of governmentality. *Journal for the Theory of Social Behaviour, 32*(1), 41–60.

Malila, V., Oelofsen, M., Garman, A., & Wasserman, H. (2013). Making meaning of citizenship: How 'born frees' use media in South Africa's democratic evolution. *Communication, 39*(4), 415–431.

Malinga, T. D. (2021, January 7). When the ANC's elephants fight… *City Press.* https://www.news24.com/citypress/voices/when-the-ancs-elephants-fight-20210107-2

Maples-Yap, M. (2020). *Signs, token, and influencers: A Foucauldian approach to Mommy Blogs.* Masters thesis, University of Uppsala.

Martin, M. E., & Solomon, H. (2016). Understanding the phenomenon of "state capture" in South Africa. *Southern African Peace and Security Studies, 5*(1), 21–35.

Mpofu, S. (2017). Disruption as a communicative strategy: The case of #FeesMustFall and #RhodesMustFall students' protests in South Africa. *Journal of African Media Studies, 9*(2), 351–373.

Mzekandaba, S. (2020, June 11). TikTok changes the social media rules in South Africa. *ITWeb*. https://www.itweb.co.za/content/raYAyqodE5gvJ38N

Nkoala, S. M. (2013). Songs that shaped the struggle: A rhetorical analysis of South African struggle songs. *African Yearbook of Rhetoric, 4*(1), 51–61.

Olivier, B. (2003). Discourse, agency and the question of evil. *South African Journal of Philosophy, 22*(4), 328–347.

Olivier, B. (2005). Lacan and the question of the psychotherapist's ethical orientation. *South African Journal of Psychology, 35*(4), 657–683.

Olivier, B. (2009). Discourse, agency and the question of evil. In *Philosophy and psychoanalytic theory. Collected essays* (pp. 1–31). Peter Lang Academic Publishers.

Olivier, B. (2010). Foucault and individual autonomy. *South African Journal of Psychology, 40*(3), 292–307.

Pring-Mill, R. (1987). The roles of revolutionary song – A Nicaraguan assessment. *Popular Music, 6*(2), 179–189.

Rabinow, P. (1994). Michel Foucault: Essential works of Foucault 1954–84. In P. Singer (Ed.), *Ethics* (p. 1). Oxford University Press.

Sam, C. H. (2019). Shaping discourse through social media: Using Foucauldian discourse analysis to explore the narratives that influence educational policy. *American Behavioral Scientist, 63*(3), 333–350.

Singh, S. K. (2019). Political marketing: A review of recent general elections of India. *International Journal of Scientific & Technology Research, 8*(11), 3537–3542.

Sipuka, S. (2020, September 3). Corruption has become SA's other 'pandemic'. *DispatchLive*. https://www.dispatchlive.co.za/news/opinion/2020-09-03-corruption-has-become-sas-other-pandemic/

Tannous, N., Belesiotis, P., Tchakarian, N., & Stewart, R. (2019, November). Public engagement with politics, information and news–South Africa. *Africa Check*. https://africacheck.org/sites/default/files/media/documents/2020-11/Public-engagement-with-politics-information-news-South-Africa_fin.pdf

The Kiffness. (2020, August 2). [WATCH VIDEO]. A song for the ANC (Pink Floyd – Another Brick in the Wall Parody). https://www.youtube.com/watch?v=sGpp4mRCLrI

van Staden, M., & van Niekerk, L. (2018). *Uncovering the value of influencer marketing through social network analysis and brand positioning insights*. Southern African Marketing Research Association (SAMRA). http://www.samra.co.za/

wpcontent/uploads/Van-Staden-Van-Niekerk_Uncovering-the-value-of-influencer-marketing.pdf

Wasserman, H. (2020, March 15). Laughter in the time of a pandemic: Why South Africans are joking about coronavirus. *The Conversation*. https://theconversation.com/laughter-in-the-time-of-a-pandemic-why-south-africans-are-joking-about-coronavirus-133528

We Are Social. (2019, April 28). *The state of digital in April 2019: All the numbers you need, and a few big surprises*. https://wearesocial.cn/blog/2019/04/28/digital-2019-q2-global-digital-statshot/

Wellman, M. L., Stoldt, R., Tully, M., & Ekdale, B. (2020). Ethics of authenticity: Social media influencers and the production of sponsored content. *Journal of Media Ethics, 35*(2), 68–82.

Yeh, O. (2019, April 10). TikTok added 188 million new users last quarter, growing 70% from Q1 2018. *Sensor Tower Blog*. https://sensortower.com/blog/tiktok-downloads-q1-2019

Zhu, C., Xu, X., Zhang, W., Chen, J., & Evans, R. (2020). How health communication via Tik Tok makes a difference: A content analysis of Tik Tok accounts run by Chinese provincial health committees. *International Journal of Environmental Research and Public Health, 17*(1), 192.

CHAPTER 12

Humour in the Time of COVID-19 Pandemic: A Critical Analysis of the Subversive Meanings of WhatsApp Memes in Zimbabwe

Mphathisi Ndlovu

Introduction

This chapter examines the subversive nature of Internet memes that are produced and circulated by ordinary Zimbabweans as a form of political communication within a repressive environment. Drawing upon memes circulated via WhatsApp during the period of the novel coronavirus disease (COVID-19), this chapter examines the political discourses that are expressed, reproduced and contested as Zimbabweans sought to cope with the new realities. Given the repressive nature of the Zimbabwean political environment that manifests through draconian laws (Moyo, 2009a; Mpofu, 2014), this chapter explores the creative ways in which citizens appropriated digital tools to create and circulate WhatsApp memes in counter-hegemonic fashion. Memes are reproduced and circulated not

M. Ndlovu (✉)
Stellenbosch University, Stellenbosch, South Africa

S. Mpofu (ed.), *Digital Humour in the Covid-19 Pandemic*,
https://doi.org/10.1007/978-3-030-79279-4_12

only for humorous purposes, but they also serve "some degree of social, cultural, or political critique" (Wiggins, 2019, 59). Jokes are circulated by ordinary Zimbabweans via mobile phones "to construct their counter-publics" by subverting "state power and media censorship" (Manganga, 2012, 243). Thus, Zimbabweans are using jokes to "express dissatisfaction with the deteriorating economic and political situation in the country" (Manganga, 2012, 243).

COVID-19 is a novel coronavirus that broke out in Wuhan, China, in December 2019 (Teti et al., 2020). This infectious disease was declared a pandemic by the World Health Organization (WHO) in March 2020. Its symptoms include dry cough, fever and shortness of breath. Hand hygiene and social distancing are some of the ways of curbing the spread of this virus (Teti et al., 2020, 2). As the pandemic spread across the globe causing death, illness and social disruption (Teti et al., 2020, 2), governments responded by sealing national borders and announcing lockdowns as preventive and containment measures. As of the end of November 2020, the death toll across the globe had exceeded 1.4 million, with over 63 million people having tested positive for COVID-19. The first COVID-19 case in Zimbabwe was recorded in March 2020. By the end of November, 277 people had lost their lives due to the pandemic. The COVID-19 cases had exceeded 10,000.

COVID-19 broke out at a time when Zimbabweans were grappling with socio-political and economic crises such as corruption, inflation, human rights abuses, and a deteriorating healthcare system (Chingono, 2020; Muronzi, 2020). With the outbreak of the COVID-19 pandemic, there were fears that the Zimbabwean government was not prepared to tackle this emergency health crisis (Makurumidze, 2020; Muronzi, 2020). The health system was paralysed as doctors and nurses were engaging in an industrial action over poor remuneration and lack of protective clothing (Chingono, 2020). Furthermore, the water crisis and food shortages in major cities like Harare and Bulawayo compounded fears about the spread of COVID-19, as citizens contravened lockdown regulations to queue for water at boreholes and for basic commodities at supermarkets. Against this background of the national lockdown, economic turmoil, political crisis and poor health care system, this chapter examines the use and appropriation of WhatsApp memes as a tool for communicating political satire. Internet memes have a subversive nature as they can be creatively appropriated and utilised as a tool against authoritarianism.

Context

The ruling party, Zimbabwe African National Union Patriotic Front (ZANU PF), has over the years relied on the state media like *The Herald* and the *Zimbabwe Broadcasting Corporation* (*ZBC*) to reproduce its nationalist discourses and sustain its legitimacy (Mpofu, 2016; Ranger, 2005). The private press, or the "independent" media, tends to propagate anti-government or counter-hegemonic discourses (Moyo, 2005, 112). Within these "competing journalisms" (Chuma, 2008, 21), there is, on the one hand, the "patriotic journalism" performed by the state media that serves to propagate ZANU PF's renditions of history and national identity (Ranger, 2005, 13). On the other hand, there is the "oppositional press" (Moyo, 2005, 11), or "opposition journalism" (Chuma, 2008, 27), that serves to "delegitimize ZANU PF and the state" (Chuma, 2008, 27). In the early 2000s, the *Daily News* embodied the "opposition press" (Moyo, 2005, 114) as it was deemed the "voice of the voiceless". After the persecution that included the bombing of its offices, the newspaper was shut down in 2003 (Moyo, 2005). Draconian laws such as the Public Order and Security Act (POSA) and the Access to Information and Protection of Privacy Act (AIPPA) had adverse effects on the operations and performance of the media in Zimbabwe by curtailing free speech and restricting the democratic space (Mpofu, 2014, 119).

Given the repressive environment in Zimbabwe, the Internet has emerged as a space for counter-hegemonic discourses. Marginalised communities are relying on new digital technologies to express themselves freely and articulate discourses that are tabooed in public spaces, such as the *Gukurahundi* genocide (Mpofu, 2015; Ndlovu, 2018). Thus, the Internet has a subversive potential as news websites (Mpofu, 2015; Ndlovu, 2018), the *Forum* social networking mailing list (Mhlanga & Mpofu, 2014) and *Inkundla* online platform (Moyo, 2009b) were appropriated by users to construct Ndebele historical memories such as the *Gukurahundi* genocide. Studies have examined the role of diasporic media as alternative public spheres that played a role in mediating the Zimbabwean crises (Moyo, 2007; Mano & Willems, 2008). Zimbabwean activists in the diaspora are using humour not "merely to mock or ridicule but to conscientize people, and to raise attention for and awareness of the situation" in the homeland (Kuhlmann, 2012, 295). Drawing upon data from cartoons and satirical messages disseminated through the Internet, Kuhlmann (2012, 295) argues that political humour in the Zimbabwean diaspora has a "counter-discursive function and serves as a 'medium of communicating dissent'". Clandestine radio stations emerged as alternative spaces that challenge "state authoritarianism" (Moyo, 2012, 485).

Social media platforms such as Twitter and Facebook have been at the centre of Zimbabwe's protest movements as they are creatively appropriated and used by activists to challenge state authoritarianism (Gukurume, 2017; Chitanana, 2020; Mpofu & Mare, 2020). Protest movements such as #ThisFlag, #ThisGown and #Tajamuka demonstrate the potency of digital activism in Zimbabwe (Gukurume, 2017; Chitanana, 2020). As such, social media tools are utilised by citizens to "reclaim their political voices and spaces" (Gukurume, 2017, 49). Thus, social media tools enable citizens to circumvent the surveillance and strategies of repressive governments (Gukurume, 2017, 51). However, Internet shutdowns that occurred in 2016 and 2019 in Zimbabwe demonstrate the manifestation of "digital authoritarianism" (Mare, 2020, 4244). Most Zimbabweans utilise their mobile phones for Internet connectivity (Mare, 2020, 4251). There is a growth in the Internet penetration rates in Zimbabwe as they rose from 9.8 percent in 2008 to around 50 percent in 2016 (Mare, 2018, 96). As of December 2019, the Internet penetration rate in the country is at 56.5 percent (MISA, 2020, 16). The most popular social networking site used by Zimbabweans is WhatsApp and is followed by Facebook (Mare, 2018, 96). WhatsApp contributes to "over 44 percent of all mobile internet usage in the country" (MISA, 2020, 19). The market share of mobile service providers is dominated by the privately owned Econet Wireless Zimbabwe (69.7 percent) and two state-enterprises, Telecel (8.9 percent) and NetOne (21.4 percent) (Mare, 2020, 4251).

Political Satire, Internet Memes and Protest Cultures

Laughter has "subversive effects" (Okawa, 2013, 16) as humour has always been used as a "tool against oppression since ages" (Kulkarni, 2017, 13). Satire plays a key role in "contesting the state-centric rendition of life in Zimbabwe" (Siziba & Ncube, 2015, 516). The late former President Robert Mugabe tended to be constructed by the state media as a "superhuman", who was invincible and "unscathed by the ravages of age" (Siziba & Ncube, 2015, 516). However, Mugabe's tumble and fall at the Harare International Airport in 2015 subverted and thwarted this narrative (Siziba & Ncube, 2015, 516). Satirical memes were produced and circulated via WhatsApp, Facebook and Twitter, which sought to ridicule and resist the myths around the "fetishization" of the former president's power (Siziba & Ncube, 2015, 516). These memes or "fictional constructions" served to depict Mugabe as the "architect of Zimbabwe's fall" and to dispel the "myth of him as a god who is immune from human weaknesses" (Siziba & Ncube, 2015, 517).

Källstig and Death (2020, 1) examine the "ambivalent mockery" evident in stand-up comedy as Trevor Noah's performances subvert "white, western and Eurocentric discourses of global politics". In repressive societies such as Zimbabwe, stand-up comedy acts as a form of resistance against the hegemonic forces (Källstig & Death, 2020, 1). Drawing upon data from the Zimbabwean comic strip *Chikwama*, which appeared on the privately owned *Daily News* in the early 2000s, Willems (2011) argues that laughter can enable ordinary people to negotiate and cope with the sociopolitical and economic crises unfolding in their country. The strip *Chikwama* demonstrates that postcolonial laughter cannot "always be treated as a form of resistance" as it "does not always address those in power" (Willems, 2011, 141). Instead, laughter can have a self-reflexive mode as the oppressed "mock their own powerlessness and lack of agency in the face of a system that they perceive as immutable" (Willems, 2011, 141).

Memes communicate information "through humour and satire" (Kulkarni, 2017, 13). The key feature of memes is their "ability to rapidly spread on social media" (Siziba & Ncube, 2015, 518). As such, Internet memes denote popular forms of humour (Ngwira & Lipenga, 2018). More importantly, memes constitute sites of struggle between hegemonic and alternative discourses (Denisova, 2019, 10). The growth of memes in the digital sphere is linked with the "rise of emoticons" (Denisova,2019, 9). Dominant scholarship examines the role of memes as forms of political communication (Makhortykh & Aguilar, 2020). The focus on memes and politics tends to be on marginalised groups (Wiggins, 2019, 59). The concept of a meme was propounded by Dawkins (1976) to describe "cultural units... disseminating virally" (Makhortykh & Aguilar, 2020, 343), or the "viral spread of an idea" (Ngwira & Lipenga, 2018, 25). A meme denotes something that "spreads throughout a culture" (Wells, 2018, 241). As such, Internet memes can be defined as "context-bound viral texts that proliferate on mutation and replication" (Denisova, 2019, 10). In this vein, Internet memes denote digital content units which combine "visual and verbal elements to steer affective reactions" (Makhortykh & Aguilar, 2020, 343). A meme is, thus, a cultural unit that can be imitated, mimicked, remixed and repackaged (Ngwira & Lipenga, 2018, 25). It constitutes an "imitable text" that can be appropriated, adjusted and circulated by Internet users (Denisova, 2019, 10). As cultural commodities, memes express people's lived practices (Wiggins, 2019, 7).

The idea of "meme" has "mutated" since its introduction due to the advent of the Internet (Wiggins, 2019, 1). The Internet has created a conducive environment for people to generate and circulate memes (Wells 2018, 241). Technological affordances of the Internet enable users to "take photos, augment both image and video, quickly edit and upload" (Wiggins, 2019, 58). Thus, new digital technologies enable an "unparalleled ease of creating and remixing digital content" and the viral distribution of memes (Makhortykh & Aguilar, 2020, 343). Given their affective potential, Internet memes emerge as a form of "political commentary" that provokes "high-arousal emotions" (Makhortykh & Aguilar, 2020, 344). Internet memes can "catch the attention of a reader in a way that an article cannot" (Wells, 2018, 241). Given their potential of articulating "emotionally charged messages", memes are intertwined with protest cultures (Makhortykh & Aguilar, 2020, 344). Thus, Internet memes are deployed, discursively, to serve political purposes (Wiggins, 2019, 57). The *Obama Joker* meme and the "remixing of the Batman villain for Trump in 2016" are some of the examples of the deployment of Internet memes for political agendas (Wiggins, 2019, 57). Other studies examine Internet memes as "lived religion" in that they express and communicate about religious identities (Aguilar et al., 2017, 1498).

The advent of the Internet has reinvigorated the potency of political humour such as memes (Pearce & Hajizada, 2014). New digital technologies are enabling oppositional forces to disseminate memes as a form of dissent in authoritarian Azerbaijan (Pearce & Hajizada, 2014, 67). At the same time, memes can express toxic populist and extremist messages (DeCook, 2018) with the purpose of "stigmatising political opponents and scapegoating minorities" (Makhortykh & Aguilar, 2020, 344). Drawing upon anti-government protests in Ukraine and Venezuela, Makhortykh and Aguilar (2020) explore how pro- and anti-government communities utilised Internet memes for their political agendas. Jenkins (2014) develops a framework for a rhetorical analysis of Internet memes by focusing on modes as collective expressions. A visual rhetorical study analyses "image-texts in context" (Jenkins, 2014, 442). Although Internet memes help people to cope with hardships, Ngwira and Lipenga (2018, 21), in their study of Malawian humour in the digital age, observe that

Internet memes promote inferiority complex as these everyday jokes "demean, devalue and underrate anything Malawian". Thus, Malawian humour is "self-directed" as it represents a "country laughing at itself" (Ngwira & Lipenga, 2018, 21).

Theoretical and Conceptual Framework

This study analyses Internet humour through the lens of Bakhtin's carnivalesque (Tembo, 2011; MacMillan, 2020). Bakhtin's theorisation of the carnivalesque is derived from his seminal work *Rabelais and His World* (Tembo, 2011, 344). It provides a framework for making sense of the transgressions and subversive nature of WhatsApp memes. The carnivalesque is associated with the medieval carnival that was intertwined with the lived experiences of ordinary people (MacMillan, 2020, 259). Carnivals were associated with laughter as dominant elites and official hierarchies were mocked, challenged and "inverted" (Badarneh, 2011, 308). The carnivals were related to the "feast of fools" in which "social hierarchies of everyday lives" could be "overturned" (MacMillan, 2020, 260). Thus, the carnivalesque is centred on the "themes of the carnival twist, mutate, and invert social conventions" (Tembo, 2011, 344). The carnival rituals involved the ridiculing of elites and attacks on the status quo (MacMillan, 2020). Thus, Bakhtin's understanding of the carnivalesque involved a "temporary suspension of the normal order, breaking down barriers, norms, prohibitions and etiquettes as well as reversing the existing hierarchical distinctions" (MacMillan, 2020, 260). Political jokes circulated via WhatsApp can be considered as carnivalesque texts that challenge the status quo as mockery and ridicule are used.

The concept of counter-publics also provides a framework for analysing the subversive potential of WhatsApp memes in authoritarian contexts. By counter-publics, I mean the "parallel discursive arenas" used by members of the subaltern to construct and circulate alternative discourses (Fraser, 1992). These counter-publics articulate the views that are excluded in the mainstream public spheres (Fraser, 1992; Asen, 2000). Asen (2000) provides a comprehensive engagement on the idea of "counter" in "counter-publics". He argues that the "counter" is not about places, people or topics (Asen, 2000). Instead, counter-publics denote "participants' recognition of exclusion from wider public spheres and its articulation through alternative discourse practices and norms" (Asen, 2000, 427). Thus, they constitute the collectives that "emerge in the recognition of various exclusions from wider publics of potential participants, discourse topics, and speaking styles and the resolve that builds to overcome these exclusions" (Asen, 2000, 438). As such, this chapter considers Internet spaces like WhatsApp as counter-publics that challenge the hegemonic ZANU PF narratives. However, this research does not consider all WhatsApp platforms as counter-publics. Rather, WhatsApp sites can be considered as counter-publics only if there is a recognition by participants of exclusion from the dominant spaces (Asen, 2000). Asen's (2000) conceptualisation suits this research as some of the WhatsApp memes that are selected for analysis are challenging the hegemonic discourses.

Methodology

Data were drawn from memes that were shared via WhatsApp groups and individual statuses. The researcher is a member of some of these WhatsApp groups where memes were circulated. Through a process of online ethnography (Mpofu, 2019, 113), the researcher was able to monitor WhatsApp groups and individual statuses in order to select memes on COVID-19. The scope of study is 7 months (April to November 2020). Purposive sampling was employed to select WhatsApp memes for analysis from over 100 texts related to COVID-19. These memes were categorised according to thematic issues. Fourteen memes were selected for analysis as they reflect the lived experiences of Zimbabweans during the COVID-19 era. The focus of the analysis was on image-texts that mediated the pandemic. Critical discourse analysis (CDA) was used to analyse the image-texts. CDA provides theories and methods that enable researchers to examine the intersection of language, meaning and power (Jorgensen & Phillips, 2002; Richardson, 2007). It provides analytical tools to examine how language is used to reproduce, sustain and challenge asymmetrical power relations (Jorgensen & Phillips, 2002; Richardson, 2007). From the various models of CDA, Fairclough's (1995) three-dimensional model was employed to analyse the intersection of texts, discursive practice and social practice. WhatsApp messages are private conversations, and hence permission was sought from participants to use the memes for research purposes. Furthermore, the identities of WhatsApp users who circulated the memes are protected.

WhatsApp Memes and the Everyday Lives

Memes express people's ways of life as these imaginations and meaning-making practices are generated by social groups in situated contexts. Cultural artefacts not only "articulate the meanings of particular social practices and events", but also "define the ways we make sense of them, how they are experienced and lived" (Grossberg, 2005, 158). WhatsApp memes, as cultural artefacts, reflect the fears, hopes and prejudices of Zimbabweans during the COVID-19 era. Zimbabweans used humour to cope with the uncertainties brought about by COVID-19. In this vein, there are memes that articulate the socio-economic dynamics in Zimbabwe. With the outbreak of COVID-19, there were discourses on the "new normal" and the changes brought about by the pandemic. However, some memes show that these changes did not really affect the unemployed. First, there are memes that highlight that the stay-at-home orders affected the daily routines of privileged communities and the working class, rather than the unemployed. The humorous text—"when you find out your normal daily lifestyle is called quarantine"—serves to highlight the struggles of the unemployed in Zimbabwe.

Second, other memes depict the locals' views on return migration:

> *Gone are the days when people show off with "I just came back from UK or USA". Show Brag now and get quarantined.*

Some social commentators attributed the spike in the country's COVID-19 cases to citizens returning home from countries such as South Africa and the United Kingdom. An analysis of expressions "show off" and "brag" demonstrates that Zimbabweans in the diaspora are depicted as pompous. The fear of being "quarantined" is represented as a way of subduing the so-called gloating returning citizens.

Other memes reinforce stereotypes and prejudices against social groups such as women and Muslims. Laughter does not always serve counter-hegemonic purposes (Willems, 2011), and as such, humour may perpetuate the widely held preconceived assumptions about certain groups. One of the memes is derogatory as a black woman's hairstyle is disparaged as the novel coronavirus. In using the image of COVID-19 to depict a female's hairstyle, this meme serves to demean and devalue a black woman's worth. It further reinforces the patriarchal and racist discourses that demean black women's bodies. The concept of intersectionality describes the experiences and suffering of black women by highlighting the multidimensional forms of oppression and discrimination such as race and gender that are intertwined (Rodgers, 2017, 36). In degrading a black woman's beauty as a pandemic, such memes promote and reinforce "coloniality of being" (Ndlovu-Gatsheni, 2013, 11). Whiteness is reproduced as it gains an "ontological density far above blackness" (Ndlovu-Gatsheni, 2013, 11). Ngwira and Lipenga (2018, 21) concur that self-derogatory jokes in the digital age may serve to perpetuate an "inferiority complex which reiterates colonial matrices of meaning". In spite of memes being reified as forms of dissent and protest culture, in this context, they may serve to reinforce gendered and racial stereotypes. Black women's hair constitute a site of political struggle as female bodies tend to be mocked, regulated and controlled. Another meme depicts Muslim women covering their head and body with hijabs or garments. The expression "*they knew all along and never told us*" is an assumption that hijabs are meant to be used as face-masks to limit the spread of COVID-19. Thus, such stereotypical statements undermine religious identities.

WhatsApp Memes as "Silent Resistance"

The rapid spread of the COVID-19 pandemic has left over a million people dead and resulted in drastic changes in people's daily routines across the globe. The socio-economic impacts of COVID-19 have been huge. The household income for the majority was severely affected by the stay-at-home orders as industries and informal markets had to be closed. There were disruptions in people's daily sources of income. Given the lockdown regulations, the poor communities such as informal traders had to come to terms with the realities of losing their sources of income. Against this backdrop, Internet users reproduced and circulated COVID-19 memes via WhatsApp to express the struggles of these marginalised, excluded and poor communities. Thus, memes articulate the socio-economic plight of the poor by depicting lockdown regulations and other COVID-19-induced measures as elitist. The following WhatsApp memes express the socio-economic plight of the subordinated groups in Zimbabwe. First, there are memes that articulate the challenges of online learning in the midst of the novel coronavirus:

I'm not against online teaching, but what about us?
Data for her online learning, or bread to feed her?

In this regard, online learning is represented as elitist as it excludes low-income students. The first meme on online learning depicts two female learners who appear to be in a rural setting. The image of the female rural learners symbolises disenfranchised and subordinated communities. It expresses the plight of low-income students during the COVID-19 pandemic. The rhetorical question "what about us?" is a cry for inclusion as learners from low-income families usually do not have Internet access at home. The second meme represents the realities of the experiences of low-income learners and their families during the COVID-19 pandemic. With schools closed, low-income students struggled to partake in online lessons due to lack of resources. The disadvantaged learners do not have access to computers and Internet. For these low-income families, food is a priority than Internet data for online learning.

Given the digital divide and socio-economic disparities, the marginalised groups tend to be left out in the Information Society. As such, Nyamnjoh posits that the Information Superhighway is "yet to be travelled by enough Africans" (1996, 8). Moreover, the Internet "remains largely an urban phenomenon" (Moyo, 2007, 85). Thus, the meme depicts a struggle between the affluent groups in the urban setting and the subordinated communities in rural areas. The marginalised communities are using digital tools such as WhatsApp for everyday resistances against the power bloc. Through the memes, the weak and subordinated are challenging the dominant system. Memes are creatively appropriated and used for counter-hegemonic purposes. Through the process of "excorporation" (Fiske, 1989, 15), the downtrodden are using the resources (Internet) associated with the privileged groups to construct their own subcultures. Fiske (1989, 15) uses the term "excorporation" to describe the process by which the "subordinate make their own culture out of the resources and commodities provided by the dominant system". In this vein, the meme is not only a critique of the elitist education system in Zimbabwe, but also repudiates the dominant capitalist system. Rather than a public good, education is depicted as having been commodified and driven by market forces. The memes, hence, constitute subversive tools that enable the subordinated groups to engage in a "guerrilla warfare" without challenging the "powerful in open warfare" (Fiske, 1989, 19).

Other memes depict the plight of vulnerable communities confined to their homes. Given that most of the people in Zimbabwe's urban areas rely on informal economic activities, the lockdown measures threatened the livelihoods of these citizens. Thus, the lockdown regulations meant to curb the spread of the novel coronavirus may have adverse effects on the vulnerable communities who live from hand to mouth.

The WhatsApp memes depict the predicament of the vulnerable communities as they are caught between a rock and a hard place. One meme depicts COVID-19 and hunger as the two forces that have put low-income families in a predicament. Another meme represents a family inside a house, with children seemingly hungry and begging their mother for food: "*mama we are hungry*". A police officer is patrolling the streets to enforce the lockdown regulations. Using a loudspeaker, the male police officer orders the family to remain indoors. This meme depicts the plight of the poor communities as they have to deal with COVID-19, hunger and law enforcement authorities. The impoverished communities are confined to their homes, as contravening lockdown regulations will expose them to the deadly COVID-19. At the same time, these starving families have to deal with the wrath of law enforcement agents. Furthermore, the stay-at-home order means the vulnerable communities who survive on informal trade are unable to put food on the table. As such, memes constitute a form of "silent resistance" (Siziba & Ncube, 2015, 517) as they articulate the plight and predicament of the subordinated groups during the time of COVID-19. Through WhatsApp memes, the counter-publics are formed and solidified as the subordinated groups articulate "recognised exclusions" (Asen, 2000, 437). Counter-publics are formed when there is a recognition by participants of "exclusion from wider public spheres" (Asen, 2000, 427). Thus, WhatsApp memes provide a platform for the disenfranchised communities to articulate "alternative discourses, practices and norms" (Asen, 2000, 427). In depicting the lockdown measures as anti-poor, there is a recognition by the subaltern of the power imbalances and socio-economic disparities in the country.

In addition, there are memes that rely on humour to depict the plight of the poor:

> *Kungcono ubaba afe nge flue esebenzela imuli ukuthi ingafi ngendlala kulokuthi imuli ife ngendlala ubaba ecatshele I flu.*

This meme is written in isiNdebele and loosely translates, "It is better for a man to succumb to influenza whilst working for his family so that they do not starve, than for his family to perish due to starvation whilst he is hiding from the flu". In this meme, COVID-19 is depicted as a non-lethal influenza. Discourses of masculinity are mobilised to project an ideal man as a provider and protector. Men are being encouraged to the contravene lockdown regulations and provide food for their families. Within this hunger/COVID-19 dichotomy, a "real man" is depicted as the one who risks contracting the virus in order to provide for his family. As such, discourses on masculinity are summoned and reproduced in a way that challenges the status quo.

Memes as a Form of Political Commentary

Humour has a subversive potential as alienated and marginalised groups share memes and jokes to mock the political elites and other privileged groups:

> *What if CORONA VIRUS is a LATIN word meaning ZANU PF?*
>
> *Orphaned Zimbabweans waiting for President Cyril Ramaphosa's address like*

These memes depict ZANU PF as a pandemic that has caused hardships and untold suffering on Zimbabweans. By pandemic, the meme denotes ZANU PF as a disease, plague or scourge to Zimbabweans. Thus, the subalterns are engaged in a subversive practice of "semiotic guerrilla warfare" (Eco, 1986) as WhatsApp memes are used to ridicule and resist ZANU PF's hegemony. Furthermore, the meme mocks the government by lamenting that Zimbabweans are "orphaned". In representing "orphaned" Zimbabweans as waiting for guidance from South Africa's president, the meme is challenging ZANU PF's leadership and legitimacy. In authoritarian societies, political jokes have the "common feature of calling into question the legitimacy of the political system" (Badarneh, 2011, 307). Zimbabweans are depicted as parentless and having been adopted by the government of South Africa. Thus, laughter serves as a way to "puncture the pomposity of the powerful" (Källstig & Death, 2020, 1). ZANU PF officials like Patrick Chinamasa have tended to mobilise the rhetoric of "Zimbabwe is not a province of South Africa" (Kwaramba and Madzimure, 2020) as a discursive shield against criticism from their neighbours concerning human rights violations. Political humour targets repressive regimes by venting "social, economic, and other frustrations" (Badarneh, 2011, 307). Thus, these political jokes enable individuals to release their "constrained and suppressed desires and freedoms" (Badarneh, 2011, 397).

Other memes are ridiculing President Mnangagwa and his predecessor, Mugabe:

> *If you could end COVID-19 by sacrificing one African president, which one would you choose and why Mnangagwa?*
>
> *It's likely that if he was alive, he would have named himself The Commander of Corona.*

In authoritarian regimes, the disempowered and aggrieved communities celebrate COVID-19 as the "great equaliser" or an omnipotent force meting out justice on the seemingly invincible politicians. ZANU PF officials such as Mnangagwa are implicated in the *Gukurahundi* genocide and other human rights crimes in the country. As such, there is a meme that depicts COVID-19 as a weapon that can be wielded against the oppressors. Siziba and Ncube (2015, 523) posit that humour constitutes a "source of cynical critique" when the oppressed are "confronted by an insurmountable crisis" where their oppressors "cannot be dislodged". Furthermore, humour serves as a "needed distraction for liveability in a gloomy context" (Siziba & Ncube, 2015, 523).

The meme is a mockery of the late and former President Mugabe's obsession with titles and power. As the head of state, Mugabe recreated himself as a "god, chief and king" (Siziba & Ncube, 2015, 523). He held numerous titles such as "the Commander in Chief of Zimbabwe's armed forces, the Chancellor of the University of Zimbabwe and all state Universities and the President and First Secretary of ZANU PF" (Siziba & Ncube, 2015, 522). The referential strategy "commander of corona" serves to highlight Mugabe's thirst for and obsession with power. Thus, the meme serves to ridicule and scorn the powerful for their obsession with titles.

Furthermore, there are memes that challenge the global order rooted in Western modernity. Through these memes, the idea of using Africans as guinea pigs to test COVID-19 vaccines is rejected. Remarks by French doctors that trials for COVID-19 vaccines should be conducted in Africa sparked outrage (BBC, 2020). Viewing Africa as a testing ground for COVID-19 vaccines was denounced as racist by Didier Drogba and other prominent figures. A meme was circulated that represents a black woman holding a knife on a white male doctor who seemingly was about to conduct vaccine testing on a black man. Within this narrative, the heroine (black woman) saves the victim (black man) from the villain (white male doctor). The message "*no vaccine testing on us*" reinforces this pan-Africanist narrative. This Afrocentric discourse serves to unmask and dismantle the dark history of Western modernity. It is a critique of Western scientific advancements that are entrenched in coloniality.

Conclusion

This chapter sought to explore the role of Internet memes as forms of political jokes. Memes not only provide humour but also reflect the lived experiences of citizens. Drawing upon WhatsApp memes on COVID-19, the chapter examined the intersection of humour and the everyday life in the context of a pandemic. Bakhtin's theory of the carnivalesque and the concept of counter-publics were employed to analyse the subversive nature of memes in authoritarian environments such as Zimbabwe. Findings demonstrate the complex nature of Internet memes as forms of political satire. First, memes constitute sites of resistance as humour is used to ridicule and challenge ZANU PF party. Second, some memes draw upon Afrocentric discourses to challenge the hegemonic Western perspectives. As forms of dissent, WhatsApp memes reinforce the decolonial perspectives that critique the dominant Eurocentric modernity and coloniality. Third, memes express the socio-economic predicaments of the disadvantaged communities who are excluded from online learning. However, WhatsApp memes also serve to reinforce stereotypical depictions of social groups such as black women. Patriarchal and racist are perpetuated through WhatsApp memes that ridicule and disparage the bodies of black women.

This chapter builds upon scholarship on digital humour by focusing on how WhatsApp memes mediate the lived experiences of ordinary citizens in Zimbabwe. In times of pandemics, Internet humour plays a pivotal role in enabling communities to cope and come to terms with the public health crisis. Despite the multifaceted nature of COVID-19, dominant debates have focused on epidemiological responses. As such, this chapter draws our attention to the subversive nature of digital humour in helping citizens to cope with the impacts of the coronavirus pandemic.

References

Aguilar, G. K., Campbell, H. A., Stanley, M., & Taylor, E. (2017). Communicating mixed messages about religion through internet memes. *Information, Communication & Society, 20*(10), 1498–1520.

Asen, R. (2000). Seeking the "counter" in counterpublics. *Communication Theory, 10*(4), 424–446.

Badarneh, M. A. (2011). Carnivalesque politics: A Bakhtinian case study of contemporary Arab political humor. *Humor, 24*(3), 305–327.

BBC. (2020). Coronavirus: France racism row over doctors' Africa testing comments. April 3. https://www.bbc.com/news/world-europe-52151722. Accessed 21 Aug 2021.

Chingono, N. (2020, April 9). Doctors Sue Zimbabwe government over lack of COVID-19 protective equipment. *The Guardian*. https://www.theguardian.com/global-development/2020/apr/09/doctors-sue-zimbabwe-government-over-lack-of-COVID-19-protective-equipment. Accessed 12 Oct 2020.

Chitanana, T. (2020). From Kubatana to #ThisFlag: Trajectories of digital activism in Zimbabwe. *Journal of Information Technology & Politics, 17*(2), 130–145.

Chuma, W. (2008). Mediating the 2000 elections in Zimbabwe: Competing journalisms in a society at the crossroads. *Ecquid Novi, 29*(1), 21–41.

Dawkins, R. (1976). *The selfish gene*. Oxford University Press.

DeCook, J. R. (2018). Memes and symbolic violence: #proudboys and the use of memes for propaganda and the construction of collective identity. *Learning, Media and Technology, 43*(4), 485–504.

Denisova, A. (2019). *Internet memes and society. Social, cultural, and political contexts*. Routledge.

Eco, U. (1986). *Towards a semiological guerrilla warfare*. Harcourt.

Fairclough, N. (1995). *Critical discourse analysis. The critical study of language*. Longman.

Fiske, J. (1989). *Understanding popular culture*. Routledge.

Fraser, N. (1992). Rethinking the public sphere: A contribution to the critique of actually existing democracy. In C. Calhoun (Ed.), *Habermas and the public sphere* (pp. 109–142). MIT Press.

Grossberg, L. (2005). History, politics and postmodernism. Stuart Hall and cultural studies. In D. Morley & K.-H. Chen (Eds.), *Stuart Hall. Critical dialogues in cultural studies* (pp. 151–173). Routledge.

Gukurume, S. (2017). From Kubatana to #ThisFlag: Trajectories of digital activism in Zimbabwe. *Journal of Information Technology & Politics, 17*(2), 130–145.

Jenkins, E. S. (2014). The modes of visual rhetoric: Circulating memes as expressions. *Quarterly Journal of Speech, 100*(4), 442–466.

Jorgensen, M., & Phillips, L. J. (2002). *Discourse analysis as theory and method*. Sage.

Källstig, A., & Death, C. (2020). Laughter, resistance and ambivalence in Trevor Noah's stand-up comedy: Returning mimicry as mockery. *Critical African Studies*. https://doi.org/10.1080/21681392.2020.1743191

Kuhlmann, J. (2012). Zimbabwean diaspora politics and the power of laughter: Humour as a tool for political communication, criticism and protest. *Journal of African Media Studies, 4*(3), 295–314.

Kulkarni, A. (2017). Internet meme and political discourse: A study on the impact of internet meme as a tool in communicating political satire. *Journal of Content, Community & Communication, 6*(3), 13–17.

Kwaramba, F., & Madzimure, J. (2020). Zim not a province of SA – Zanu PF. September 12. *The Herald*. https://www.herald.co.zw/zim-not-a-province-of-sa-zanu-pf/. Accessed 21 Aug 2021.

MacMillan, C. (2020). Welcome to the carnival? Podemos, populism and Bakhtin's carnivalesque. *Journal of Contemporary European Studies, 25*(2), 258–273.

Makhortykh, M., & Aguilar, J. M. G. (2020). Memory, politics and emotions: Internet memes and protests in Venezuela and Ukraine. *Continuum: Journal of Media and Cultural Studies, 34*(3), 342–362.

Makurumidze, R. (2020). Coronavirus-19 disease (COVID-19): A case series of early suspected cases reported and the implications towards the response to the pandemic in Zimbabwe. *Journal of Microbiology and Immunology and Infection, 53*(3), 493–498.

Manganga, K. (2012). The use of jokes and mobile telephony to create counter-publics in Zimbabwe. *Journal of African Media Studies, 4*(2), 243–255.

Mano, W., & Willems, W. (2008). Emerging communities, emerging media: The case of a Zimbabwean nurse in the British *Big Brother* show. *Critical Arts, 22*(1), 101–128.

Mare, A. (2018). Politics unusual? Facebook and political campaigning during the 2013 harmonised elections in Zimbabwe. *African Journalism Studies, 39*(1), 90–110.

Mare, A. (2020). State-ordered internet shutdowns and digital authoritarianism in Zimbabwe. *International Journal of Communication, 14*, 4244–4263.

Media Institute of Southern Africa (MISA). (2020). *An analysis of social media use in the SADC region 2014–2020*. MISA.

Mhlanga, B., & Mpofu, M. (2014). The virtual parallax: Imaginations of Mthwakazi Nationalism – Online discussions and calls for self-determination. In A. M. G. Solo (Ed.), *Handbook on research on political activism in the information age* (pp. 129–146). IGI Global.

Moyo, D. (2005). *The "independent" press and the fight for democracy in Zimbabwe: A critical analysis of the banned Daily News* (pp. 109–128). *Westminster Papers in Communication and Culture*.

Moyo, D. (2007). Alternative media, diasporas and the mediation of the Zimbabwean crisis. *Ecquid Novi: African Journalism Studies, 28*(1), 81–105.
Moyo, D. (2012). Participation, citizenship and pirate radio as empowerment: The case of *Radio Dialogue* in Zimbabwe. *International Journal of Communication, 6*, 484–500.
Moyo, L. (2009a). Repression, propaganda and digital resistance: New media and democracy in Zimbabwe. In F. O. Mudhai, F. Banda, & W. J. Tettey (Eds.), *African media and the digital public sphere* (pp. 57–72). Palgrave.
Moyo, L. (2009b). Constructing a home away from home: The internet, nostalgia and identity politics among Zimbabwean communities in Britain. *Journal of Global Mass Communications, 2*(1), 66–85.
Mpofu, S. (2014). Memory, national identity and freedom of expression in the information age: Discussing the taboo in the Zimbabwean public sphere. In A. M. G. Solo (Ed.), *Handbook on research on political activism in the Information Age* (pp. 114–128). IGI Global.
Mpofu, S. (2015). When the subaltern speaks: Citizen Journalism and genocide 'victims' voices online. *African Journalism Studies, 36*(4), 82–101.
Mpofu, S. (2016). Zimbabwe's state controlled public media and the mediation of the 1980s genocide 30 years on. *Journal of African Media Studies, 8*(2), 145–165.
Mpofu, S. (2019). For a nation to progress victims must 'move on': A case of Zimbabwe's social media discourses of Gukurahundi genocide silencing and resistance. *African Identities, 17*(2), 108–129.
Mpofu, S., & Mare, A. (2020). #ThisFlag: Social media and cyber-protests in Zimbabwe. In M. N. Ndlela & W. Mano (Eds.), *Social media and elections in Africa* (pp. 153–173). Palgrave Macmillan.
Muronzi, C. (2020). Coronavirus to push Zimbabwe to the brink? *Business Live*. April 2. https://www.businesslive.co.za/fm/features/africa/2020-04-02-coronavirus-to-push-zimbabwe-to-the-bring/. Accessed 21 Aug 2021.
Ndlovu, M. (2018). Speaking for the dead: Testimonies, witnesses and the representations of Gukurahundi atrocities in new media. *Journal of African Cultural Studies, 30*(3), 293–306.
Ndlovu-Gatsheni, S. J. (2013). Why decoloniality in the 21st century. *The Thinker, 48*, 10–15.
Ngwira, E., & Lipenga, K. J. (2018). A country laughing at itself: Malawian humour in the Digital Age. *English Studies in Africa, 61*(2), 21–35.
Nyamnjoh, F. B. (1996). Africa and the Information Superhighway: Silent majorities in search of a footpath. *Africa Media Review, 10*(2), 1–21.
Okawa, R. (2013). Humour in exile: The subversive effects of laughter in Sam Selvon's The Lonely Londoners and Gisèle Pineau's L'Exil selon Julia. *Journal of Postcolonial Writing, 49*(1), 16–27.

Pearce, K., & Hajizada, A. (2014). No laughing matter humor as a means of dissent in the digital era: The case of authoritarian Azerbaijan. *The Journal of Post-Soviet Democratization, 22*(1), 67–85.

Ranger, T. (2005). *The rise of patriotic journalism in Zimbabwe and its possible implications* (pp. 8–17). *Westminster Papers in Communication.*

Richardson, J. E. (2007). *Analysing newspapers. An approach from critical discourse analysis.* Palgrave Macmillan.

Rodgers, S. T. (2017). Womanism and Afrocentricity: Understanding the intersection. *Journal of Human Behavior in the Social Environment, 27*(1–2), 36–47.

Siziba, G., & Ncube, G. (2015). Mugabe's fall from grace: Satire and fictional narratives as silent forms of resistance in/on Zimbabwe. *Social Dynamics, 4*(3), 516–539.

Tembo, N. M. (2011). Subversion and the carnivalesque images of resistance in Ngugi wa Thiong'o's Wizard of the crow. In G. Collier (Ed.), *Spheres public and private: Western genres in African Literature* (pp. 337–361). Editions Rodopi.

Teti, M., Schatz, E., & Liebenberg, L. (2020). Methods in the Time of COVID-19: The Vital Role of Qualitative Inquiries. *International Journal of Qualitative Methods, 19*, 1–5.

Wells, D. D. (2018). You all made dank memes: Using Internet memes to promote critical thinking. *Journal of Political Science Education, 14*(2), 240–248.

Wiggins, B. (2019). *The discursive power in digital culture. Ideology, semiotics and intertextuality.* Routledge.

Willems, W. (2011). Comic Strips and "the Crisis": Postcolonial laughter and coping with everyday life in Zimbabwe. *Popular Communication, 9*(2), 126–145.

CHAPTER 13

Humour in the Age of Contagion: Coronavirus, 'Janata Curfew' Meme and India's Digital Cultures of Virality

Imran Parray

Introduction

The proliferation of social media networks and microblogging platforms powered by Web 2.0 has transformed the way citizens around the world express opinions and engage in larger political events and conversations. An undercurrent of this newfound and unfiltered mode of expression is exchange of humour, which is embedded in text, talk and visuals, often directed at political leaders and aimed at criticising and mocking their policies and actions at moments of sociopolitical, economic or health crises. This chapter undertakes a critical analysis of the 'Janata Curfew' meme,[1] a collection of images and videos circulated on social media platforms in India and beyond, which mocked Prime Minister Narendra Modi after he advised his fellow Indians to clap hands and bang plates as a sign of respect

I. Parray (✉)
Department of Communication and Journalism, Institute of Home Economics, University of Delhi, New Delhi, India
e-mail: imran.parray@ihe.du.ac.in

S. Mpofu (ed.), *Digital Humour in the Covid-19 Pandemic*,
https://doi.org/10.1007/978-3-030-79279-4_13

for medical workers fighting coronavirus. Because of the multiplicity and interactivity of communication patterns in India's digital cultures with an ever-growing presence of citizens on the Internet,[2] Modi's message became an instant satirical hit among users on Twitter, Facebook, WhatsApp and TikTok at the time when medical experts had warned that Indian government was short of necessary medical infrastructure, resources, strategies and skills to fight the deadly pandemic (Sharma, 2020).

As it turned out, Modi's public address was viewed by many online users as political rhetoric to hide his government's inefficiencies. What followed was a barrage of visuals mocking the prime minister and his right-wing Bharatiya Janata Party government, giving rise to a new popular meme and a site of huge political contestation. The chapter seeks to study the 'Janata Curfew' meme as a symbolic totality that crystallised a number of connotative meanings foregrounded in humour, ridicule, satire and irony. It will analyse signs and codes employed in the visual content, arguing that online users in India derive humour and satire from cultural industries such as the nation's film industry, Bollywood, and the existing socio-economic and political tensions. Besides humour, however, the 'Janata Curfew' meme offered a moment of reflection for digitally connected citizens on the state of governance in India and the archaic, rhetorical, superstitious and irrational political communication deployed by high-level political leaders. Furthermore, it will be demonstrated how armies of users—humans as well as bots—seek to engage with such memes and indulge in both symbolic resistance and violence. As a consequence, it's argued, the lines between humour, ridicule, comedy, trolling and threats blur in India's emergent digital cultures.

Humour in the Times of COVID: Metalising Political Protest

Apart from ushering in fear and anxiety, which is symbolic of the 'risk society' (Beck, 1992) we live in, the COVID-19 pandemic has also given rise to humour and laughter, expressed via a multimedia display of visuals and written text (Nicholls, 2020). The place of humour at the time of a global grieving—1.64 million deaths have been recorded so far—at once invokes the impulses of Superiority theory and Release release theory (Carr, 2020; Fessell, 2020; Nicholls, 2020). In both circumstances, humour has become a vital communicative act, a catharsis for those who are caught in an endless cycle of quarantine and enforced lockdown but connected with others through the technology of the Internet. However, a deeper explanation in the overall rise of humour in both the West and the developing world is the demonstration of 'gross political ineptitude' by political leaders and citizens' distrust of the system (Nicholls, 2020). Humour has been also directed at government-mandated initiatives to promote behavioural change, a sense of inclusion and solidarity (Carr, 2020).

As Boss and t-Hart (2008) show, humour possesses a unique power to frame social and political protest. Humour acts as a political expression that helps people cope up with their political struggles (Rehak & Trnka, 2019). It is thus a method through which people resist power.

In the context of India, much of the humour circulated online surrounding the 'Janata Curfew' meme took recourse to satire, offering citizens a moment of psychological release by mocking leaders (in this case Modi). Added to this practice of satire for the sake of satire was the production of cartoons and memes that sought to speak "truth to power" in many different ways (Nicholls, 2020). In fact, the process of production, reproduction and recirculation of humour serves as, what Philipose (2020) calls, a "counter-power", the deployment of which tends to momentarily 'destabilise' structures of power and deepen democratic deliberation. Such expressions of humour online can land artists in trouble as is the case in India where the government has initiated contempt proceedings against those mocking the system and its utilities.

Announcing 'Janata Curfew': Coronavirus in India and Official Response

The first COVID case in India was detected on 27 January 2020 in the southern state of Kerala, when a 20-year-old woman, who had a travel history to Wuhan, China, complained of dry cough and sore throat at General Hospital in Thrissur. Shortly after identifying the symptoms, authorities admitted the woman to an isolated ward where samples for examination were collected. After three days, a government laboratory confirmed that the woman had contracted the virus. After undergoing treatment for over 20 days in a COVID facility, she was discharged from the hospital on February 20 (Andrews et al., 2020). Despite this initial success story, the cases of contagion and death were already on the rise, as shown in Figs. 13.1 and 13.2.

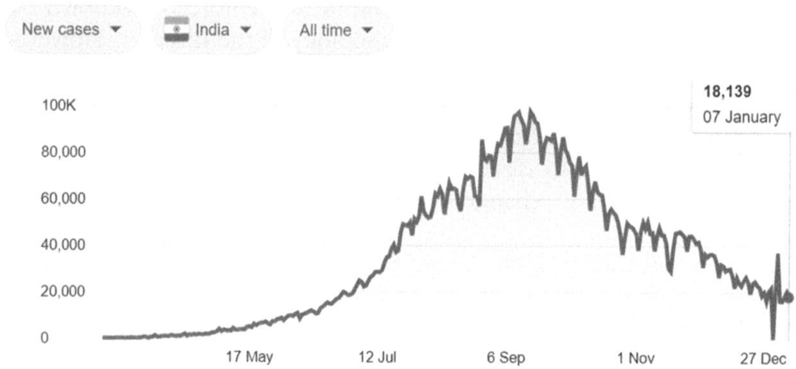

Fig. 13.1 A matrix of COVID-19 cases in India. (Source: Data repository for the 2019 Novel Coronavirus Visual Dashboard operated by the Johns Hopkins University Center for Systems Science and Engineering (JHU CSSE))

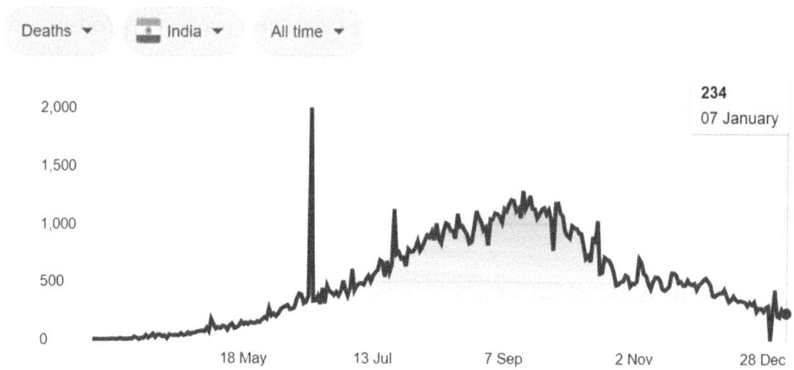

Fig. 13.2 A matrix of COVID-19 deaths in India. (Source: Data repository for the 2019 Novel Coronavirus Visual Dashboard operated by the Johns Hopkins University Center for Systems Science and Engineering (JHU CSSE))

According to official estimates, more than 10 million people contracted coronavirus in India while more than 140,000 have died so far (Ministry of Health and Family Welfare, 2020). India ranks second worst-affected country in the world after the USA (Asrar, 2020). Critics of Modi including opposition parties slammed the BJP-led government for mishandling the crisis while expressing irony that the state was busy hosting the US President Donald J. Trump when hundreds of thousands of migrant labourers were facing widespread suffering and death in the wake of the rising number of cases. Critics suspected that the government was using the pandemic 'to convert democracy into autocracy'. A member of the parliament from All India Trinamool Congress Derek O'Brien thus remarked, "you need humility ... This government needs humility" (PTI, 2020). O′ Brien's comment alludes to a certain liminality in moral governance where the government is expected to at once possess humility and reason (Button, 2005). The Indian government was criticised for lacking both. While its citizens were confronted by a broken and inadequate healthcare system, politicians of the nationalist party continued to invoke religious mantras for the containment of the virus like drinking cow urine (Singh, 2020). It was this callous and unscientific approach of the government towards COVID-19 that—to turn India's Chief of Defence Staff Bipin Rawat's expression on its head—taught India a 'lesson' (Hindustan Times, 2020). On the economic front, Modi's 'irrational' steps were widely criticised, with the leaders of opposition saying the country was plunging into recession while unemployment was increasing (Press Trust of India, 2019). The first national lockdown in India was imposed by Modi for 21 days on 24 March. At that point, 600 cases of COVID were identified while 10 had died. Since the imposition of lockdown, the Indian economy has plunged into a deep economic crisis with the gross domestic product shrinking by a record 23.8 per cent as per the Reserve Bank of India assessment (Wallen, 2020). This situation has pushed an estimated 400 million Indians into poverty. Among India's 500 million workforce, around 90 per cent are employed in the informal sector such as construction. The work of this workforce suddenly came to a grinding halt. As Wallen (2020) reports, small and medium enterprises were forced to close their ventures. Sundar and Nilsen (2020) write that Modi's "callous indifference to the travails of ordinary Indians and preference for symbolic gestures over a sustained and substantive public health response transformed the pandemic into a humanitarian crisis".

Instead of delivering, Modi has "exploited the pandemic for repression, political gain, and corporate profiteering" (Sundar & Nilsen, 2020). This kind of a political performance is seen to fit well with "decades of neoliberal economic policy" that the BJP has combined with its "politics of Hindu majoritarian nationalism to distribute vulnerabilities along hierarchies of class, caste, and regional and religious identity" (Sundar & Nilsen, 2020). For instance, as Sundar and Nilsen point out, the imposition of the lockdown helped the government to quell the protest movement against the anti-Muslim Citizenship Amendment Act.

By March 2020, the fast spread of the coronavirus had already assumed the character of a pandemic. In response, the majority of world leaders started imposing lockdowns to contain the contagion from spreading. On 19 March 2020, India's Prime Minister Narendra Modi announced what he called 'Janata Curfew', asking citizens to stay indoors at a later date, that is, March 22. Modi's announcement on national television was just a case of world leaders making themselves politically relevant at a time when bodies politic of modern nation-states were under enormous challenges to tackle the microbial onslaught on the human populations. However, what was interesting in Modi's message was his plea to citizens to "stand in the balconies of their houses for five minutes … and clap as a sign of thanks for emergency workers" (Indian Express, 2020). This suggestion by the head of the government, as critics later commented, was a joke in the face of the predicament, which was about to overwhelm India given the country's huge population and citizens' deep sense of socialisation. To this end, Modi and his government were found not only inefficient but also indifferent to deal with an impending healthcare crisis, while his initiative, PM Cares, has been seen by critics as a 'murky venture,' nothing short of a 'black hole' (Newslaundry, 2020) and 'a scheme to pad the BJP's war chest' (Sundar & Nilsen, 2020). Modi's message—which his supporters from across the country would follow as a duty and in particular celebrities from the worlds of cinema and cricket would appear on balconies and post pictures with their families clapping and banging plates—thus became an instant attraction for meme-hungry users in India's digital landscape.

The prime minister's words—like other revelations of "nonsense and grotesquery on part of our Dear Leaders" (Nicholls, 2020, 313)—propelled a multimedia storm with memes of different kinds beginning to appear and circulate on multiple channels. Taken together, this collection of pictures, graphics and videos assumed the character of a master meme that carried a common theme and target: Modi's irrational self. What followed the appearance of this meme, apart from its fast spread like a contagion, was its continued repackaging with newer humour configurations in text and visuals emerging from different vantage points. It is argued that this totalising meme can be viewed as a political comment at a historical moment in India that has been defined by massive citizens' protests against the populist policies of the Modi government marked by the controversial Citizenship Amendment Act and the proposed National Register of Citizens. On the other hand, what was explicit in this collection of memes was references to Bollywood films and soap operas in conveying underlying meaning, which signified the similarity of melodrama in Indian politics and film industry. The overall meme can thus be said to contain, following Terry Eagleton, the shades of both the comic and the serious, creating an incongruity effect.

Invoking Bollywood: Finding Resonance in Popular Cinema and Soap Operas

The totalising meme—that brought to the fore multiple ironies evinced in photographs, graphics, cartoons, videos and so on—mainly derived its voice from Bollywood and the soap opera industry of the country. Since laughter and comedy have played a significant role in shaping Bollywood (Ganjoo, 2020), much of the humour employed in the meme was derived from popular Bollywood films. Thus, in the recirculated photographs and graphics, film and soap opera characters were likened to Modi in order to emphasise the rhetoric and melodrama that he is accused of often employing in his speeches. Figure 13.3 shows a satirical image in which Modi is compared with a female character of a soap opera. Modi is shown humiliating coronavirus (embodied by another female actor) with his speech, while China (embodied by a male actor) is seen consoling the heart-broken female (the virus). After breaking coronavirus's heart through his clapping antidote, the male actor (China) turns to Modi embodying a female character and expresses, "Rula diya na bechari ko" (Made this poor soul cry). The edited image, widely circulated on the Internet, is significant in at least two ways: First, it establishes a spatial relationship between China and coronavirus as if the two share the same future together. Secondly, it links Modi's speech to melodrama because Indian soap operas are often melodramatic and full of exaggeration.

A widely circulated visual that was part of the overall meme drew on a Bollywood film, Singham, directed by Rohit Shetty and starring Ajay Devgan. In the edited image, where the entire meaning is reconstructed through the addition of text on an original image grab, the main villain (coronavirus) is seen crying before the protagonist Inspector Bajirao

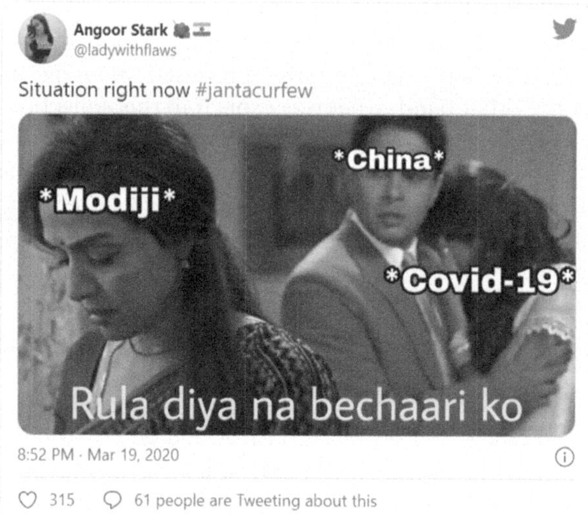
Angoor Stark
@ladywithflaws
Situation right now #jantacurfew
China
Modiji
Covid-19
Rula diya na bechaari ko
8:52 PM · Mar 19, 2020
315
61 people are Tweeting about this

Fig. 13.3 In this edited image, Modi is shown as a soap opera character (original picture is that of Bollywood film actress Hema Malini) confronting a third female character (coronavirus), while China (handsome male) is seen consoling the virus after a silly bashful by the Indian prime minister. (Source: Twitter)

Singham (reference is to Modi) who seems to have nabbed the politician-criminal (coronavirus). If this individual meme is humanised, it simply goes like this: after hearing Modi's strategy to counter it, coronavirus cries, saying, "cheating karta hai tu" (you are cheating). This mockery of the prime minister's plan is further expanded through the invocation of a reality television show, 'Kaun Banega Crorepati,' hosted by famous Indian film actor Amitabh Bachchan who keeps clapping hands and asking members of the audience to do so (See Fig. 13.4).

Taken together, this collection of pictures seems to mock and satirise Modi's suggestion of clapping. To this end, Twitter users compared Modi's speech with the popular kids cartoon show "If You're Happy and You Know It", in which the main character suggests children to "clap" their hands. The invocation of this show has an uncanny resemblance with Modi's suggestion to clap and bang plates.

This slice of the totalising meme portrays Modi as a charmer at the time when the country was underequipped to handle the COVID-19 crisis and

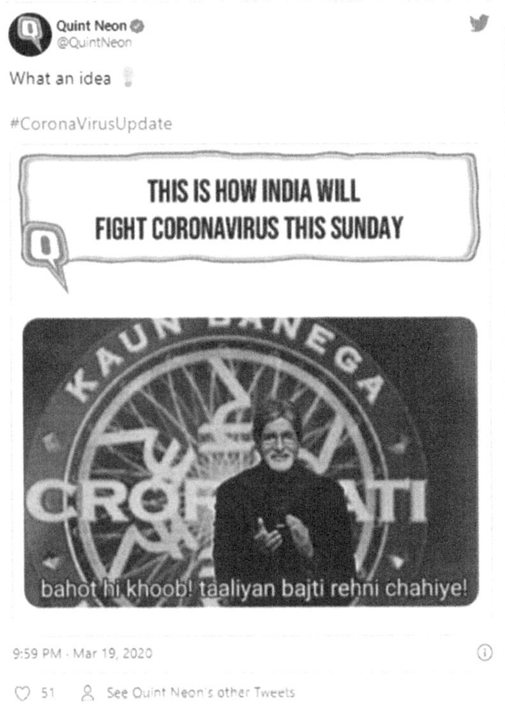
Quint Neon
@QuintNeon
What an idea
#CoronaVirusUpdate
THIS IS HOW INDIA WILL FIGHT CORONAVIRUS THIS SUNDAY
KAUN BANEGA CROREPATI
bahot hi khoob! taaliyan bajti rehni chahiye!
9:59 PM · Mar 19, 2020
51
See Quint Neon's other Tweets

Fig. 13.4 The picture shows Amitabh Bachchan on the sets of KBC, a popular reality show, clapping and asking audience members to keep clapping. It satirises the Modi government's ineffective plans to contain the virus. (Source: Twitter)

when the head of the government was supposed to offer concrete solutions like ensuring optimum healthcare facilities. Instead, Modi's speeches appeared theatrical and filmy where he appealed to multiple topics of sentiment, thereby moving the situation away from critical treatment. In response to this, the Internet users sought to ridicule the prime minister while taking recourse to humour, which allowed citizens to resurrect an old and complex relationship between humour and ridicule (Billig, 2005).

'Apne Baap Ko Mat Sikha': Political Comment Wrapped in Humour

Apart from individual-specific references to Modi and his politico-scientific rationality as a leader of the so-called world's largest democracy, various parts of the master meme drew on the existing sociopolitical tensions in the country. The term 'curfew' in Modi's announcement of the 'Janata Curfew' struck a familiar chord with users from Indian-administered Kashmir where the Indian state often imposes long and harsh curfews to tackle the indigenous struggle for freedom.[3] In one widely shared visual from a film in which the popular Indian actor Akshay Kumar utters to someone an oft-repeated phrase "*apne baap ko mat sikha*", which is a *desi* way to assert one's superiority in terms of age and wisdom over the other. It loosely translates as "Don't teach your dad".

Through this film dialogue, online users from the conflict region sought to not only mock the prime minister about what they felt was a worn-out exercise for them but also highlighted that curfews were commonplace in the disputed Himalayan territory. Such an engagement, constructed on humour, satire and parody, catapults users to a position of both as critics of political power and as creators of popular artwork in the digital realm. As such this meme has purely political overtones because the political relationship between Kashmiris and the Indian state has been rather complex. This complexity has torn down the place. Local journalists, activists and members of the public in Kashmir are often targeted for their journalistic work or activism. Therefore, recourse to humour on the Internet is ideal. Announcements like 'Janata Curfew' thus propel their desire to engage in humour not only as passive participants in recirculating memes but also as creating newer and remodelling the existing ones, thereby exercising their agency as active agents in the wider processes of production and transformation of viral ideas.

Giving Coronavirus a Voice: 'I Can't Survive This; I Will Die'

Another dimension of the 'Janata Curfew' meme was its constant pursuit to give voice to coronavirus in order to imagine and frame its possible reactions to Modi's plan. A viral visual showed popular actor Nawazuddin Siddique (metaphoric of coronavirus) stuck in an unfriendly place with danger lurking ahead. The danger referred to in this picture is the clapping and banging of plates, a component of the prime minister's plan. Coronavirus, embodied by Siddique in this image, is shown to fear for his life because it might not survive the clapping. This predicament facing COVID is further reflected in other visuals in which coronavirus is seen to surrender to the noise of banging plates. Together, these visuals ridicule

Modi and express irony over his political leadership that sought to hide in rhetoric, superstition and irrationality.

Humour as 'Counter-Power': Confronting the State with Laughter

Memes have been identified as a powerful tool to counter the state and initiate a political protest (Mina, 2019). Humour and laughter serve as a powerful tool in social protest (t'Hart, 2007). Responding to Modi's call for Janata Curfew, India's most popular and controversial stand-up comedian, Kunal Kamra, tweeted a picture of himself showing his middle finger to the prime minister's plan. He captioned the image: "Prepping for tomorrow". Kamra has been a fiercest critique of the BJP-led government. In his Janata Curfew satire post, he tweeted on 21 March: "I'm showing a middle finger to the PM's marketing stunt at a time like this, epidemic seems to be unreported & our economy in anyway in state of panic… He should realise that there is no election around the corner & propose policies instead of these stunts." Such kind of humour laced with serious comment has its limits in India. In November 2020, the government of India initiated a series of contempt proceedings against Kamra, who, according to the nation's Attorney General K.K. Venugopal, had insulted the Supreme Court of India and its chief justice (The Wire Staff, 2020). Kamra, in his satirical tweets, had posted images that showed the Supreme Court painted in saffron, the colour symbolic of the ruling right-wing Bharatiya Janata Party. In the edited image, Kamra had inserted the BJP flag atop the court.

These images and captions accompanying them were viewed by the government as an assault on the federal court's independence. Kamra's criticism of the federal court came in the wake of the grant of bail to the television anchor, Arnab Goswami, who was arrested by the police in the southern state of Maharashtra for his abetment in the suicide of an architect and his mother in 2018. Kamra and many others in India raised questions over the special legal treatment accorded to Goswami—who is considered a BJP mouthpiece—by the Supreme Court, while the court uses a different yardstick for those who are languishing in Indian jails without trial.

Crossing Lines: On the Limits of Humour

A core argument of this chapter is that the lines between humour, ridicule, comedy, trolling and threats are blurring in India's emergent digital cultures. It is in this context that emphasis is placed on recent memes directed against Kamra. A viral visual showed a tweet by a user, Divyanshu Saxena, abusing the artist after the Supreme Court issued another contempt notice on December 18 against the comedian.

Although such tweets apparently violate community standards, social media platforms themselves (e.g., Facebook) have been accused of being complicit in allowing such communicative acts in extreme speech, which serve Modi's populist politics (Thakurta & Sam, 2019; Purnell & Horwitz, 2020).

Apart from abuses on general occasions, the Janata Curfew meme also gave rise to a few memes on Twitter in which a particular identity of movie characters was likened to coronavirus. Another viral post showed an elderly Muslim man being used as a metaphor for coronavirus. Since all others in the scene are silent in observance of the curfew call, it is the Muslim body which is at once vilified as virus and non-observant of Modi's programme. Such memes, it is argued, can deepen the existing prejudices against minority communities in India because of the reach of social media. This meme acted as a prequel to an upcoming action movie. The vilification of the Muslim body took a more serious turn when in May 2020 leaders of the BJP claimed that Tablighi Jamaat, a Muslim organisation, was responsible for the spread of the virus. Such claims provided members of the right-wing BJP "yet another excuse to viciously scapegoat Muslims" (Sundar & Nilsen, 2020). It has been observed that this scapegoating is part of the state apparatus of oppressing the Muslim community in the country.

Conclusion

The chapter explored the Janata Curfew meme as a symbolic totality in which multiple narratives emerged as a consequence of users' engagement with circulation, production and reproduction of humour. The humour that followed was directed at both Modi's rationality and his government's policies. The Bollywood and soap opera industry offered a great cushion within which the meme was located. Furthermore, existing political issues also foregrounded the production of humour and its consumption.

However, this production of humour carries with itself the danger of trespassing other zones which are detrimental not only for democracy but for humanity itself.

Notes

1. A meme, following Richard Dawkins' conceptualisation, is referred to as the viral spread of an idea (Dawkins, 2006). At the heart of the term is the Greek concept 'minema', which translates as imitation. Thus, meme as an idea "transforms from a single event to a shared social phenomenon through the process of imitation, copying, mimicking, remixing or repackaging" (Taecharungroj & Nueangjamnong, 2015). The Internet is viewed as a great site where memes carrying contagious cultural ideas undergo this process.
2. India, with a population of around 1.4 billion, has been described as a 'cell phone nation' (Jeffrey & Doron, 2013). The mobile telephony is viewed to have led to a significant transformation in politics, business and the ordinary life. The sheer numbers are baffling. Towards the end of 2019, there were 687.62 million Internet users in the country (TRAI, 2020). This number, according to certain estimates, is expected to further increase to one billion users by 2025 (Statista, 2020).
3. After the revocation of Article 370 of the nation's Constitution, which granted the state of Jammu and Kashmir a semi-autonomous status with the Indian Union, the Government of India, fearing widespread protests, imposed months of curfew and a communication blockade, which was described as the world's longest ever communications shutdown.

References

Andrews, M. A., Binu, A., Rajesh, K. R., Jijith, K., Suryakala, R., Biju, K., Muraly, C. P., & Santhosh, P. V. (2020). First confirmed case of COVID-19 infection in India: A case report. *Indian Journal of Medical Research, 151*(5), 490–492.

Asrar, S. (2020, December 19). India's 10 million coronavirus cases explained in 10 charts. *TimesofIndia.com*. https://timesofindia.indiatimes.com/india/indias-10-million-coronavirus-cases-explained-in-10-charts/articleshow/79816240.cms

Beck, U. (1992). *Risk society: Towards a new modernity*. Sage.

Billig, M. (2005). *Laughter and ridicule: Towards a social critique of humour*. Sage.

Boss, D., & t'Hart, M. (2008). *Humour and social protest*. Cambridge University Press.

Button, M. (2005). "A Monkish Kind of Virtue"? For and against humility. *Political Theory, 33*, 840–868.

Carr, M. (2020). Why is there laughter during the COVID-19 pandemic? *Autism Spectrum News*. https://autismspectrumnews.org/why-is-there-laughter-during-the-COVID-19-pandemic/. Accessed 12 Aug 2020.

Dawkins, R. (2006). *The selfish gene*. Oxford University Press.

Fessell, D. (2020). Laughter leaves me lighter: Coping with COVID-19. *JAMA, 323*, 2476–2477. https://doi.org/10.1001/jama.2020.9283

Ganjoo, M. (2020). Laughter through the ages: Role of comedy films in shaping Bollywood. *Global Media Journal: Indian Edition, 12*, 1–17.

Hindustan Times. (2020, April 16). 'COVID-19 has taught India a lesson…': CDS General Bipin Rawat. *YouTube*. https://www.youtube.com/watch?v=KBXu45hX710

Indian Express. (2020, March 20). Memes, jokes on social media after PM Modi announces 'Janata Curfew' to slow COVID-19 spread. *Indian Express*.

Jeffrey, R., & Doron, A. (2013). *Cell phone nation: How mobile phones have revolutionized business, politics and ordinary life in India*. Hachette India.

Meghnad, S. (2020). A black hole called PM Cares fund. *Newslaundry*. https://www.newslaundry.com/2020/04/02/a-black-hole-called-pm-cares-fund. Accessed 20 July 2020.

Mina, A. X. (2019). *Memes to movements: How the world's most viral media is changing social protest and power*. Beacon Press.

Ministry of Health and Family Welfare. (2020). COVID-19 India as on: 03 January 2021. *Government of India*. https://www.mohfw.gov.in/

Nicholls, C. (2020). Online humour, cartoons, videos, memes, jokes and laughter in the epoch of the coronavirus. *Text Matters: A Journal of Literature, Theory and Culture, 10*, 274–318.

Philipose, P. (2020). Backstory: Journalism and the power of laughter. *The Wire*. https://thewire.in/media/backstory-journalism-satire-kunal-kamra. Accessed 21 Nov 2020.

Press Trust of India. (2019, December 10). Country facing recession, unemployment due to Modi govt's 'irrational' policies: Sunil Jhakar. *Business Standard*. https://www.business-standard.com/article/pti-stories/country-facing-recession-unemployment-due-to-modi-govt-s-irrational-policies-sunil-jhakar-119121001364_1.html

PTI. (2020, September 16). Opposition questions Modi govt's handling of COVID-19 pandemic. *Times of India*. https://timesofindia.indiatimes.com/india/opposition-questions-modi-govts-handling-of-COVID-19-pandemic-seeks-compensation-for-migrants-who-died-during-lockdown/articleshow/78151818.cms

Purnell, N., & Horwitz, J. (2020). Facebook's hate-speech rules collide with Indian politics. *The Wall Street Journal*. https://www.wsj.com/articles/Facebook-hate-speech-india-politics-muslim-hindu-modi-zuckerberg-11597423346. Accessed 15 Aug 2020.

Rehak, J. K., & Trnka, S. (2019). *The politics of joking: Anthropological engagements*. Routledge.

Sharma, N. C. (2020). India's overburdened health infra is ill-prepared to handle epidemics. *Livemint*. https://www.livemint.com/news/india/is-india-equipped-to-handle-health-epidemics-like-coronavirus-11580199650282.html. Accessed 29 Jan 2020.

Singh, S. S. (2020, July 18). Drink cow urine to fight virus: Bengal BJP chief. *The Hindu*. https://www.thehindu.com/news/cities/kolkata/drink-cow-urine-to-fight-virus-bengal-bjp-chief/article32119516.ece

Statista. (2020). *Number of internet users in India from 2015 to 2020 with a forecast until 2025*. https://www.statista.com/statistics/255146/number-of-internet-users-in-india/. Accessed 8 Nov 2020.

Sundar, A., & Nilsen, A. G. (2020, August 1). COVID-19 in Narendra Modi's India: Virulent politics and mass desperation. *The Wire*. https://thewire.in/health/COVID-19-in-narendra-modis-india-virulent-politics-and-mass-desperation

T'Hart, M. (2007). Humour and social protest: An introduction. *International Review of Social History, 52*, 1–20.

Taecharungroj, V., & Nueangjamnong, P. (2015). Humour 2.0: Styles and types of humour and virality of memes on Facebook. *Journal of Creative Communications, 10*, 288–302.

Thakurta, P. G., & Sam, C. (2019). *The real face of Facebook in India*. Paranjoy.

The Wire Staff. (2020). For the second time, AG gives nod to contempt proceedings against Kunal Kamra. *The Wire*. https://thewire.in/law/attorney-general-initiate-contempt-proceedings-against-kunal-kamra-latest-tweet. Accessed 20 Nov 2020.

TRAI. (2020). *The Indian telecom services performance indicators: July–September, 2019*. Telecom Regulatory Authority of India.

Wallen, J. (2020, November 12). COVID plunges India into recession for first time in history. *The Telegraph*. https://www.telegraph.co.uk/global-health/science-and-disease/covid-plunges-india-recession-first-time-history/

CHAPTER 14

The Use of Meme and Hashtags on Twitter Towards Government Response During the COVID-19 Curfew Announcement from 1 June to 14 June 2020

Keziah Wangui Githinji and Joyce Omwoha

Introduction

The Coronavirus Disease (COVID-19) is a respiratory illness which easily spreads from one person to another. It spreads through contact with droplets produced through the coughing or sneezing of a person or a contaminated object or surface. Recent studies indicate that some people infected with COVID-19 don't have symptoms and are likely to play a role in its spread (World Health Organization, 2020). Wuhan, China, reported the

K. W. Githinji (✉)
United States International University Africa, Nairobi, Kenya
e-mail: kwangui@usiu.ac.ke

J. Omwoha
Department of Journalism and Media Studies, The Technical University of Kenya, Nairobi, Kenya
e-mail: joyce.omwoha@tukenya.ac.ke

S. Mpofu (ed.), *Digital Humour in the Covid-19 Pandemic*,
https://doi.org/10.1007/978-3-030-79279-4_14

first case of COVID-19 in the late 2019, leading to a global spread (KEMRI, 2020). The outbreak of COVID-19 created a global health crisis with a deep impact on how humanity perceives their everyday lives and the world. The safety measures put in place to contain the spread of the virus require social distancing by refraining from doing what is human, which is to find solace in the company of others. Since 31 December 2019 and as of February 2020, 103,448,210 cases of COVID-19 infections (in accordance with the applied case definitions and testing strategies in the affected countries) have been reported, including 2,236,453 deaths (WHO, 2021). According to the World Health Organization, as of 25th August 2021, there are 230,794 positive cases and 4564 deaths reported in Kenya.

The first COVID-19 case in Kenya was reported on 12 March 2020 in Nairobi, a case of a Kenyan citizen who travelled back to Nairobi from the United States via London, United Kingdom, on 5 March 2020. Confirming this was the National Influenza Centre Laboratory at the National Public Health Laboratories of the Ministry of Health (KEMRI, 2020). Since the first case was reported, the Kenyan government imposed quarantines and movement restriction around and into the country. The measures contributed to a slow virus spread, though it led to a near-collapse of Kenya's economy. Odhiambo et al. (2020) note that since the first case of COVID-19 was reported in Kenya on 13 March 2020, the country, just like other countries in the world, has been experiencing massive destruction of the economy in terms of GDP decline and job losses.

Since the outbreak, the Kenyan authorities had been conducting random temperature screenings in spaces frequented by the public. Once an individual displays signs or symptoms of coronavirus, he can self-isolate or expect to receive such a directive from a health worker. The Kenyan authorities take such individuals into a State health facility, when they cannot self-isolate. According to the Government of Kenya, anyone testing positive for COVID-19, presenting mild symptoms, should self-isolate at home. To contain the COVID-19 outbreak, Kenya's President Uhuru Kenyatta set up a curfew and restricting public gatherings. On 25 March 2020, the government closed schools, airports, mosques and churches; public gathering restricted, tightening of border controls and imposing of curfew in urban areas. This may have helped in slowing the spread of the virus. While the livelihoods of millions of Kenyans who live in urban and rural areas, depending on face-to-face interaction, were interfered with, many moved to social media, not only to communicate with the world but also to denounce the chaotic and harsh police enforcement of public health directives (Chiba, 2020).

According to the new Kenya Economic Update, COVID-19 damaged the livelihoods of Kenyans, especially youth, women and refugees. One in three Kenyan workers were working in firms facing risks of permanent or temporary closure and reduced revenues, thus impacting the vulnerability of household incomes. COVID-19 pandemic induced social and economic disruptions, eroding progress in poverty reduction in Kenya, forcing an estimated 2 million Kenyans into poverty. The World Bank country director Keith Hansen reported that "COVID-19 poses an unprecedented shock to the economy, disrupting economic activity". He continues: "the government, with the help of partners, needs to ensure that the shock remains temporary, by targeting support to the most vulnerable affected households" (World Bank, 2021).

After the initial curfew, the government added more days but extending the curfew hours from 4 am to 9 pm effective from 7 June 2020. It was a week before the announcement that Kenyans on social media showed different memes trying to convince the president not to extend the curfew period and hours. The most popular hashtag being #FreedomDay. In his speech on 6 June 2020 to announce the extension of the curfew, President Kenyatta mentioned the trending meme on Twitter #FreedomDay. This brought humour to his speech and to the internet too. According to a BBC report, published on 9 June 2020, about 1.2 million Kenyans had lost their jobs since the pandemic hit the country, with many more having to take pay cuts. The BBC report noted too that many businesses closed down and families were struggling to make ends meet. With these, Kenyans anticipated for a day of freedom from lockdown so that they can go back to their work stations and improve the economy as they make a livelihood; therefore, the hashtag #FreedomDay was coined to bring attention to government and to build conversations on Twitter around the socio-economic impacts of the lockdown and curfew to the citizens. Humour, depicted in the hashtags and memes around freedom day, included one of the most shared video clip in Swahili compiled by comedian Mtume Orroson, showing him in conversation with the president, using old sound bites of Mr. Kenyatta completely out of context.

Below is an excerpt (BBC, 2020):

Comedian: Uhuru, when will you set us free?
President: After three weeks ...

Comedian: This is so wrong … you've placed us under curfew then sent police to beat us up.
President: It's not me … I have not sent anyone …
Comedian: Could you at least open up the clubs only—just for a single day so I can sanitise (my throat) with one beer. What do I do when all clubs are shut?
President: Use the back door …
Comedian: Heeey! What if your cops arrest me?
President: You'll have to defend yourself … and these guys don't mess around!

> In the same context, a famous tweet by a tweeter user The Impeccable @ RealDerrow, followed by a meme in the form of a video read, "Tomorrow issa day that the Lord has made … we shall rejoice and be glad in it. Happy friday. #WorldEnvironmentDay2020 #BlackLivesMatter #CurferKenya #mutaikagwe #FreedomOfExpression."

The video contained the song "Freedom Is Coming Tomorrow", a soundtrack from the movie Sarafina. The content of the video was various dace moves from the movie, funny dance moves by children politician and comedians, plus a compilation of sound bites from President Kenyatta's previous speeches.

Humour, especially in African context, has often been analysed as a source of political resistance and social commentary. Comedians and social commentators use different avenues—memes, impromptu everyday humour, cartoons, televised satire shows and stand-up comedy—in challenging the subvert status quo and politicians. For instance, Nigerian cartoonists, in the midst of coronavirus, have used cartoons specifically to comment on the irony of politicians seeking medical help abroad instead of using their own local healthcare services (Mwambari & Martin, 2020).

Countries in Africa frequently feature in media for outbreaks and health crises, the most recent one being the Ebola epidemic in the Democratic Republic of Congo and West Africa. Both explicit and implicit narratives framed these epidemics, often pointing to "traditional" social practices contributing to transmission, hence making it "their own fault". Europe narratives about COVID transmissions have pointed the blame on governmental and structural issues (Mwambari & Martin, 2020). Mwambari and Martin (2020) continue by asserting that during the West African Ebola outbreak, many countries in the global North imposed restrictions and, in some cases, full bans from Ebola-affected areas. Memes, act as a social commentary during COVID-19 pandemic, pointing to the disease's prominence yet it seems more of a problem in the global North (Mwambari & Martin, 2020).

A study conducted by Pearce and Hajizada (2014) reveals that humour involved in a meme can be a tool or a means of protest, containing a statement of disagreement to the government (Pearce & Hajizada, 2014). Hatab (2016) echoes by noting that memes are used in conveying messages of disagreement, disseminated through the internet. The spread of memes containing disapproval is also used as messages for reaching a wider audience. Hatab (2016) further illustrates that the humour used during the Tunisia revolution between 2010 and 2011 was a mobilization through social media, in which political satire was widely used in starting up a conversation or discourse in social media through humour in languages that contain puns, synonyms, antonyms, lexical ambiguity and rhyme.

Meme involves the perspective of social groups; memes shape the mindset and forms of behaviour (Gal et al., 2016). A study conducted by Boxman-Shabtai and Shifman (2016) showed that memes tend to show global content rather than pure local content. Memes using themes of animals, sex and gender tend to dominate digital humour in the form of memes. Hashtags on the other hand are used to highlight keywords, phrases and tweets, with the intention of categorizing tweets so that they can be searched easily.

Hashtags are used as symbols of dark humour; humour representing a horrible situation or a shocking phenomenon, which is said to illuminate the dark areas of society but includes satire.

In this study, we looked at the use of memes and hashtags on Twitter towards government response during the COVID curfew announcement from 1 June to 14 June 2020. The research answered the following questions:

Q1 Why are memes and hashtags used as forms of communication on Twitter?

Q2 How did Kenyans on Twitter use hashtags and memes to communicate to the government before the president's curfew announcement on 6 June 2020?

Q3 In what way were memes and hashtags used to express Kenyans' perception towards the president's curfew extension?

Meme Concept

Memes come from an ancient Greek word meaning "something imitated". Speech acts are studied in the pragmatics field research, which describes pragmatics as the study of "what speakers mean" and emphasizes that communication depends on "not only recognizing the meaning of words in an utterance, but recognizing what speakers mean by their utterances" Yule (2006, 112). The meme concept is an academic concept coined by Richard Dawkins in 1976. It is a gene-centred approach to cultural evolution defined as a "unit of cultural transmission". The meme concept is everywhere on the internet; it relates to certain kinds of jokes, images or trends (Castaño Díaz, 2020). Memes are a common way for people to communicate online. Internet users frequently use memes to respond to each other on social networking sites or other online forums. When creating memes with specific semiotic resources used, the internet community interprets the resources to facilitate between the internet community and the meme creator.

Internet memes are a ubiquity of social media across different technological devices such as mobile phones, tablets, computers, mobile phones and ordinary devices, re-shaped by internet mobile technology. Due to new media, a meme can take the form of audio-visual material through animations and videos, and still-images. Examples of audio-visual memes include Downfall of "Hitler reacts to …", a modified video sequence from the German drama, *Constantine Film*, German 2004. The film section features Adolf Hitler losing his temper and scolding his commanders, who all become the focus of the parodies. For instance, "Ben Affleck cast as Batman" and "Twilight the Movie" (2009) are some of the examples of video memes that individuals use and are also on social media.

Memes are a shorthand for humour; they are created with the awareness of each other and are circulated through the internet by many users. When memes are created, they can easily be retweeted and circulate on social media (cf. Huntington, 2016: 78; Shifman, 2013: 41). Memes are used as online humour and typically regarded as involving constant transformation, which is what distinguishes them from virals, which spread across digital media in a form that is unchanged (e.g. Dynel, 2016a; Shifman, 2013; Wiggins, 2019).

Educational establishments and banks use memes for marketing purposes; thus, the trend invites a systematic media scrutiny and poses as a mature cultural phenomenon (Bury, 2016). Despite the enshrined legitimacy, internet memes are still in infancy. Electronic ephemera and online sources have the most dynamic and comprehensive sources of information on internet memes as opposed to academic publications. Websites present a rich source of primary data on internet memes; however, Davison (2012) recognizes there are many notable online meme sources. The internet memes lack an accurate definition, especially as a cultural device proving to be inconsistent (Cannizzaro, 2020).

Studies argue that humour is a crucial method of communication quite important for emotional and mental well-being. There are other studies linking the notion of the internet and humour therapy (Louie & Kost, 2010; Dionigi & Canestrari, 2018; Cropley & Galloway, 2001).

Twitter

Twitter is a social media tool allowing users to receive and send messages of no more than 140 characters in length, called "tweets". In August 2014 Twitter had 271 million users, and as it grows in popularity, it has become a tool for disseminating research and teaching among college professors (Priem et al., 2012), and as of 2021, Twitter has 330 million users (Schl, 2021). Twitter users follow other users so as to subscribe to their content (thought tweets). As a Twitter user one can create their own tweets or retweet the information tweeted by other users. Retweeting means information is efficiently shared with many people. Many people initially wondered how they could use it, but it has now become the social media platform of choice for many. The nature of tweets is mostly for smartphone users who are not interested in reading long content items on screen. The tweets can be disseminated by either an individual, group or organization. Insights into non-academic aspects of one's life can help make one an interesting person to follow. If one is tweeting on behalf of an organization, project or group, then they may choose only to send research-related tweets. ESRC (2020) says that Twitter is an informal communications tool and encourages people to embrace a personal, friendly, and humorous approach to tweeting (ESRC, 2021). Twitter presents new research sites providing billions of data points to research. Twitter is a great avenue for consideration for public data due to its prominence in social computing research (Fiesler & Proferes, 2018). It's popular due to its availability. Compared to Twitter, Facebook has more users, though it has more strict limits in its application programming interface (API; Fiesler et al., 2017).

Twitter is a successful platform for research, resulting in knowledge and studies on topics such as disease tracking (Lamb et al., 2013; Signorini et al., 2011), disaster events (Kogan et al., 2016; Sakaki et al., 2010; Palen & Starbird, 2011), election prediction and stock market (Bollen et al., 2011; Tumasjan et al., 2010), hence classified as elitist. It has resulted in scholars and researchers using Twitter content (profile information and tweets) in examining all sorts of aspects of human interaction. Prior research shows Twitter users have restricted understandings of how the public content might be used (Felt, 2016; Zimmer & Proferes, 2014). As compared to other social media platforms, Twitter users imagine many people are reading their tweets and that may not be the reality (Bernstein et al., 2013; Litt, 2012; Marwick & boyd, 2011). According to Proferes (2017), some Twitter users may not realize that what they tweet is viewable. The users that have under-protected accounts, meaning their tweets are only viewed by their followers, though, may endure privacy violations through retweets (Meeder et al., 2010). Unfortunately, Twitter privacy is an issue, as information may leak accidentally through users, such as tweeting under the influence (Mao et al., 2011).

Background and Context

Twitter Users in Kenya

The social media statistics highlight that social media takes the following percentage of users: Facebook 37.84%, Twitter 24.85%, Pinterest 23.74%. The above statistics are social media statistics as of November 2020. Studies show that Kenya has the second most active Twitter users in Africa (Stats, 2020), with active users famously known as Kenyans of Twitter (KOT). When it comes to Twitter usage, South Africans are the most prolific with 5,939,226 tweets, considering it is the continent's biggest economy. Kenya is the second most active country with 2,476,800 tweets. Nigeria has only 1,646,212 tweets from its 160 million people, followed by 1,214,062 and Morocco with 745,620 tweets. About 20–40 years is the age of Twitter users in Africa, while 57% of the tweets are from mobile phones. Kenya's politician Raila Odinga and President Paul Kagame of Rwanda are Twitter users, including President Uhuru Kenyatta from

Kenya. Kagame got into an infamous Twitter spat in 2012 with journalist Ian Birrell of *The Guardian* of London, with the two trading tweets about human rights and repression in the central African nation. Kagame's foreign minister initiated the cyber-conversation that went global. The fact that politicians use social media allows Twitter users to engage with them. There is a lack of hierarchy and Twitter users can ask their leaders questions and comment without any form of fear. In relation to this study, the Twitter users used memes concerning the curfew, hoping the information would reach the president and the government leaders concerning not extending the curfew. Kenyan fighters and soldiers of an extremist Somali Islamist group have been at loggerheads with each other. Representatives from both parties have taken the battle onto Twitter, with insults, taunts and accusations being directly traded in an infrequent engagement on the internet. "How Africa Tweets" is a research done that found Twitter is helping in joining new links within Africa. Beatrice Karanja, head of Portland Nairobi, said: "We saw the pivotal role of Twitter in the events in North Africa last year, but it is clear that Africa's Twitter revolution is really just beginning" (Joe et al., 2020).

Kenyan politicians are using Twitter as a means of communication to the public, especially the youth, and have realized the power of social media. According to a Kenyan news article published on 20 April 2020, it shows that William Ruto, the deputy president in Kenya, has 2.9 million followers. He is the second most popular person on Twitter after President Kenyatta. Dr. Ruto built his base by interacting with Kenyans on his day-to-day activities, he has been using social media to attack his perceived and real political enemies. President Kenyatta had many followers, but after being bullied, he deactivated his account. According to the *East African Standard* publication on 22 March 2019, President Kenyatta's account was closed after communication from State House stating that the president's social media accounts had been hacked. Being the most followed African leader on Twitter, the blackout sparked speculation that his handle, @UKenyatta with 3.62 million followers, may have been debarred by the microblogging site. This is after a tweet on corruption from @UKenyatta handle that, according to Kenyans online, was seen as targeting his deputy William Ruto. The last tweet from President Kenyatta's account before it was suspended read:

> *If you are corrupt we will fight you. You can be my brother or my sister or my closest political ally but if you are corrupt we will fight you. I won't be clouded*

> *by ethnicity or status in my quest to leave behind a united nation and I will continue championing for Kenya's unity.*

Raila Odinga, an active politician for about three decades, accompanied with his parable peppered speeches as a means of communication. He has 2.5 million followers and has transferred his popularity "on the ground" on Twitter. As much as he communicates in parables, he has not changed this style on social media. The embattled Nairobi governor Mike Sonko has 1 million followers. He has managed to divert traffic to his Twitter pages through interacting with his followers in simple Sheng and Swahili languages, posting controversial or exciting videos, or basing his critics. Former senate's majority leader Kipchumba Murkomen has 1 million followers. He is a close ally of DP Ruto and a government critic, earning popularity on Twitter. He has often used the platform to invite his followers into his farm and living room. Hassan Joho, the charismatic Mombasa governor, has 896,000 followers. He has endeared his followers with his opulence, class and refined taste of fashion (Joe et al., 2020). Hence, this becomes clear that politicians and leaders are active on Twitter and can communicate easily with their followers.

Theoretical and Conceptual Framework

This research is predicated upon the social exchange theory, which is defined by George Homans (1961) as being influenced by sociological perspective and social psychology. The theory states that a relationship between two people is created through a process of cost-and-benefit. This means for each individual the effort is poured into a person-to-person relationship. The theory views exchange as a social behaviour that may result in both social and economic outcomes. Online social networking is an ideal application of social networking theory. Researchers find that a positive social influence to use an online community increases online community self-disclosure; reciprocity increases self-disclosure; online community trust increases self-disclosure; privacy risk beliefs decrease self-disclosure.

Social media reflects the opinions and beliefs of the users; the Twitter users in Kenya reflect their opinions and beliefs concerning the lockdown. The theory helps in explaining how the political and non-political memes on Twitter are used to reflect the perception of Twitter users concerning the lockdown. The study examined the specific impacts of memes' visual/textual form and political nature on affect and perceptions of memes' persuasiveness. In doing so, this study also examined the role of humour through memes reflecting their political opinions concerning the lock-down extension.

Methodology

COVID-19 case was first reported in Kenya in March 2020, and it was at this time that the government declared a curfew of 21 days up to 6 June 2020 from 5 am to 7 pm. After the curfew the government added more days, but extended the time from 4 am to 9 pm effective from 7 June 2020. It was a week before the announcement that Kenyans on social media created and shared different memes in order to convince the President of Kenya to postpone the curfew. President Kenyatta on 6 June 2020, during the announcement of the extension of the curfew, mentioned a trending meme on social media, to be specific, Twitter #FreedomDay. Hence, the researcher will look at the memes on social media, to be specific, Twitter #FreedomDay, focusing on one week before the announcement of the extension of the curfew and one week after the announcement on 6 June 2020.

Purposive sampling (also known as judgement, selective or subjective sampling) is a sampling technique in which a researcher relies on his or her own judgement when choosing members of a population to participate in the study (Black, 2010). It was done for the study from 1 June 2020 to 14 June 2020, the research covered tweets and retweets of memes seven days after the announcements, which portrayed the response of the Kenyans concerning the government's response and the comments towards the memes. The researcher looked at the Twitter comments and highlighted several hashtags with regard to the announcement. The researcher used random sampling for data collection to analyse memes and attached hashtags. On Twitter, hashtags and memes can reach many people through retweets and tweets. The researcher interpreted the meaning of the users through memes concerning the president's decision towards the curfew and a reaction seven days after the extension of the curfew.

Data Presentation and Analysis

The amount of memes currently circulating on the internet and social media is enormous. Meme creation platforms such as Memegenerator.net make it possible for anyone to create a meme. However, while the numbers of possible meme types are unlimited, the number of standard meme types is actually quite small (Shifman, 2013, 342). A standard meme refers to a meme that becomes well known and is frequently used by the internet community as a whole. This chapter looked at the use of memes and hashtags on Twitter towards government response during the COVID-19 announcement from 1 June to 14 June 2020.

The intention of the speaker is described as what the speaker wants the reader or hearer to recognize in a communication. The politicians in Kenya have resorted to Twitter because they realized the power of communicating to the masses on Twitter. As opposed to speaking to the public openly during, for instance, rallies, Twitter helps the politician reach a large number of people with any form of geographical boundary. The other advantage is a politician is able to get direct feedback from his or her followers, which may assist in knowing the mentality of individuals pertaining to certain issues.

Memes as a voice clearly show that they represent the opinions of the user. The intention of a speaker can be described as that which the speaker wants the hearer or reader to recognize in a communication. For instance, when we interpret the meaning of a text (written or spoken) of a Twitter user, we do not only consider the words or utterances used to communicate the message, but also rely on what we think the writer or the speaker intended to communicate.

Therefore, social exchange theory proposes that social behaviour is usually as a result of an exchange process. The aim of the exchange is to either minimize costs or maximize benefits. People aim in weighing the potential risks and benefits of social relationships. Focusing on the theory that grounds this research, the aim of the different memes and hashtags used on Twitter was to get President Kenyatta's attention, to convince him not to extend the curfew, on the one hand, and, on the other hand, to air the citizen's grievances and frustrations. Therefore, the users used these memes with his photo attached to get his attention. Below are examples of some of the memes used with President Kenyatta's face before 7 June 2020.

In one meme President Uhuru was called His excellency, Their daddy, Commander-in-Chief, Uhuru *mwenyewe, msee wa mashati* (a man with beautiful shirts), Chancellor *wa Ma-Uni* (chancellor of universities), and it ends by stating he should not disappoint the citizens. Humour is used in the form of praising the president's appearance and intellect, urging him not to disappoint Kenyans by extending the curfew. In another meme he was shown looking at his watch, interpreted as him waiting for the right time to make the dreaded announcement. The first meme illustrates the need to pamper the president so that he would relax the restrictions on movement and curfew. Here, Kenyans are hoping that he there will be no curfew extension. The anxiety of the Kenyans on Twitter (KOT) was based on the fact that they were expecting the president not to extend the curfew.

A tweet by Arap Liwliw (@arap_liwliw). His Excellency president Uhuru Kenyatta was expected to address the nation at 3 pm, State House Time. The hashtags that followed this meme were: #UhuruDontLiftLockdown #UhuruDONTOpen #CurfewinKenya. Part of the curfew instruction was restriction to public places, including bars, and there was a meme showing President Kenyatta drinking beer and this was a way of asking him to open taverns. The president himself is known for allegedly loving his alcoholic drinks and this is an outcry for the opening of social places so that people like him can enjoy themselves.

Here, the authors use the social exchange theory that views exchange as a social behaviour that may result in both social and economic outcomes. The theory helps to explain how online social networking is an ideal application of the social networking theory. A positive social influence to use an online community increases online community self-disclosure; reciprocity increases self-disclosure; online community trust increases self-disclosure; privacy risk beliefs decrease self-disclosure.

Humour on Twitter

Humour is known as a universal phenomenon exhibited by most cultures. Humour primarily consists of jokes that are either written or spoken words and actions which generate mirth and elicit laughter; the actions can be described in words (Critchley, 2002; Ritchie, 2004). Given that qualitative research is characterized by a heavy dependence on data that are word based (interviews, observer notes, documents, manuscripts etc.), this therefore posits that humour analysis has potential as an investigative qualitative research tool. There are dozens of different definitions of humour. Romero and Cruthirds (2006, 59) define humour as "amusing communications that produce positive emotions and cognitions in the individual, group, or organization", and Crawford (1994, 57) defines humour as any communication generating an effective response or positive cognitive from listeners. Just as.

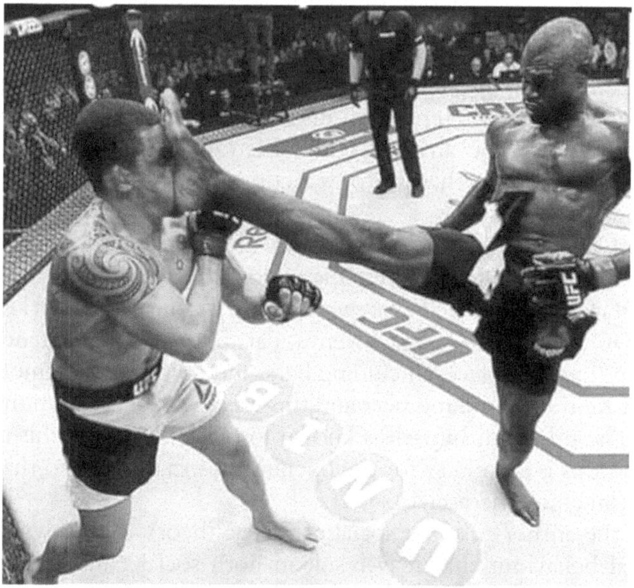

Fig. 14.1 @snnyamaoUhuruKenyatta right on the face of Kenyans...! #wanjohi #CurfewinKenya'

After the infamous 6th June announcement, many Kenyans on Twitter showed their disappointment concerning the curfew extension.

"Fellow Kenyans" was the president's famous statement while addressing the nation. Registering their disappointment to the president, Kenyans created the meme of a boy who seems to be crying bitterly, telling the president not to refer to Kenyans as "fellow Kenyans" anymore because his act of extending the curfew indicates that Kenyans and the president are no longer on friendly terms.

Figure 14.1 shows a meme shared by @snnyamao on his Twitter account with an image of kick boxers fighting, captioned, "#UhuruKenyatta right on the face of Kenyans...! #wanjohi #CurfewinKenya", magnifying the betrayal and pain of curfew extension by President Uhuru on 6 June 2020. It was likened to a kick on the citizens' face. As the meme went viral, this was a clear indication that the announcement that President Uhuru gave was received with disappointment.

Figure 14.2 is a meme referencing slay queens. Humour is made using slay queens as an example. A slay queen is a girl who lives a lavish life at the

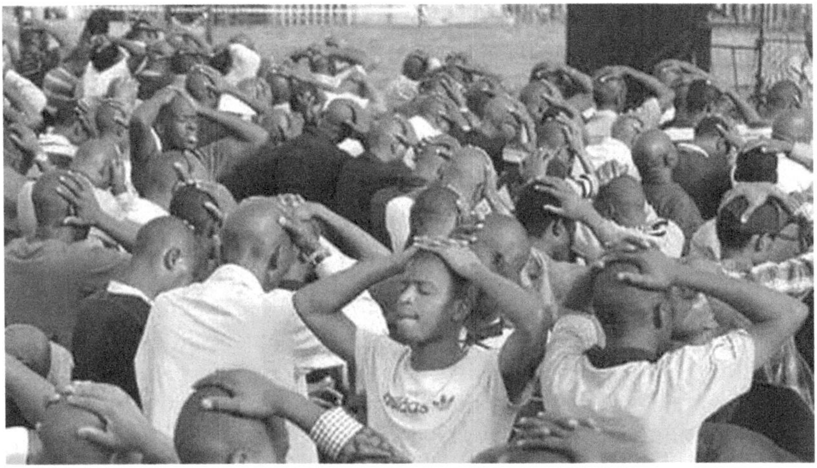

Fig. 14.2 Kelly Nivex @ndubinivex June 6. "Current Situation for slay queens with curfew extension" #UhuruKenyatta #6thjune #wanjohi

cost of an older man, mostly a married man. With the lockdown and curfew, their movement have been restricted; hence, they are not in a position to sustain their lifestyles. The meme illustrates displeasure on the president's unfavourable announcement, which affected the economic lives of some citizens.

COVID-19 humour exists too with daily reports on the infection numbers and the death toll, which may be considered as dark humour (Bischetti et al., 2020); the humour is about—or at least, produced or inspired by the context of—grave topics, illness and deaths (Dynel & Poppi, 2018). Even though the appreciation, that is, funniness versus aversiveness, of COVID-19 humour must rely on various factors, some of them being the distance from the epicentre (Bischetti et al., 2020) and the very nature of a given specimen (e.g. whether or not it addresses the topic of death or disease per se), the prevalence of this humour on social media indicates its social significance.

People resisted lockdown through memes and blamed experts for ill advising the president. In a tweet with a man carrying stones ready to fight, Fidel Castro @I_amfidel tweeted, "Another 30 days of premium tears. Wanjohi has acknowledged the meme industry #wanjohi #Another30 #UhuruDontLiftLockdown #UhuruKenyatta #6thjune." The comment here is that people were at war against experts who advised the president to extend the lockdown. The meme is accompanied by hashtags just showing the disappointment Kenyans have on Twitter—for instance, #Another30, which in a humorous way depicts another 30 days of what Kenyans termed as suffering.

The meme that attracted the hashtag #premiumtears, a clear indication that the decision made by the president is a disappointment to the Kenyans on Twitter, showed a jean button on which was written "it will end in tears". The disappointment of Kenyans on Twitter concerning the curfew extension is represented by tears (Omondi, 2020); premium tears, experienced after the memes failed to sway the president to lift the lockdown and curfew. What is worth noting is that all the memes on Twitter were used to contain aspects of humour; the messages are clearly highlighted so that the communication process takes place.

Hashtags on Social Media

A hashtag is symbolized by the sign (#) and is usually used on Twitter to call attention to social media users for multi-participation in certain topics so as to mobilise those interested to join the conversation. On Twitter, "#" is used at the beginning of an unbroken word or phrase, creating a hashtag. The use of hashtags in a tweet often is linked to all other tweets that include it. Inclusion of a hashtag gives a tweet conversation longevity and a tweet context. Therefore, hashtags are used for the purpose of the tweet conversation longevity and a tweet context. Hashtags are important on Twitter for helping users organize and sort their tweets. They indicate that the content is relevant to a certain topic, with the aiming of getting the tweet in front of an interested audience.

According to the social exchange theory, defined by George Homans, a relationship between two people is created through a process of cost-and-benefit. The theory views exchange as a social behaviour that may result in both social and economic outcomes. Online social networking is an ideal application of the social networking theory. Researchers find that a positive social influence to use an online community increases online community self-disclosure; reciprocity increases self-disclosure; online community trust increases self-disclosure; privacy risk beliefs decrease self-disclosure. In Kenya, the official government communication on Twitter is @StateHouseKenya with 1.2 million followers. The author of this chapter selected the #FreedomDay in order to narrow down on the memes and hashtags used between 1 June and 14 June 2020. President Uhuru, in his speech on 7 June 2020, said: "I have seen your 'freedom day' memes, let us have patience." This was proof that the president was able to see the memes on Twitter, making reference to them in his address Other hashtags that came up related to #FreedomDay are as follows:

> ***#June6th*** #StaySafe ***#CurfewinKenya #tuwabebe #wabebe #UhuruAddress #UhuruDontLiftLockdown #wanjohi #lockdownextension #UhuruDONT-Open #UhuruKenyatta right on the face of Kenyans…!***

Also the institutions or individuals that were tagged during this ***#FreedomDay*** are:

@UhuruKenyatta, @ministry of education, @magoha. Magoha served as the Minister of Education at this time. This chapter analysed memes portraying the attitude of Kenya on Twitters regarding the curfew. The majority of the memes do not want President Kenyatta to extend the curfew. The main reason most Kenyans on Twitter did not want President Kenyatta to extend the curfew was mostly because most of them wanted to stay late in social gatherings. Hence, that became a problem to many Kenyans on Twitter. Before the president's statement concerning COVID-19, the majority of the Kenyans on Twitter used memes to communicate to the president not to extend the curfew through using hashtags such as ***#June6th***#StaySafe ***#CurfewinKenya #tuwabebe #wabebe #UhuruDontLiftLockdown #wanjohi #lockdownextension #UhuruDONTOpen #UhuruKenyatta right on the face of Kenyans…!***

Minimal memes leaned towards telling the president to extend the curfew and lockdown. Below are some of the tweets that the Twitters in Kenyan sent. An account known as Kenyans On Twitter retweeted a message from Uhuru Kenyatta concerning 6th June as a response to the memes of Twitter users in Kenya before he made an announcement:

> **Kenyans On Twitter Retweeted**
> Uhuru Kenyatta **Commentary**
> @UhuruKE
> ***Morning Kenyans, I am aware today is #June6th even without all the reminders :). For the love of God, relax. Please remember, my number one responsibility is keeping all Kenyans alive. I will address the nation later in the day. Again, relax and*** #StaySafe

Conclusion

Per COVID statistics on 7 June 2020, Kenya has recorded a high of 167 positive cases out of the 2833 samples tested in the last 24 hours. The total number of positive cases while this study was carried out stood at 2767. At that point, the government had tested 97, 340 samples. Out of the 167 cases 125 were males and 42 females, where the youngest was 11 months old and the oldest was 75 years. About 21 days later, 29 June 2020, out of the 41 counties that have reported COVID-19 positive cases, Nairobi still led with 3031, followed by Mombasa with 1445, Busia 407, Kajiado 242 and Kiambu 222. Most of the remaining 36 counties reported cases below 100 (Ministry of Health, 2020). The COVID cases continued increasing but based on the statistics given, the lockdown and curfew prevented the cases from going as high as was expected. Hence, as much as Kenyans complained on Twitter about the president's curfew extension to observe COVID measures and restrictions, it was instrumental towards reducing the number of infections. Modern memes are perceived as a humorous image that is copied, with slight variations, and quickly shared across the internet. Funny pictures and jokes are enjoyed by all, but are they actually important in social media communication? This study revealed that memes provide a unique snapshot into the cultural events of a moment in time. Some memes rotate for years, while others live a short, but often explosive life. Memes offer users the opportunity to make a reference to an established inside joke that the entire internet is a part of. Memes carry more power than meets the eye. Contemporary popular culture has chosen to baptize the phenomenon which sees certain digital media texts going "viral" and being collectively remixed as "internet memes". This choice of term is indebted to Dawkins' theory of culture-as-memes as proposed in his book *The Selfish Gene*, and later supported by scholars of emetics.

This chapter has highlighted how Kenyans on Twitter have used memes and hashtags on Twitter towards government response during the COVID-19 curfew announcement from 1 June to 14 June 2020. Most Kenyans before 6 June 2020 did not want the president to extend the curfew and were not afraid to show it through memes. After the curfew extension, many Kenyans on Twitter were disappointed, and it reflected on the memes they used. Disappointment notwithstanding, memes and hashtags offered comic relief that helped the society to heal and cope with the negative effects of the pandemic, which include deepened inequalities, loss of jobs, ill health, domestic violence and death.

References

BBC News. (2020, June 9). Why Kenyans are begging their president for freedom. *BBC News*. Accessed 10 Feb 2020. https://www.bbc.com/news/world-africa-52977771

Bernstein, M. S., Bakshy, E., Burke, M., & Karrer, B. (2013). Quantifying the invisible audience in social networks. In *Proceedings of the ACM conference on human factors in Computing Systems (CHI)* (pp. 21–30). ACM.

Bischetti, L., Canal, P., & Bambini, V. (2020). *Funny but aversive: A large-scale survey on the emotional response to COVID-19 humor in the Italian population during the lockdown*. Lingua. In Press. https://doi.org/10.1016/j.lingua.2020.102963

Black, K. (2010). *Business statistics: Contemporary decision making* (6th ed.). John Wiley & Sons.

Bollen, J., Mao, H., & Zeng, X. (2011). Twitter mood predicts the stock market. *Journal of Computational Science, 2*(1), 1–8.

Boxman-Shabtai, L., & Shifman, L. (2016). Digital humor and the articulation of locality in an age of global flows. HUMOR, 29(1), 1–24. https://doi.org/10.1515/humor-2015-0127

Bury, B. (2016). Creative use of internet memes in advertising. [online] *Worldscientificnews.com*. Available at: http://www.worldscientificnews.com/wp-content/uploads/2016/06/WSN-57-2016-33-41.pdf. Accessed 7 Feb 2021.

Cannizzaro, S. (2020). *Internet memes as internet signs: A semiotic view of digital culture*. Retrieved 3 December 2020, from https://core.ac.uk/download/pdf/132197888.pdf

Castaño Díaz, C. (2020). *Defining and characterizing the concept of Internet Meme*. Retrieved 3 December 2020, from http://www.scielo.org.co/scielo.php?script=sci_arttext&pid=S2011-30802013000200007

Chiba, Y. (2020). Kenya's case of COVID-19. *Csis.org*. Retrieved 3 December 2020, from https://www.csis.org/analysis/kenyas-case-COVID-19

Crawford, C. B. (1994). Theory and implications regarding the utilization of strategic humour by leaders. *The Journal of Leadership Studies, 1*(4), 53–67.

Critchley, S. (2002). *On humour*. Routledge.

Cropley, A., & Galloway, G. (2001). Humour and mental health: Implications for psychotherapy. *The Journal of Psychology, 2*(2), 3–14.

Davison, P. (2012). The language of internet memes. In M. Mandiberg (Ed.), *The social media reader*. New York University Press.

Dionigi, A., & Canestrari, C. (2018). The use of humor by therapists and clients in cognitive therapy. *European Journal of Humour Research, 6*(3), 50–67.

Dynel, M. (2016a). "I has seen Image Macros!" Advice Animals memes as visual-verbal jokes. *International Journal of Communication, 10*, 660–688.

Dynel, M., & Poppi, F. I. M. (2018). In tragoedia risus: Analysis of dark humour in post-terrorist attack discourse. *Discourse & Communication, 12*(4), 382–400.

Felt, M. (2016). Social media and the social sciences: How researchers employ Big Data analytics. *Big Data & Society, 3*(1), 1–15.

Fiesler, C., & Proferes, N. (2018). "Participant" Perceptions of Twitter Research Ethics – Casey Fiesler, Nicholas Proferes, 2018. *SAGE Journals.* Retrieved 7 February 2021, from https://journals.sagepub.com/doi/10.1177/2056305118763366

Gal, N., Shifman, L., & Kampf, Z. (2016). "It Gets Better": Internet memes and the construction of collective identity. *New Media & Society, 18*(8), 1698–1714. https://doi.org/10.1177/1461444814568784

Grundlingh, L. (2018). Memes as speech acts. *Social Semiotics, 28*(2), 147–168.

Hatab, W. A. (2016). The Arab Spring: A new era of humor consumption and production. *International Journal of English Linguistics, 6*(3), 70–87.

Homans, G. (1961). The Humanities and the Social Sciences. *American Behavioral Scientist, 4*(8), 3–6. https://doi.org/10.1177/000276426100400802

How to use social media. Beta.ukri.org. (2021). Retrieved 27 September 2021, from https://beta.ukri.org/councils/esrc/impact-toolkit-for-economic-and-social-sciences/how-to-use-social-media/

Huntington, H. E. (2016). Pepper Spray cop and the American dream: Using synecdoche and metaphor to unlock internet memes' visual political rhetoric. *Communication Studies, 67*(1), 77–93.

Joe, A., Masinde, Y., Joe, A., Squad, K., Joe, A., & Masinde, Y. et al. (2020). Study shows Kenya has second most active Twitter users in Africa – KenyanVibe. *KenyanVibe.* Retrieved 3 December 2020, from https://www.kenyanvibe.com/how-africa-tweets-study-shows-kenya-has-second-most-active-users-Twitter-users-in-africa/

KEMRI. (2020). *General Information About COVID-19.* Retrieved 17 October 2021. https://www.kemri.org/coronavirus-disease-2019-covid-19/

Kogan, M., Palen, L., & Anderson, K. M. (2016). Think local, retweet global: Retweeting by the geographically-vulnerable during Hurricane Sandy. In *Proceedings of the ACM conference on Computer-Supported Cooperative Work & Social Computing (CSCW)* (pp. 981–993). ACM.

Lamb, A., Paul, M. J., & Dredze, M. (2013). Separating fact from fear: Tracking flu infections on Twitter. In *Proceedings of the HLT-NAACL* (pp. 789–795). ACL.

Litt, E. (2012). Knock, knock. Who's there? The imagined audience. *Journal of Broadcasting & Electronic Media, 56*, 330–345.

Louie, R., & Kost, G. (2010). A Point-of-Care Test for H1N1 Influenza—Louie et al. reply. *Disaster Medicine And Public Health Preparedness, 4*(2), 100–101. https://doi.org/10.1001/dmphp.4.2.100-b

Mao, H., Shuai, X., & Kapadia, A. (2011). Loose tweets: An analysis of privacy leaks on Twitter. In *Proceedings on the ACM workshop on privacy in the electronic society* (pp. 1–12). ACM.

Marwick, A., & boyd, d. (2011). To See and Be Seen: Celebrity Practice on Twitter. *Convergence: The International Journal of Research Into New Media Technologies, 17*(2), 139–158. https://doi.org/10.1177/1354856510394539

Meeder, B., Tam, J., Kelley, P. G., & Cranor, L. F. (2010). RT @IWantPrivacy: Widespread violation of privacy settings in the Twitter social network. In *Web 2.0 security and privacy* (pp. 28–48). IEEE.

Ministry of Health. (2020). *Ministry of Health.* Retrieved September 27, 2021, from https://www.health.go.ke/

Mwambari, D., & Martin, L. (2020). *Humour ignores social distancing: Postcolonial Irony and COVID-19 in Africa | African Arguments.* African Arguments. Retrieved 7 February 2021, from https://africanarguments.org/2020/05/humour-ignores-social-distancing-postcolonial-irony-and-COVID-19-in-africa/

Nairobi and Mombasa bears the bulk of COVID 19 infections Nairobi, Monday June 29, 2020 – MINISTRY OF HEALTH. (n.d.). https://www.health.go.ke/nairobi-and-mombasa-bears-the-bulk-of-covid-19-infections-nairobi-monday-june-29-2020/

Odhiambo, J., Weke, P., & Ngare, P. (2020). Modeling Kenyan economic impact of corona virus in Kenya using discrete-time Markov chains. *Journal of Finance and Economics, 8*(2), 80–85.

Omondi, I. (2020). Premium tears: Kenyans react to Uhuru'S extension of COVID-19 Restrictions – Citizentv.Co.Ke. *Citizentv.co.ke* [online]. Available at: https://citizentv.co.ke/news/premium-tears-kenyans-react-to-uhurus-extension-of-COVID-19-restrictions-334895/. Accessed 3 Dec 2020.

Palen, L., & Starbird, K. (2011). Twitter-based information distribution during the 2009 Red River Valley flood threat. *Bulletin of the American Society for Information Science and Technology, 36*(5), 13–17. https://doi.org/10.1002/bult.2010.1720360505

Pearce, K., & Hajizada, A. (2014). Humor as a means of dissent in the digital era: The case of authoritarian Azerbaijan. *Demokratızatsiya, 22*(1), 67–85.

Priem, J, Costello, K, & Dzuba, T. (2012). *Prevalence and use of Twitter among scholars.* http://www.figshare.com/articles/Prevalence_and_use_of_Twitter_among_scholars/104629. Accessed 3 Dec 2020.

Proferes, N. (2017). Information flow solipsism in an exploratory study of beliefs about Twitter. *Social Media + Society, 3*(1), 2056305117698493.

Ritchie, G. (2004). *The linguistic analysis of jokes.* Routledge.

Romero, E. J., & Cruthirds, K. W. (2006). The use of humour in the workplace. *Academy of Management Perspectives, 20*(2), 58–69.

Sakaki, T., Okazaki, M., & Matsuo, Y. (2010). Earthquake shakes Twitter users: Realtime event detection by social sensors. In *Proceedings of the 19th international conference on World Wide Web, WWW 2010*, Raleigh, North Carolina, USA, April 26–30, 2010.

Sehl, K. (2021). Katie Sehl, Author at Social Media Marketing & Management Dashboard. *Social Media Marketing & Management Dashboard*. Retrieved 27 September 2021, from https://blog.hootsuite.com/author/katie-sehl/

Shifman, L. (2013). *Memes in digital culture*. MIT Press.

Signorini, A., Segre, A. M., Polgreen, P. M. (2011). *The Use of Twitter to Track Levels of Disease Activity and Public Concern in the U.S. during the Influenza A H1N1 Pandemic*. PLoS ONE 6(5): e19467. https://doi.org/10.1371/journal.pone.0019467

Stats, G. (2020). *Social Media Stats Kenya | StatCounter Global Stats*. StatCounter Global Stats. Retrieved 3 December 2020, from https://gs.statcounter.com/social-media-stats/all/kenya

Tumasjan, A., Sprenger, T. O., Sandner, P. G., & Welpe, I. M. (2010). *Predicting Elections with Twitter: What 140 Characters Reveal about Political Sentiment*. In: Proceedings of the Fourth International AAAI Conference on Weblogs and Social Media. Retrieved 15 October 2021. https://www.aaai.org/ocs/index.php/ICWSM/ICWSM10/paper/viewFile/1441/1852

What is Twitter and why should you use it? – Economic and Social Research Council. Esrc.ukri.org. (2020). Retrieved 3 December 2020, from https://esrc.ukri.org/research/impact-toolkit/social-media/Twitter/what-is-Twitter/

Who.int. (2021). *Coronavirus disease (COVID-19): How is it transmitted?* [online] Available at: https://www.who.int/emergencies/diseases/novel-coronavirus-2019/question-and-answers-hub/q-a-detail/coronavirus-disease-COVID-19-how-is-it-transmitted. Accessed 7 Feb 2021.

Wiggins, B. E. (2019). *The discursive power of memes in digital culture: Ideology, semiotics, and intertextuality* (1st ed.). Routledge. https://doi.org/10.4324/9780429492303

World Bank. (2021). *Kenya economic update: COVID-19 erodes progress in poverty reduction in Kenya, increases number of poor citizens*. [online] Available at: https://www.worldbank.org/en/country/kenya/publication/kenya-economic-update-COVID-19-erodes-progress-in-poverty-reduction-in-kenya-increases-number-of-poor-citizens#:~:text=%E2%80%9CKenya%20has%20made%20considerable%20progress,Practice%20of%20the%20World%20Bank. Accessed 7 Feb 2021.

World Health Organization. (2020). *Kenya: WHO Coronavirus Disease (COVID-19) Dashboard With Vaccination Data*. Covid19.who.int. Retrieved 27 September 2021, from https://covid19.who.int/region/afro/country/ke/

Yule, G. (2006). *The study of language* (3rd ed.). Cambridge University Press.

Zimmer, M., & Proferes, N. (2014). A topology of Twitter research: disciplines, methods, and ethics. *Aslib Journal of Information Management, 66*(3), 250–261. https://doi.org/10.1108/ajim-09-2013-0083

Tweets by Twitter Users and YouTube Uploads

Mtume Orroson. (2020). Uhury ametudisappoint ama namna gani. https://youtu.be/-EyjMalxKXE. Accessed 31 Jan 2021.

Ahmed Mohamed@Asmali Ahmed Mohamed ((ASMALi)) (@Asmali77) / Twitter. Accessed 10 Feb 2021.

The Impeccable @RealDerrow THE IMPECCABLE on Twitter: "Tomorrow issa day that the Lord has made...we shall rejoice and be glad in it. Happy friyay 😎 #WorldEnvironmentDay2020 #COVID19 #UhuruKenyatta #Uhurustoughchoices #BlackLivesMatter #CurfewKenya #mutaikagwe #FreedomOfExpression https://t.co/A1aszaA1yE" / Twitter. Accessed 31 Jan 2021.

Jacktone Onguso Jacktone Oguso on Twitter: "It has ended in Premium tears for many ,but if president #UhuruKenyatta had reopened the lockdown then the spread of Covid19 would have gone out of hand (mngepelekea wazae hii virusi ocha in droves).Closing for another 31 days is good #UhuruAddress" / Twitter. Accessed 2 Feb 2021

Abdirizack Somo Abdirizack Somo on Twitter: "Msee wa mashati kali kali, uhunye, the son of our 1st president will shortly address his fellow kenyan's and he will give another dose (14days) #PresidentUhuruKenyatta https://t.co/qelLSlixaD" / Twitter. Accessed 31 Jan 2021.

His Majesty His Majesty on Twitter: "@dailynation @ntvkenya Curfew, haina shida, but lockdown yawa, why dont u consider feeding pple in nairobi, imagine the hawkers who used to roam country bus, the shops that depended on it, the grounded matatus, and still the land lord awaits, please reconsider daddy, msee wa mashati kali kali 😎😎😂😅" / Twitter. Accessed 2 Feb 2021.

Arap Liwliw Arap Liwliw (@arap_liwliw) / Twitter. 10 February 2021.

Kahinde Wasiu KEHINDE WASIU ADIO on Twitter: "S.N. Nyamao 🇰🇪 (@snnyamao) Tweeted: Kim Jong Un must be a worried man... https://t.co/uRyUR2HRXB (https://t.co/CT6ZVTqfBJ) One of the greatest leader of all time reportedly hospitalised" / Twitter

Kelly Nivex Kelly Nivex on Twitter: "Current Situtation for slay queens with curfew extension #UhuruKenyatta #6thjune #wanjohi https://t.co/xmDTQ0Eskh" / Twitter. 10 Feb 2021.

Fidel Castro Fidel Castro (@I_amfidel) / Twitter. 10 Feb 2021.

Kenyans On Twitter (KOT) Kenyans On Twitter (@kot) / Twitter. 10 Feb 2021

CHAPTER 15

Dark Humour, Ubuntu and the COVID-19 Pandemic: A Case of Subaltern Humouring of Political Elite Deaths on Social Media

Shepherd Mpofu

Introduction

The COVID-19 pandemic, as expressed in almost all chapters in this volume, saw world economies show decline, many people losing their lives or loved ones, and environments being changed from normal to the 'new normal'. In the process, the spread of fake news about the virus and subsequent vaccines, and humorous celebration of the death of those considered public enemies found fertile ground on social media and other alternative public spheres. COVID-19 affected most countries around the globe, especially at the start of 2020, and in the process, they went on lockdown, whereby people's livelihoods, economies and educational and social lives were impacted as some lost their means of income (Matsilele, 2021). In the process some companies, especially technology companies and courier companies, made booming profits as people's homes became

S. Mpofu (✉)
University of Limpopo, Polokwane, South Africa
e-mail: shepherd.mpofu@ul.ac.za

S. Mpofu (ed.), *Digital Humour in the Covid-19 Pandemic*,
https://doi.org/10.1007/978-3-030-79279-4_15

offices and 'working from home' became an oft-repeated phrase and ritual. Citizen creativity, or as Hartley (2010) prefers to call it, silly citizenship, as most chapters here demonstrate, became the order of the day as people tried to cope with the pandemic, to critique government and political leaders, and to share thoughts, news and fears about the pandemic and, later on, about the vaccine. In some cases Global South citizens made jokes about the global order to the effect that the pandemic was an equalizer and therefore the vaccine was going to be created quicker than that of Ebola since it affected the Global North as well. In fact, many lives were lost in many Western countries due to the pandemic and the vaccine was created within a year. This was in comparison to the lack of urgency by especially the Global North in finding a cure for Ebola, which affected mostly West African countries (Mwambari & Martin, 2020). As Mwambari and Martin observe: '[D]uring the West African Ebola epidemic too, people were victimized on a global scale. The outbreak led to a mass hysteria in the global North, leading many countries to impose restrictions and, in some cases, full bans from Ebola-affected areas' (2020). The humorous engagements with the pandemic offered truthful critiques to the global order, demonstrating an understanding and keen observation of the functioning of the world by ordinary Africans.

The COVID-19 pandemic, according to the World Health Organization (WHO) (2020), is the first pandemic globally to take place in a digital age and therefore making the distribution of information problematic in a context where even citizens are in a position to act as journalists and spread information. Thus, as citizen journalists, citizens are able to use hand-held technological gadgets such as cameras and cell phones, or fly drones enabled with video capturing, storage and other software to gather, edit and disseminate news. Citizen journalism, even though a slippery term to define (Mpofu, 2015; De Burgh, 2005; Deuze, 2005; Steensen, 2011; De Beer, 2004), is seen as a participatory culture that has redefined the profession and practice of journalism (Mpofu, 2019a, b, c; Mutsvairo, 2016). Citizen digital storytelling and expression saw the rise of fake news, conspiracy theories and humorous engagement with each other and the political leaders.

This spread of conspiracy theories and fake news was not limited to the Global South; neither was it an isolated event. The then US President Donald Trump was accused of peddling false information and conspiracy theories (Mahdawi, 2020; Bomey, 2020). Trump was against the wearing of masks, did not promote social distancing and had a negative attitude towards lockdown for political motives. However, he was vocal in announcing the soon coming of the COVID-19 vaccine. In Zambia the government embarked 'on a crackdown against people spreading false information concerning the COVID-19' (Anon, 2020); in Mauritius the Information and Communication Technology Act was used to punish those who spread false news. In South Africa those who spread false news were also arrested under the laws promulgated to contain the spread of the virus by controlling human behaviour and economic activity through various stages of lockdown. Elijah Muthui Kitonyo, a Kenyan man was arrested after he

> published the fake news on a fabricated Twitter account. A tweet said the Kenyan health ministry lied about the first confirmed case in the country coming from the US via London. It said the patient was coming from Rome. The directorate of criminal investigations confirmed the arrest, adding that contravention of Kenya's cyber laws could result in a fine of R830,000, a 10-year jail sentence, or both. (Senne, 2020)

The spread of fake news and governments' reactions cast into sharp light the debates on freedom of expression and the role of citizens in moderating their conversations without the heavy-handed interventions from authorities. Amnesty International (2020) reports that two bloggers were arrested in Tunisia as they faced

> several criminal charges of 'insulting state officials', 'causing disturbances to the public' and defamation. They have been charged for posting videos on social media alleging that the government has failed to provide adequate compensation to people struggling financially and address shortage of basic food supplies in the market amid COVID-19 pandemic. (2020)

In some cases, people shared sarcastic or comic posts on social media and were arrested for spreading fake news (Sophie, 2020). The attacks on freedom of expression by the state also extended to professional journalists in countries such as Zimbabwe, Nigeria, Egypt and Somalia. The pandemic led to the weaponization of the pandemic and undermining of human rights in some countries.

Besides the sharing of fake news and disinformation, social media were used by politicians and everyday citizens to share commentary about COVID-19 in serious or humorous ways. Social media, as Davis et al. argue, 'have fostered new forms of ... communication and participation. These communicative forms take on the conventions of internet culture, which include wit, parody, sarcasm, co-optation, and playful memification as "economics of laughter have become inextricably entangled with civic processes"' (2018, 3900). This chapter asks and answers the following questions: How were the good and bad leaders humorously mourned? What readings, in the context of ubuntu, of dark humour can be made on the way South African and Zimbabwean politicians were mourned? Next I explore the practice of citizen journalism and effects thereof in relation to humour and COVID-19 pandemic.

Subalterneity, Citizen Dissidence and Ubuntu

Social media have played different roles in politics, including as a space for resistance against the government atrocities and memory suppression (Ndlovu, 2017a, b; Ndlovu, 2018; Theocharis et al., 2015; Mpofu, 2014, 2015, 2019a, b, c), as sites for resistance and protest planning (Shirky, 2011; Mpofu, 2017), and as citizens' sites for critiquing the government of the day and expressing themselves during elections (Stein, 2013; Poell, 2014; Jungherr et al., 2016; Mpofu, 2019b) and undermining or rebelling against governments (Matsilele & Ruhanya, 2020; Guobin, 2009; Cross, 2016; Matsilele, 2019). Dissidents are seen as traitors and enemies of the state especially if they depart from the political elite authored script of what it means to be a citizen. These alternative media platforms have provided avenues for the subaltern, 'those groups in society who are lacking autonomous political power' (Smith, 2010, 39), 'leading to their alienation' (Mpofu, 2015, 83). Ordinary citizens are alienated in most countries, especially in the Global South, leading to them creating subaltern communicative avenues, the subaltern public spheres (Fraser, 1992), to undermine the authority's use of mainstream media to communicate biased viewpoints, creating, in the process, narratives that rail against the grain. In some cases governments' control and laws during the COVID-19 lockdowns were considered unreasonable, suppressing people's voices and rights—hence the use of alternative spheres to undermine the laws. Mpofu adds:

> The process of acquiring a voice where there is official silencing by the state could be empowering, therapeutic and humanizing. Silencing not only demarcates discursive boundaries but also delegitimizes the actions, aspirations and voices of the subaltern. In cyberspace these ostracized communities have found an avenue for self-expression through unique voices produced with the help of technology.

This chapter deals with death and dark humour, something inimical to some aspects of ubuntu that some leaders, especially in Zimbabwe, tried to forcibly instil in the mourning of the bodies that political elite deemed to matter (Agamben, 1998), those of politicians who died of the COVID-19 pandemic. Ubuntu is an 'African moral view binding Africans together in a way of living a life of humanity and empathy towards other people, especially outsiders' (Zondi & Makhoba, 2018). The humane and dignified treatment of other people cuts across the board, but in Africa, it seems, ubuntu has to apply to ordinary people amongst themselves, as political leaders seem to exempt themselves from demanding, from themselves, treatment of ordinary people in an *ubuntuistic* fashion. For instance, one may be curious of the South African government's 1997 White Paper on Social Welfare defining ubuntu as:

> The principle of caring for each other's well-being will be promoted, and a spirit of mutual support fostered. Each individual's humanity is ideally expressed through his or her relationship with others and theirs in turn through a recognition of the individual's humanity. Ubuntu means that people are people through other people. It also acknowledges both the rights and the responsibilities of every citizen in promoting individual and societal well-being. (Koma, 2020)

Contrast this with the definition, if you may, of this term by Biko, who said that ubuntu is married to economic liberalization and fighting against poverty. He added: 'It is only through the active engagement of all South Africa's citizens in this war on poverty that we can rediscover the spirit of ubuntu. South Africans have to embrace people centricity as a guiding principle for a national battle for shared prosperity' (2013, 27). Ubuntu, to eradicate poverty and marginalization, has to reside, first and foremost, in those in political leadership, as they make life-impacting decisions. Be that as it may, the crux of my argument here is the brand of ubuntu that politicians demand be extended to them in the event that they die or when people share rumours of their death in celebration and mockery should be equal to the one they afford their *subjects*. Politicians, in some contexts, are hated by ordinary people because they abrogate their political duties by indulging in corruption and looting state resources, as happened in Zimbabwe and South Africa, as funds to help during COVID-19 were misused. Citizen mockery of the politicians stem from this. The question therefore becomes: who are worthy humans to be extended the dignity and treatment of ubuntu. The political elite and the subaltern clash on this in some contexts. It is this contest and context that deploys ubuntu, subalterneity and dark humour in the time of the COVID-19 pandemic.

Journalism as Storytelling

For a long time 'journalism has hitherto been viewed as a lecture, online news media have upset this 'status quo' and introduced citizen journalism, which has shown that journalism can be a conversation as well where audiences interact both with journalists and amongst themselves' (Mpofu, 2016, 89). Journalism, just like citizen journalism, has no established boundaries in terms of definition (Mpofu, 2019a, b, c). Deuze (2005, 446) says that there are possibly five key 'ideal-typical values' that characterize journalism and these are public service, objectivity, autonomy, immediacy and ethics. Further, Mpofu says of Deuze's characterizations:

> [T]hese define 'real journalism' and locate power of definition and authenticity in the occupational ideologies and values of journalism in a straight-jacketed manner. But then there is need to critique the extent of this power bestowed upon 'real' journalism in relation to ownership, commerce, politics, social pressures and technology ... The myth of public service as a measure of 'real' journalism is problematic when it excludes 'other' forms of journalism that are not considered mainstream especially coming from those Stuart Allan has called accidental journalists or just citizen witnesses, meaning citizen journalists.

Rutigliano (2008, 45) defines citizen journalism using four critical points: '1) it is not produced by a traditional news organization; 2) it is produced by a group; 3) it is open to audience contributions and participation; 4) it strives to cover marginalized communities through recruitment of members of these communities and coverage of these communities.' Key to citizen journalism is the communal culture and rituals followed in covering those in the margins.

For Mpofu (2015, 87) and for the purposes of this research, 'citizen journalism is that form of storytelling which moves from seeing journalism ... as a conversation ... where "everyday people".. assume power to take charge and be influential in telling their stories from their own perspectives, through blogs, reader comments, e-mail listservs, etc.' This concept is not without criticisms. Lindner (2015, 555) argue that 'certainly has the potential to contribute to a democratized public sphere, much of the popular commentary and scholarship on the subject has veered toward the hyperbolic and romantic'. There are many themes that drive the relevance of citizen journalism in different and specific contexts (Mutsvairo & Salgado, 2020) and in playing different roles (Mutsvairo and Muneri, 2019), including dissidence and whistleblowing (Matsilele, 2019, Matsilele & Ruhanya, 2020; Mpofu & Matsilele, 2020). These accidental journalists, the citizens, were born largely due to the rise of and advances in new information and communication technologies (Mpofu & Barnabas, 2016; Banda, 2010; El-Nawawy & Khamis, 2013; Goode, 2009; Mpofu, 2015). There are criticisms of citizen journalism bordering on ethics, truthfulness and the potential to spread hate speech (Mutsvairo et al., 2014). Mpofu magnifies the issue of ethics by saying: 'While citizen journalism has dismantled gatekeeping and other ethics-enhancing codes used by traditional media to protect audiences, this has left audiences exposed to unethical journalistic practices which infringe on people's security and privacy' (2016, 91).

Fake news can pose a danger of an ill-informed citizenry. There was news spread via social media platforms such as blogs, Twitter, WhatsApp and Facebook suggesting that the virus came from 5G internet network. This led to the destruction of 5G towers in South Africa. A ruling party councillor, Sifiso Mngadi, circulated a voice note via WhatsApp to locals in the KwaZulu-Natal province where he said: 'As leaders of eThekwini we need to take action against this disease. It is not Covid. We are getting this thing from 5G towers, [some] installed during this period in preparation of the second wave' (cited in Pitt, 2021). Fake news was spread about the deaths of some ministers in Zimbabwe, sparking debates on ubuntu and ethical leadership.

Methodology

Data for this qualitative study were gathered from social media platforms such as Facebook and Twitter, and also from newspaper archives through digital ethnography. Digital ethnography was born out of the ubiquity of the internet and related technologies that have acted as extensions of organizations and people's lives. This trend makes it difficult for social scientists to ignore digital methods in research (Murthy, 2008). As this chapter is written during lockdown necessitated by the COVID-19 pandemic, digital ethnography and other online data gathering methods such as online videos, online questionnaires, online interviews and analyses of weblogs and social media networking sites have become all the more important. Digital ethnography can be covet, that is, stealth and invisible (Ebo, 1998), or overt, that is visible, depending on the research design and aims of the researcher. In this instance, I collected data without participating in any of the debates taking place on social media sites that I used. My lurking was unobtrusive and passive (Mare, 2018; Denzin, 1999; Kozinets, 2002). This does not in any way suggest that there was neutral engagement, nor does it suggest that there are neutral engagements in digital ethnography bereft of any power relations between the researcher and the subjects or the researched members of society. My data gathering and analyses, however I may try to be methodologically astute, remain biased, subjective and informed by personal histories, biases, perceptions and agendas. Data used were conveniently sampled to fit the theme of this chapter, as there were many different reactions to the deaths of the political elite than black humour, the central focus here. The digital divide, that is the disparity between those communities with access and without access to the internet and enabling technologies, affects the *globality* of researches carried out using digital ethnography. Therefore, the views and data gathered may not be representative of every member of the community, even though we argue that textual engagements are part of human interaction and culture and have integrity, and therefore could be studied on their own. On the other hand, as Murthy (2008) observes, digital ethnography allows for the inclusion of the disabled and even those not confident to speak in public or participate on offline forums and focus group interviews.

This chapter uses a narrative analysis of the jokes about the deaths of politicians in Zimbabwe and South Africa. Narrative analysis helps us gain an understanding of the world and processes of production of data in that context. Most importantly this allows us to engage and know what realities people make of their world through telling their own stories. Storytelling helps in sharing world views and in the construction of identities (Rosenwald & Ochberg, 1992). As a researcher, I am in a dilemma whereby I have to make sense of the people's narratives while they are making sense of their own world. To this end, meaning can be considered ambiguous because it is born out of a process on multi-interactionism between many parties to meaning-making. To this end Reissman says: 'Meaning is fluid and contextual, not fixed and universal. All we have is talk and texts that represent reality partially, selectively, and imperfectly' (1993, 15).

Humour in Pandemics

Humour serves different purposes in life and society (Abel, 2002; Berlyne, 1972; Boyd, 2004; Brown, 2013; Davis et al., 2018; Dionigi & Canestrari, 2018). COVID-19 humour leads one to reflecting on the role and use of humour in pandemics. Park and Park (2010), in an article titled 'Fear and Humour in the Art of Cholera', recall: '[It] has long been recognized that in times of such adversity humour can play a significant role in aiding communities to cope with the fear of disease and death' (2010, 481). They observe that, in the context of art, which focused on the cholera pandemic of the nineteenth century, fear and humour work in tandem. The humour, mainly carried through newspaper cartoons, served different purposes, including highlighting 'the disagreement between doctors on the diagnosis and treatment of cholera, public mistrust of the medical profession and their ineffective treatment, and political attacks on government policies' (2010, 481). The authors conclude with a futuristic outlook to pandemics in the age of technology and say: '[As] future pandemics appear, even in this era of multimedia, there remains an important role for art in documenting not only the physical suffering but also the use of humour as a coping mechanism to alleviate fear of disease and death' (483).

Rosa (2012, 735) explores the use of humour in Portugal during the swine flu pandemics in 2009–2010, where she argues that 'humour is a valuable resource to study social trends and shared meanings, while providing information about the way social meaning is attached to specific risk events'. Newspapers used humour to 'stress the cyclic nature of health risks, reducing the impact of dramatic information on the audience' (2012, 735). Newspapers use editorial humour such as cartoons to engage with the public, providing 'cognitive maps to decode everyday life' (Rosa, 2012, 738). Mainstream media are different from social media, which are the focus of the present study, and Rosa demonstrates that there is an establishment of authority on pontificating on the pandemic in a formal mainstream newspaper. In addition, editorial gatekeeping processes allow for credible information to be shared, something that is not present in social media and citizen journalists' engagements with the world. Mainstream media also propose the way an issue has to be approached, 'suggesting an interpretation and a course of action' and they go further to define normative agenda that allows readers to evaluate' media content leading to the promotion of a 'desire for action, capitalizing symbolic resources to a particular cause' (Rosa, 2012, 737). This humorous engagement with a pandemic is socially responsible and building, since the one who is a comedian, especially a cartoonist in the newspaper, is similar to a columnist.

A similar study to Rosa's (2012) was done by Lobanov (2021), who looked at humour in newspapers during the Spanish flu of 1918–1919. Lobanov's archival research unravelled how 'the Spanish flu generated humour as a tool to explore the social world in conditions of heightened disgust and wide-spread political instability'. Lobanov concludes that humour is important in society and helps us understand human capabilities in tragic moments.

In contrast to Rosa, who studied humour regarding the swine flu in newspapers, Cynthia Chew and Gunther Eysenbach did an infodemiological study, whereby they looked at the swine flu, spread of information and also some aspects of humour from the perspective of Twitter. The researchers realized that among the tweets containing the words 'swine flu', 'swineflu' and 'H1N1' shared during 1 May–12 December 2013, 12.7% were humorous. Accompanying this were cases of disinformation owing to lack of gatekeeping measures in social media applications such as Twitter.

Nwabueze et al. (2017) has also written on newspaper cartoons focusing on the Ebola virus in Nigeria. They preface their argument by noting that cartoons satirize and tell stories at the same time and are 'effective channels for the formation of public opinion on salient social issues' (2017, 1). Cartoons and cartoonists are important players in the newspaper industry, as they act as the soul of society in those democratic spaces or independent newspapers where freedom of expression is constrained by those in power. Cartoons become 'effective tools for criticizing wrong actions in the society and calling the attention of the public and their leaders to burning national issues of national interest and development' in those contexts (Nwabueze et al., 2017, 1). Respondents to the study observed that the cartoons were informative and funny at the same time. In addition, they also observed that some cartoons were too technical, their interpretation becoming inaccessible to audiences. Besides, the authors conclude that the cartoons also had a fear frame and horrific elements which 'brought about heightened fear among Nigerians on the devastating effect of the Ebola virus' (Nwabueze et al., 2017, 4).

COVID-19 and Dark Humour

There is inchoate literature on humour on the COVID-19 pandemic of which this book project forms a seminal part. Some aspects of academic research on humour have been addressed in chapters written by Mpofu in this volume, and these will not be worth reiterating. However, it is important to make a few observations and also to engage with people's understandings of humour during the pandemic. Most importantly, humour in pandemics served as political critique as well as for healing purposes. Saricali et al. conclude in their research that 'the effect of fear of COVID-19 on hopelessness was partly mediated by mindfulness and humor, and which was supported by bootstrapping. Therefore, higher fear of COVID-19 was associated with lower mindfulness and humor. In turn, lower mindfulness and humor were related with higher hopelessness' (2020, 1). Those who feel hopeless during pandemics are highly suicidal (Bhuiyan et al., 2020; Beck et al., 2006). This humour comes mostly from ordinary people, where they demonstrate their understanding of a multiple facets of global and world orders, power, politics, social relations and identities. Ordinary people and politicians used social media to share humorous moments during the pandemic. On its Facebook page, a South African radio station, *Cape Talk*, ran a story where they solicited reader and listener comments where they asked: 'Should we laugh about and spread jokey memes about COVID-19?' A number of participants on the page responded in all manners: humorously, seriously and everything in between.

Below I reproduce some of the comments from the readers:

A. Sometimes the best way to deal with scary things is to joke about them. As they say. Laughter is the best medicine. Let's not take that away too. If you don't like the memes don't look at them.
B. Don't worry ... The virus won't last long ... After all. It was made in China ...
C. The more dramatic/sensational the reporting/the impact, the more jokes are made. Whether crude or not, laughing is a very human way to get rid of stress. Necessary, though not always sensitive.
D. They are not laughing at people who are sick. Stop being petty.
E. This is how we deal with shit ☺
F. It's stupidity too make jokes about it ... They won't joke and laughs if the virus hit them ... Too me it's so common

G. Great, we need some humour to ease the crazy hysteria surrounding this virus that's blown out of proportion.
H. People will always joke about tragedies. It's a coping mechanism. It makes the enormity of the situation easier to deal with. It is also the mechanism by which the ego 'insists that it cannot be affected by the traumas of the external world' (Freud).
I. Humour is a way to deal with stress, risk, uncertainty. Especially in SA. Quite natural. Sometimes quite clever actually.

These demonstrate an understanding of humour and its role during the pandemic that is not contrary to findings in researches on the role of humour during moments of crises. While some cringe at the idea of sharing humour during pandemics, some find it unproblematic, as this assists in advancing the well-being of society in the face of adversity. The following sections discuss dark humour in relation to political deaths.

Death humour is dark humour relating to both dark humour, whereby people make light death news, or joke about death in a way that is irreverent. Added to that it is humour in memory of the dead, good or bad. This is the humour that is crude and meant to attack the dead, especially if they held power in society and were deemed to be working for an evil system. For the purposes of this study I use the deaths and rumours of death of ministers and political leaders in Zimbabwe and South Africa. These countries are deliberately chosen because of the author's familiarity with the political contexts. I have been following news and political events around COVID-19 and politics in Zimbabwe.

Zimbabwe's President as a Joker

At the beginning of March, Zimbabwe's President Emerson Mnangagwa, while attending a national clean-up campaign, gave a speech in which he seemed to boast about building a mortuary which he considered the coldest:

> When I was a member of parliament for Kwekwe, I constructed a state-of-the-art mortuary with 12 bays, very cool inside. I told people in Mbizo that there is a prize for the family that brings its dead first. At that time, there was already someone who had passed on at the hospital and that family won the prize (Newzimbabwe.com, 2020)

The statement, made when the country was in the middle of a pandemic, was read as disturbing and unbecoming of a president, for he took death lightly. The following were reader reactions to a video posted on the NewZimbabwe.com Facebook page:

A: Madness fix the economy how many jokes will u make before u die your self
B: I know an idiot when I see one … this man is a natural one!!!
C: The guy actually too well upstairs … his stupid jokes are disgusting
D: He builds a cool mortuary and set a race for people to die by not letting the doctors having enough apparatus and a good working environment. Shame and sorry maningi (trans. Too much)
E: You have said it all, your interest is on death of people only with no constructive idea. Shame on you. You don't deserve to be a president, not even a chief.
F: I have a problem with media give us a full video with its content then we can judge the no matter how bad the man is but give us a full content not small clips that you show people for your personal gain

In defence of Mnangagwa's pronouncement, the country's Secretary for Information, Publicity and Broadcasting Services Nick Mangwana (2020) argued, in a state-controlled public but Zanu-Pf mouthpiece newspaper article, that people did not understand the president's dark humour, which was meant to be taken lightly; hence, they were trying to silence him. Silencing the president, Mangwana argued, was tantamount to dehumanizing him, as '[r]epressing laughter is dehumanizing the human race. Laughter is one thing that separates us from animals in that most animals do all that human beings do except to laugh. Not even a hyena. It just makes a laughing sound but that is not a laugh. So those who want to repress the President's humour, are you not trying to dehumanize him?' (Mangwana, 2020). Mangwana further argued: 'None of the jokes made by President Mnangagwa was transgressive. The President tackles taboo subjects with humour, thought-provoking ideas and laughter.' He faulted those accusing the president of being insensitive in his joke, of having lower cognitive capabilities, for 'if you are cognitively gifted, you won't need to employ a lot of effort to get a dark joke. This is when you hear those less gifted using pejorative terms like "morbid, nasty, twisted, sick or grotesque". But humour processing depends very much on one's cognitive ability' (Mangwana, 2020). Mangwana (2020) went on to argue: 'Dark humour empowers people to speak about sensitive, serious and unsettling subjects by according oneself permission to be negative in a healthy way.' For Mangwana, Mnangagwa's joke about death and rewarding the first person to die with some money meant that the president was human too, as leaders need not to be too serious all the time. This made Mnangagwa appear folksy, and

> [j]ocularity humanizes those at the top making them approachable. It makes the 'servant leadership' genre of leadership a reality. After all the word, 'humour' itself is derived from the Latin word, which meant fluid and flexible. So to suggest that the President should stop joking is probably proffering fools' wisdom. He should continue to enjoy the sagacity of humour even in the face of his phenomenal responsibility of turning this country around. If the President was to ask for my advice, I would suggest that he keeps dancing and keeps joking and if he feels like singing, by all means sing. That's just what humans do and in Zimbabwe, he is the first among equals. Someone once said, 'dark humour is like food, not everyone gets it'. (Mangwana, 2020)

In response in the comment sections some readers maintained that the president's joke was not welcome. One respondent wrote: 'Mangwana, the electorate did not vote for a comedian. The president's job is a very serious position and as such is no place for clowning around. The economy and society is suffering while you defend such nonsense. Please be serious for a change.' Another responded: 'Making jokes at the expense of the suffering masses? It just tells you how out of touch this guy is. He's not fit even to be chairman of a burial society let alone a country.' Mnangagwa's political opponents decried the president's remarks, with the Movement for Democratic Change Alliance leader, Nelson Chamisa, arguing: 'In other countries, Mnangagwa's talk on mortuaries would have gotten him impeached a long time ago. When you see a president talk like that, celebrating things like that, it shows you he is out of touch with reality and that his days are numbered.' If political leaders use dark humour, can citizens do the same when it's the politicians on the other side of the *audience*? I discuss this below.

Jackson Mthembu: The Death of a Good Man

The aim here is to demonstrate the relevance and accessibility of the humour shared in grieving the loss of good men. It is a moment, as Erica Buist says in her article in the *Guardian* newspaper, to 'fuck death ... it doesn't need our respect' (2018). Jackson Mthembu was a senior member of the South African ruling African National Congress. He was also a minister in the presidency and had been at the forefront of the government's COVID-19 communications campaign. At one time he mistakenly called the ventilators used in intensive care units (ICU) as vibrators, sex toys. He later realized the joke, and humorously corrected himself. He died of COVID-19 on 21 January 2021. Mourners from across the political spectrum celebrated Mthembu as a giant who worked tirelessly for the country (see South African Government, 2021; Gottschalk, 2021). Speaking directly to the concept of ubuntu resident in politicians, or as it is supposed to be resident in politicians, President Cyril Ramaphosa said:

> He laughed like someone who really loved to laugh. He laughed at many things, some of which he probably shouldn't have ... Mthembu was a kind and gentle soul, but when it came to corruption, self-serving leadership, brazen abuse of power, you would see another side of him. He was never deceived by the false smiles and empty promises of those who sought to enrich themselves at the expense of the poor. He called them out and did not care if they were more powerful than he was. (McCain, 2021)

A fellow minister added, appealing to the humorous side of Mthembu, 'we will miss his jokes, we will miss his laughter. He lived a life bigger than any person is required to live' (du Plessis, 2021). This was further attested to by the nurse who helped nurse him at the hospital, who said: 'We didn't nurse a "do you know who I am" person'. Humour shared during his memorial included criticizing the government for incompetence, for example. One Noma Bolani, who was trying to log onto a Zoom platform titled *Minister Jackson Mthembu's Memorila Service*, shared a screenshot of the misspelling of memorial and commented: 'This was the first indication it wasn't going to go well.' Besides, different people shared images of Mthembu dancing outside parliament and other places, demonstrating his jovial mood. A nurse at the hospital where Mthembu died shared how he called her to come and watch Minister of Police, Bheki Cele, dancing in a video saved in Mthembu's mobile phone and later said that Cele cannot dance and 'I show him how to when I get out' of hospital. His jovial

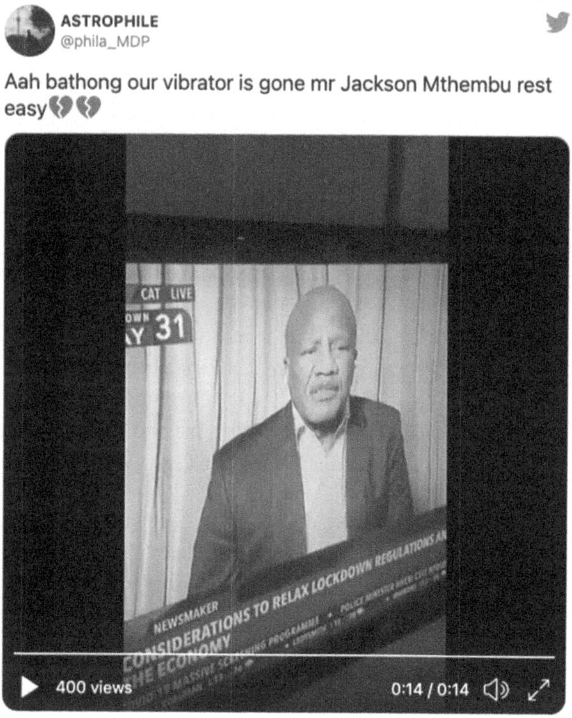
ASTROPHILE
@phila_MDP
Aah bathong our vibrator is gone mr Jackson Mthembu rest easy💔💔
CAT LIVE
NEWSMAKER
400 views
0:14 / 0:14

Fig. 15.1 A still from a video clip of Jackson Mthembu mistakenly calling ventilators vibrators posted on Twitter in remembrance of his funny and gaffe moments

mood was the centrepiece of the celebrations of his life. Another interlocutor on Twitter, shown in Fig. 15.1, mourned Mthembu, calling him 'our vibrator'. The post is humorous, and fits into dark humour, making us laugh during sombre times. Thus, the reliving of the dead's life through their funny moments and actions is important in dark humour and also makes mourning these people palatable (Lund et al., 2008).

The sharing of humour at the death of Mthembu serves two purposes, to strengthen people in the face of death, a natural thing that, even though feared, will befall anyone, and secondly, to prepare people to face the pandemic with some form of resolve and hope of winning the war set by many global governments against the pandemic. To this end Eleanor Haley says of the goodness of this humour in her essay 'The Utility of Laughter in Times of Grief':

> Not only is this type of humor good for the individual morale, but it's good for morale of larger groups as well as it makes the enemy or the challenge seem less intimidating, eases tension, makes suffering in the moment seem far more tolerable, and strengthens social bonds. (2014)

The sombre mood that accompanies most deaths is because of death's power to rob us 'of our self-esteem, our individuality … when we die, we're demoted. We become like everyone who ever died, every beast, every insect, every perished germ. This is why we don't speak ill of the dead; it's like kicking them while they're six feet down' (Buist, 2018). In the following section, those politicians who die are celebrated by the political elites from the ruling party while citizens celebrate and mock their deaths through dark humour for political purposes.

Dark Humour and Unmourning the Mournables

The case of Zimbabwe demonstrates how dark humour was used in a context where politicians are seen as not serving the public and therefore their demise is worth celebrating as comic relief. Three ministers had died of COVID-19 by the end January 2021, the same month most African governments were making plans to acquire the vaccines. Most Zimbabweans believed that the politicians in the ruling party would acquire vaccines for themselves before everyone else. The three ministers who faced their demise are the coup face and spokesperson, Sibusiso Moyo. Moyo was at the forefront of the communications between the public and a group of Zanu-Pf and the military men involved in the 2017 unconstitutional coup which overthrew the country's founding leader and dictator Robert Mugabe. After the coup Moyo was appointed foreign affairs and international trade minister. The coup was presented as an opportunity to restore Zimbabwe's legacy, which, even today, remains a myth, and establish a New Dispensation. However, it seems Zimbabwe is worse off than when Mugabe was leader due to the continuation of toxic leadership under his successor, Mnangagwa and his militarized regime. The other minister who died three days after Moyo is Joel Biggie Matiza, the Minister of Transport. Before then, Parrance Shiri, a man heavily involved in Zimbabwe's genocide, died in July 2020, sparking celebrations from the victims of the genocide and some Zimbabweans who felt let down by the current regime.

Government takes deaths of the political leaders seriously, as these are routinely declared national heroes and buried at a shrine preserved for the heroes for nation-building purposes. However, the declaration of a hero status and the space for burial are sites of contention between the ruling party, opposition parties and citizens in general (Mpofu, 2016). When Mnangagwa announced Shiri's death on Twitter one respondent wrote: 'Is the cold mortuary still available?' Another posted a quote from one of the country's rulers during colonialism, Ian Smith, with the statement: 'if blacks are to rule themselves ppl in towns will walk on sewage until they believe its normal, all the gains from colonization will vanish, infrastructure will collapse, roads will be impassable, trains will kill people until they're abandoned as an unsafe mode of transport.' Another interlocutor quoted Muchinguri's statement that COVID-19 was God's punishment of the West and yet the pandemic, funny enough struck Zimbabwe, as shown in the meme in Fig. 15.2.

Further responses to Mnangagwa's tweet wished that he also caught the virus. These are illustrative, 'I hope you went to see him without PPE ...' and 'When was the last time you two were physically close? You know it can take 3 weeks or more for symptoms to develop. Then whammo! (trans. You will soil your pants).' Most comments expressed relief at Shiri's death and wished Mnangagwa also caught COVID-19. The reactions to these comments were laughing emojis or words like lol and hahahahaha. Some people simply posted insults. There was suspension of ubuntu in this case, as politicians would later argue, where the predicament of Shiri was celebrated instead of mourned.

When Moyo died, Mnangagwa also posted an announcement on his Twitter page where he declared Moyo as a 'dedicated public servant and a true hero, and ... a friend..[who] fought his entire life so that Zimbabwe could be free'. Almost similar to the responses to Shiri's death, one citizen asked if the coldest mortuary has been opened for Moyo. Another responded with an emoji of former US president Donald Trump dancing in happiness, with a caption 'winning'. Another comment from a discussant based in the diaspora said: 'Removing criminals surrounding children of Zimbabwe. We are scattered all over the world because of you. Minus 1. Covid uri gandanga. Hosiah Chipanga. Covid 19 uri ndururani (COVID-19 you are mischievous).' Some people played around some statements from his speeches he used during the coup such as 'the situation has reached another level' and used this to mock and laugh at the level of panic within the corridors of power as the reality of the pandemic and vulnerability of the politicians became palpable.

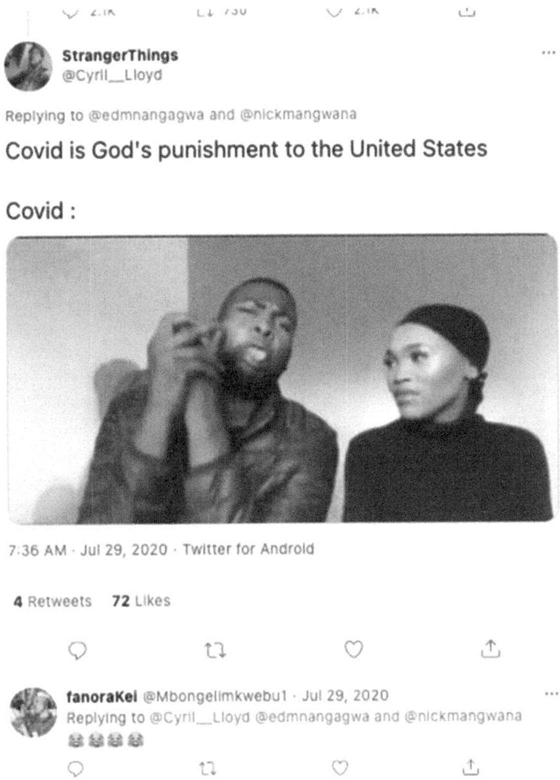
StrangerThings
@Cyril__Lloyd
Replying to @edmnangagwa and @nickmangwana
Covid is God's punishment to the United States
Covid :
7:36 AM · Jul 29, 2020 · Twitter for Android
4 Retweets 72 Likes
fanoraKel @Mbongelimkwebu1 · Jul 29, 2020
Replying to @Cyril__Lloyd @edmnangagwa and @nickmangwana

Fig. 15.2 COVID turning the tables from attacking the West to attacking Mnangagwa's inner circle after a minister said it was sent by God to kill the West for imposing sanctions on Zimbabwe

Some citizens posted what they called COVID-19 wishlist, with names and boxes to tick if those they wished dead died, as shown in Fig. 15.3. This partly led to the spread of fake news, as those ministers some wished dead were subject of fake news posts and the government had to issue statements and the state-controlled broadcaster Zimbabwe Broadcasting Television had to interview the so-called dead ministers to prove that they were alive. The spread of fake news was called inhumane by Zanu-Pf, as they deemed such as against ubuntu.

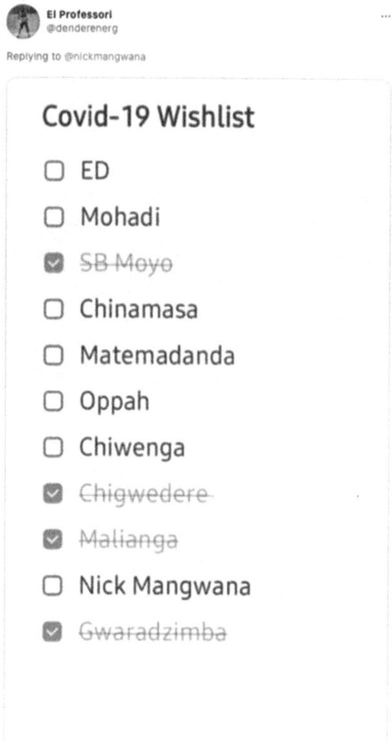

Fig. 15.3 COVID-19 death wishlist

J.B. Matiza's death was not mentioned on the presidential Twitter account, but Nick Mangwana shared the news of Matiza's death. One citizen shared a tweet on how J.B. Matiza, while campaigning for political office, went with a 'donation' of computers to a constituency, did the political speech and handover, and then left with the computers and performed the same stunt at the next constituency. This highlighted the selfish and untrustworthiness of politicians. When J.B. Matiza was declared a national hero some wondered why, because, in Zimbabwe, there is a perception that one has to have been involved in the war to be a hero. However, one respondent wrote on Twitter: 'JB Matiza is a Genetically Modified Hero'.

Discussion and Conclusion

The deaths of politicians due to COVID-19 elicited dark humour to different effects. In the South African example, Mthembu was celebrated as a hero who served the people, eschewed corruption and unified different politicians. His death served as a loss to many but at the same time to celebrate the values he might have taught South Africans. In the Zimbabwean context, however, death was used differently by opposing sides, that is, some ruling party officials and citizens opposed to them. Death symbolizes a disruption of a certain order (Harper, 2010), and for the powerful, death becomes a point of defeat and shame, especially after living lives of invincibility—hence the reprimands that are directed at citizens celebrating, mocking and spreading fake news about the deaths of politicians. A dead body is laden with meanings: 'Concrete and protean, sacred and profane, the corpse is a complex, ambiguous and enigmatic object. It is thus a source of no small amount of ambivalence that energizes human and political imagination, evoking multi-vocal meaning and inspiring diverse, if conflicting, political visions and uses among political rulers and their subjects' (Kalusa, 2017, 1138–1139).

In the context of COVID-19, it seems both opposing sides needed corpses for various political points. Ordinary citizens who celebrated the deaths of politicians due to COVID-19 used social media to celebrate that we are all equal before death and this was a moment for politicians to learn. Political leadership needed dead bodies of fellow politicians to demonstrate power during burial rituals, where the president becomes the one at the apex of national identity definition and policy announcement, giving hope and demonstrating power to command the state security apparatus to intimidate foes. Social media have enabled citizens to take advantage of existent socio-political and economic issues to engage in the economy of humour and laughter that exists in civic rituals. The following tweets from citizens are illustrative:

> With all due respect Hon, I think it's high time for leaders to reflect on their attitude toward the masses. Obviously they are doing something wrong for the masses to be excited about their deaths. Zambia mourned Mwanawansa openly in the streets. This doesn't define us let's fix it.

> Have you ever NOTICED why there is so much hatred of the ruling class, to the extent that people celebrate their death? It's not part of Ubuntu to celebrate someone's demise, but please guys correct all the mistakes starting with the justice system which is so selective to M.O.H (Ministry of Health).

Thus while the ruling elite may think the deaths of colleagues are mournable (in contrast to the thousands of ordinary citizens who die unnoticed), citizens believe otherwise, even if it means defying the precepts of ubuntu. This tension led to Mangwana accusing Zimbabwean doctors of being political assassins, that is, killing ministers. This suggests that there are lives that matter and those that do not, especially in the eyes of those in power (Butler, 2009). The heroes acre burials are used as sites for demonstrating power and commandment of the nation (Marschall, 2006) by the presidium as they make speeches and policy announcements, outsmart opposition and internal enemies or factions, threaten opponents and reprimand citizens in their burial speeches. These speeches are critical tools at governing, meant to build a sense of community and strengthen bonds between government and citizens (Zarefsky, 2008). Silly citizenship, demonstrated through robust irreverence, mockery and dark humour directed at politicians, attempts to undermine power and ridicule main actors while at the same time empowering citizens who feel fully human for their ability to throw punches at their leaders, who have for a long time suppressed them (Hartley, 2010; Vis, 2013; Highfield, 2016). Humour shared in reaction to politicians' deaths in both contexts helps with identification, that is, the construction of political subjectivity (Davis et al., 2018) and assertion of patriotism to one's nation regardless of political leadership. Most of the frustrations and contests online between Zimbabwean politicians and citizens are basically a battle for the nation, where politicians are seen as having looted the resources and citizens are fighting for the restoration of a dignified and functional economy.

From the forgoing, one may conclude that dark humour was used especially by citizens and politicians in a duplicitous way. Firstly, the Zimbabwean president joked about the cold mortuary and citizens protested online and labelled him callous, and yet when political leaders died some citizens proffered commentary via dark humour and did not reprimand each other as much as they shared the humour. Interestingly it was political leaders who reprimanded them, bringing into question when is it right to engage with COVID-19 deaths humorously and who has the right to do the same. One may argue that dark humour is accessed and read differently depending on which side of death and bereavement one stands. If it is the ordinary, *homo sacer* and bare life dying, politicians do not care and would laugh, but when citizens mock and laugh at politicians' deaths, it becomes problematic. This demonstrates that 'black humour processing is seemingly a complex information processing task that depends on cognitive and emotional aspects' (Willinger et al. 2017, 167). And death humour is a highly emotive subject that could be narrated in different ways and, in the process, unravels a lot about a given society and context.

References

Abel, M. (2002). Humor, stress, and coping strategies. *Humor: International Journal of Humor Research, 15*(4), 365–381.

Agamben, G. (1998). *Homo sacer: Sovereign power and bare life* (Daniel Heller-Roazan, Trans.). Stanford University Press.

Amnesty International. (2020). *Tunisia: End prosecution of bloggers for criticizing government's response to COVID-19.* https://www.amnesty.org/en/latest/news/2020/04/tunisia-end-prosecution-of-bloggers-for-criticizing-governments-response-to-covid19/

Anon. (2020). *Zambia launches crackdown on people spreading fake news on COVID-19.* http://www.xinhuanet.com/english/2020-03/20/c_138899158.htm

Banda, F. (2010). *Citizen journalism and democracy in Africa: An exploratory study.* Highway Africa.

Beck, A. T., Brown, G., Berchick, R. J., Stewart, B. L., & Steer, R. A. (2006). Relationship between hopelessness and ultimate suicide: A replication with psychiatric outpatients. *Focus, 147*(2), 190–296. https://doi.org/10.1176/foc.4.2.291

Berlyne, D. E. (1972). Humor and its kin. In J. H. Goldstein & P. E. McGhee (Eds.), *The psychology of humor: Theoretical perspectives and empirical issues* (pp. 43–60). Academic Press.

Bhuiyan, A. I., Sakib, N., Pakpour, A., Griffiths, M. D., & Mamun, M. A. (2020). COVID-19-related suicides in Bangladesh due to lockdown and economic factors: Case study evidence from media reports. *International Journal of Mental Health and Addiction. Advance online publication.* https://doi.org/10.1007/s11469-020-00307-y

Biko, H. (2013). *The great African society: A plan for a nation gone astray.* Jonathan Ball Publishers.

Bomey, N. (2020). *Social media teems with conspiracy theories from QAnon and Trump critics after president's positive COVID-19 test.* https://www.usatoday.com/story/tech/2020/10/02/trump-covid-conspiracy-theories-emerge-social-media-after-positive-test/5892808002/

Boyd, B. (2004). Laughter and literature: a play theory of humor. *Philosophy and Literature, 28*(1), 1–22.

Brown, G. (2013). Web culture: Using memes to spread and manipulate ideas on a massive scale. *Interface: The Journal of Education, Community, and Values, 13*, 187–193.
Buist, E. (2018). *Death doesn't need our respect. Let's celebrate life at funerals.* https://www.theguardian.com/commentisfree/2018/jul/25/celebrate-life-funerals-death-respect
Butler, J. (2009). *Frames of War: When is life Grievable?* Verso.
Cross, C. (2016). *African governments versus social media: Why the uneasy relationship?* https://theconversation.com/african-governments-versus-social- media-why-the-uneasy-relationship-73292. Accessed 20 July 2018.
Davis, J., Love, T., & Killen, G. (2018). Seriously funny: the political work of humor on social media. *New Media & Society, 20*(10), 3898–3916.
De Beer, A. S. (2004). Ecquid Novi – The search for a definition. *Ecquid Novi: African Journalism Studies, 25*(2), 186–209.
De Burgh, H. (2005). Introduction: Journalism and the new cultural paradigm. In H. de Burgh (Ed.), *Making Journalists* (pp. 1–21). Routledge.
Denzin, N. K. (1999). Cybertalk and the method of instances. In S. G. Jones (Ed.), *Doing internet research: critical issues and methods for examining the net* (pp. 107–126). SAGE.
Deuze, M. (2005). What is journalism? Professional identity and ideology of journalists reconsidered. *Journalism, 6*(4), 442–464.
Dionigi, A., & Canestrari, C. (2018). The use of humor by therapists and clients in cognitive therapy. *European Journal of Humour Research., 6*(3), 50–67.
Du Plessis, C. (2021). *Government remembers 'man of the people' Jackson Mthembu at memorial service.* https://www.news24.com/news24/southafrica/news/government-remembers-man-of-the-people-jackson-mthembu-at-memorial-service-20210125
Ebo, B. (1998). Internet or outernet? In B. Ebo (Ed.), *Cyberghetto or Cybertopia? Race, class, and gender on the internet* (pp. 1–12). Praeger.
El-Nawawy, M., & Khamis, S. (2013). *Egyptian revolution 2.0: Political blogging, civic engagement and citizen journalism.* Palgrave Macmillan.
Fraser, N. (1992). Rethinking the public sphere: A contribution to the critique of actually existing democracy. In C. Calhoun (Ed.), *Habermas and the public sphere* (pp. 109–142). MIT Press.
Goode, L. (2009). Social news, citizen journalism and democracy. *New Media & Society, 11*(8), 1287–1305.
Gottschalk, K. (2021). *Jackson Mthembu's death unites friends and rivals in tribute.* https://www.moneyweb.co.za/news/south-africa/jackson-mthembus-death-unites-friends-and-rivals-in-tribute/
Guobin, Y. (2009). *The power of the internet in China: Citizen activism online.* Columbia University Press.

Haley, E. (2014). *The utility of laughter in times of grief.* https://whatsyourgrief.com/laughter-in-times-of-grief/

Harper, S. (2010). The social agency of dead bodies. *Mortality, 15*(4), 307–322.

Hartley, J. (2010). Silly citizenship. *Critical Discourse Studies, 7*(4), 233–248.

Highfield, T. (2016). *Social media and everyday politics.* Polity Press.

Jungherr, A., Schoen, H., & Jürgens, P. (2016). The mediation of politics through Twitter: An analysis of messages posted during the campaign for German Federal Election 2013. *Journal of Computer Mediated Communication, 21*(1), 50–68.

Kalusa, W. T. (2017). The Politics of the Corpse: President Levy Mwanawasa's Death, Funeral and Political Contestation in Post-Colonial Zambia. *Journal of Southern African Studies, 43*(6), 1137–1155.

Koma, S. (2020). *Ubuntu and solidarity in the COVID-19 era.* https://www.nihss.ac.za/sites/default/files/Covid%20Articles/ubuntu_and_solidarity_in_the_COVID-19_era_-_COVID-19_0.pdf

Kozinets, R. V. (2002). The field behind the screen: Using netnography for marketing research in online communities. *Journal of Marketing Research, 39*(1), 61–72.

Lindner, A. M., Connell, E., & Meyer, E. (2015). Professional journalists in 'citizen' journalism. *Information, Communication & Society, 18*(5), 553–568.

Lobanov, N. (2021). Spanish Flu: The first modern case of viral humour. In D. Derrin & H. Burrows (Eds.), *The Palgrave handbook of humour, history, and methodology* (pp. 405–428). Palgrave.

Lund, D. A., Utz, R., Caserta, M. S., & De Vries, B. (2008). Humor, laughter, and happiness in the daily lives of recently bereaved spouses. *Omega (Westport), 58*(2), 87–105.

Mahdawi, A. (2020). *The most unhinged Trump conspiracy theory comes from – Who else? – Q A non followers.* https://www.theguardian.com/commentisfree/2020/oct/03/trump-coronavirus-conspiracy-theory-qanon

Mangwana, N. (2020). *Should the president stop making jokes?* https://www.sundaymail.co.zw/should-the-president-stop-making-jokes

Mare, A. (2018). Tracing and archiving 'constructed' data on Facebook pages and groups: Reflections on fieldwork among young activists in Zimbabwe and South Africa. *Qualitative Research, 17*(6), 645–663.

Marschall, S. (2006). Visualizing memories: The Hector Pieterson Memorial in Soweto. *Visual Anthropology, 19*, 145–169.

Matsilele, T. (2019). *Social media dissidence in Zimbabwe.* An unpublished doctoral dissertation, University of Johannesburg.

Matsilele, T. (2021). The Implications of COVID 19 on Institutions of higher learning: A case of Zimbabwe and South Africa. In G. Motsaathebe (Ed.), *Education in Africa* (pp. 93–116). Nova Science Publishers Inc.

Matsilele, T., & Ruhanya, P. (2020). Social media dissidence and activist resistance in Zimbabwe. *Media, Culture & Society*, 0163443720957886.

McCain, N. (2021). *'I have lost a dear friend' – Cyril Ramaphosa says goodbye to Jackson Mthembu.* https://www.news24.com/news24/southafrica/news/i-have-lost-a-dear-friend-cyril-ramaphosa-says-goodbye-to-jackson-mthembu-20210124

Mpofu, S. (2014). *Public and diasporic online media in the discursive construction of national identity: A case of 'Zimbabwe'.* An Unpublished PhD Dissertation. University of the Witwatersrand, Johannesburg.

Mpofu, S. (2015). When the subaltern speaks: citizen journalism and genocide "victims" voices online. *African Journalism Studies, 36*(4), 82–101.

Mpofu, S. (2016). Participation, citizen journalism and the contestations of identity and national symbols: A case of Zimbabwe's national heroes and the Heroes' Acre. *African Journalism Studies, 37*(3), 85–106.

Mpofu, S. (2017). Disruption as a communicative strategy: The case of #FeesMustFall and #RhodesMustFall students' protests. *Journal of African Media Studies, 15*(1), 351–373.

Mpofu, S. (2019a). For a nation to progress genocide victims must 'move on': A case of Zimbabwe's social media discourses of resistance. *African Identities, 17*(2), 108–129.

Mpofu, S. (2019b). Art as journalism in Zimbabwe: The case of Owen Maseko's banned Zimbabwean genocide exhibition. *Journalism Studies, 20*(1), 60–78.

Mpofu, S. (2019c). Jesus comes to South Africa: Black Twitter as citizen journalism in South African politics. *African Journalism Studies, 40*(1), 67–90.

Mpofu, S., & Barnabas, S. B. (2016). Citizen journalism and moral panics: A consideration of ethics in the 2015 South African xenophobic attacks. *African Journalism Studies, 37*(4), 115–136.

Mpofu, S., & Matsilele, T. (2020). Social media and the concept of dissidence in Zimbabwean politics. In S. J. Ndlovu-Gatsheni & P. Ruhanya (Eds.), *The history and political transition of Zimbabwe. African histories and modernities* (pp. 221–243). Palgrave Macmillan.

Murthy, D. (2008). Digital ethnography: An Examination of the use of new technologies for social research. *Sociology, 42*(5), 837–855.

Mutsvairo, B. (Ed.). (2016). *Perspectives on participatory politics and citizen journalism in a Networked Africa: A connected continent.* Palgrave Macmillan.

Mutsvairo, B., Columbus, S., & Leijendekker, I. (2014). Reconnoitering the role of (citizen) journalism ethics in the emerging networked public sphere. *African Journalism Studies, 35*(3), 3–22.

Mutsvairo, B., & Muneri, C. (2019). *Journalism, democracy and human rights in Zimbabwe.* Rowman & Littlefield Publishing Group.

Mutsvairo, B., & Salgado, S. (2020). Is citizen journalism dead? An examination of recent developments in the field. *Journalism,* 1–18. https://journals.sagepub.com/doi/10.1177/1464884920968440

Mwambari, D., & Martin, L. S. (2020). *Humour ignores social distancing: Postcolonial irony and COVID-19 in Africa*. African Arguments. https://africanarguments.org/2020/05/humour-ignores-social-distancing-postcolonial-irony-and-COVID-19-in-africa/

Ndlovu, M. (2017a). Facing history in the aftermath of Gukurahundi atrocities: New media, memory and the discourses on forgiveness on selected Zimbabwean news websites. *Peace and Conflict Studies, 24*(2), Article 3.

Ndlovu, M. (2017b). Speaking for the dead: testimonies, witnesses and the representations of Gukurahundi atrocities in new media. *Journal of African Cultural Studies, 3*(30), 293–306.

Ndlovu, M. (2018). Gukurahundi, new media and the 'discourses of silence': The reproduction of the hegemonic narratives of the Matabeleland post-colonial violence on selected Zimbabwean news websites. *African Identities, 16*(3), 275–289.

Newzimbabwe.com. (2020). https://www.Facebook.com/125973854117415/posts/2757784324269675/

Nwabueze, C., Igboeli, C., & Ubah, U. (2017). Framing of cartoons on Ebola virus disease in selected Nigerian Dailies: A content analysis. *Journal of Healthcare Communications, 2*(1/7), 1–6.

Park, M. P., & Park, R. H. R. (2010). Fear and humour in the art of cholera. *Journal of the Royal Society of Medicine, 103*, 481–483.

Pitt, R. (2021). *KZN cellphone towers torched as 5G conspiracy theories ignite*. https://www.dailymaverick.co.za/article/2021-01-08-kzn-cellphone-towers-torched-as-5g-conspiracy-theories-ignite/

Poell, T. (2014). Social media activism and state censorship. In D. Trottier & C. Fuchs (Eds.), *Social media, politics and the state: protests, revolutions, riots, crime and policing in an age of Facebook, Twitter and YouTube*. Routledge.

Riessman, C. K. (1993). *Narrative analysis*. Sage.

Rosa, G. P. (2012). The swine flu pandemics in Portugal through newspaper humour. *Journalism and Mass Communication, 2*(7), 735–747.

Rosenwald, G. C., & Ochberg, R. L. (1992). *Storied lives: The cultural politics of self-understanding*. Yale University Press.

Rutigliano, L. W. (2008). *Covering the unknown city: Citizen journalism and marginalized communities*. PhD Dissertation, The University of Texas at Austin, Austin, TX.

Sarıçalı, M., Satıcı, S. A., Satıcı, B., Göçet-Tekin, E., & Griffiths, M. D. (2020). Fear of COVID-19, mindfulness, humor, and hopelessness: A multiple mediation analysis. *International Journal of Mental Health and Addiction*, 1–14. https://doi.org/10.1007/s11469-020-00419-5

Senne. B. (2020). *Kenyan man arrested for spreading fake news on coronavirus*. https://www.timeslive.co.za/news/africa/2020-03-16-kenyan-man-arrested-for-spreading-fake-news-on-coronavirus/

Shirky, C. (2011). The political power of social media: Technology, the public sphere, and political change. *Foreign Affairs, 90*(1), 28–41.
Smith, K. (2010). Gramsci at the margins: Subjectivity and subalternity in a theory of hegemony. *International Gramsci Journal, 2*, 39–50.
Sophie, L. (2020). *[Urgent] Arrêtée pour un post humoristique: Rachna Seenauth devra s'acquitter d'une caution de Rs 7 000.* https://www.lexpress.mu/article/375016/urgent-arretee-pour-un-post-humoristique-rachna-seenauth-devra-sacquitter-dune
South African Government. (2021). *Jackson Mthembu tributes.* https://www.gov.za/JacksonMthembu-tributes#
Steensen, S. (2011). Cozy journalism. *Journalism Practice, 5*(6), 687–703.
Stein, L. (2013). Policy and participation on social media: The case of YouTube, Facebook, and Wikipedia. *Communication, Culture & Critique, 6*(3), 353–371.
Theocharis, Y., Jan van Deth, W. L., & García-Albacete, G. (2015). Using Twitter to mobilize protest action: online mobilization patterns and action repertoires in the Occupy Wall Street, Indignados, and Aganaktismenoi movements. *Information, Communication and Society, 18*(2), 202–220.
Vis, F. (2013). Twitter as a reporting tool for breaking news: journalists Tweeting the 2011 UK riots. *Digital Journalism, 1*, 27–47.
WHO. (2020). *Managing the COVID-19 infodemic: Promoting healthy behaviours and mitigating the harm from misinformation and disinformation.* https://www.who.int/news/item/23-09-2020-managing-the-COVID-19-infodemic-promoting-healthy-behaviours-and-mitigating-the-harm-from-misinformation-and-disinformation#:~:text=An%20infodemic%20is%20an%20overabundance,will%20continue%20to%20thrive
Willinger, U., Hergovich, A., Schmoeger, M., Deckert, M., Stoettner, S., Bunda, I., Witting, A., Seidler, M., Moser, R., Kacena, S., Jackler, D., Loader, B., Mueller, C., & Auf, E. (2017). Cognitive and emotional demands of black humour processing: the role of intelligence, aggressiveness and mood. *Cognitive Processing, 18*, 159–167.
Zarefsky, D. (2008). *Public speaking: Strategies for success* (5th ed.). Pearson.
Zondi, N. B., & Makhoba, K. L. (2018). What has happened to the principles of ubuntu? Exploring the concept of xenophobia in the post-apartheid literary work, Kudela Owaziyo by Maphumulo. *South African Journal of African Languages, 38*(3), 269–275.

Index[1]

[1] Note: Page numbers followed by 'n' refer to notes.

S. Mpofu (ed.), *Digital Humour in the Covid-19 Pandemic*, https://doi.org/10.1007/978-3-030-79279-4

The manufacturer's authorised representative in the EU is Springer Nature Customer Service Centre GmbH, Europaplatz 3, 69115 Heidelberg, Germany. If you have any concerns regarding our products, please contact ProductSafety@springernature.com

Printed and bound by CPI Group (UK) Ltd, Croydon, CR0 4YY
22/09/2026
02221066-0014